Medicine and Biomedical Sciences in Modern History

Series Editors
Carsten Timmermann
University of Manchester
Manchester, UK

Michael Worboys
University of Manchester
Manchester, UK

The aim of this series is to illuminate the development and impact of medicine and the biomedical sciences in the modern era. The series was founded by the late Professor John Pickstone, and its ambitions reflect his commitment to the integrated study of medicine, science and technology in their contexts. He repeatedly commented that it was a pity that the foundation discipline of the field, for which he popularized the acronym 'HSTM' (History of Science, Technology and Medicine) had been the history of science rather than the history of medicine. His point was that historians of science had too often focused just on scientific ideas and institutions, while historians of medicine always had to consider the understanding, management and meanings of diseases in their socio-economic, cultural, technological and political contexts. In the event, most of the books in the series dealt with medicine and the biomedical sciences, and the changed series title reflects this. However, as the new editors we share Professor Pickstone's enthusiasm for the integrated study of medicine, science and technology, encouraging studies on biomedical science, translational medicine, clinical practice, disease histories, medical technologies, medical specialisms and health policies.

The books in this series will present medicine and biomedical science as crucial features of modern culture, analysing their economic, social and political aspects, while not neglecting their expert content and context. Our authors investigate the uses and consequences of technical knowledge, and how it shaped, and was shaped by, particular economic, social and political structures. In re-launching the Series, we hope to build on its strengths but extend its geographical range beyond Western Europe and North America.

Medicine and Biomedical Sciences in Modern History is intended to supply analysis and stimulate debate. All books are based on searching historical study of topics which are important, not least because they cut across conventional academic boundaries. They should appeal not just to historians, nor just to medical practitioners, scientists and engineers, but to all who are interested in the place of medicine and biomedical sciences in modern history.

More information about this series at
http://www.palgrave.com/gp/series/15183

Violetta Hionidou

Abortion and Contraception in Modern Greece, 1830–1967

Medicine, Sexuality and Popular Culture

palgrave
macmillan

Violetta Hionidou
History, Classics & Archaeology
Newcastle University
Newcastle, UK

Medicine and Biomedical Sciences in Modern History
ISBN 978-3-030-41489-4 ISBN 978-3-030-41490-0 (eBook)
https://doi.org/10.1007/978-3-030-41490-0

Cover illustration: MirageC

This Palgrave Macmillan imprint is published by the registered company Springer Nature Switzerland AG.
The registered company address is: Gewerbestrasse 11, 6330 Cham, Switzerland

Acknowledgements

This book would not have been written without the generous sabbatical provision of Newcastle University. For this I am extremely grateful. I also thank Newcastle University for funding my frequent trips to Greece over the years to visit libraries and archives to collect material for this book. I am most grateful to the staff at the National Library of Greece, the Library of the Hellenic Parliament at Lenorman, Philip Robinson at Newcastle, Firestone Library at Princeton, Mykonos Library, Syros Library and Koraes Library on Hios. I also thank very much, once again, all the friends I made over the years, at the places where I researched this book. They are too many to list and I am sure there are plenty that I have forgotten, but I will mention a few nevertheless: Voula Skagia, Aristoula Koufopantelis, Maria Monioudi, Michalis Assimomitis and Hara Skavaki. They have all helped me enormously, introducing me not only to their friends and acquaintances but also to their local cultures.

I extend an especially warm 'thank you' to all of the people who have opened up their houses and hearts to me since 1993, and who, over the years, have happily talked about their pasts. This project would not have been possible without their trust, which allowed me into their homes to talk about extremely private matters. Most interviews took place thanks to funded projects: the transcription of the last set of interviews was funded by the Wellcome Trust [082800/B/07/LS/HH (Strategic Award in History of Medicine)] awarded to the Northern Centre for the History of Medicine. The Hios and Syros interviews were collected and transcribed as part of the Wellcome Trust for the History of Medicine post-doctoral Fellowship (no. 056211). The Mykonos interviews were collected as part of the Human Capital and Mobility Fellowship, funded by the EU (CHBICT930867). I am extremely grateful to all for their financial support.

I thank Vicky Manolopoulou for undertaking the data inputting of the *Sofianopoulos Clinique* register. She did so with extraordinary efficiency and good humour despite the gruesome subject matter. I also thank Elena Katselli for commenting on part of Chap. 6. It helped me improve it significantly. I am extremely grateful to Margery Mooney, who happily and readily looked after her grandchildren when I needed to undertake fieldtrips or participate in conferences. I am also very grateful to my own mother, who talked to me from an early age about her abortion experiences that spanned from the USSR to Greece, and who first brought to my attention the extensive unreliability of coitus interruptus as well as the population's unquestioned ignorance surrounding contraception. It was her incessant story-telling that made me a good listener, a priceless attribute when undertaking oral history. I dedicate this book to the women who shaped my life—my grandmother Maria, my mother Ioulia and my daughter Ilia—but also to Yuri, who has taught me a lot about the ways young men think today.

I am fortunate enough to write the final lines of this manuscript while based at the Seeger Hellenic Centre, Princeton University. I am extremely grateful to the Centre for awarding me one of their prestigious fellowships, enabling me to spend time at Princeton. It has been an extraordinary experience.

Praise for *Abortion and Contraception in Modern Greece, 1830–1967*

'Hionidou's meticulous historical study shows in exemplary fashion how political and economic change can influence attitudes toward contraception and abortion. She persuasively demonstrates how and why one ostensibly pronatalist country could increasingly accept them – even on the part of medical and religious personnel, who often both privately supported and personally practiced their use in defiance of religious and professional dogma and of official policy. This book will find readers and imitators far beyond Greece's borders.'

—Michael Herzfeld, Ernest E. Monrad Research Professor of the Social Sciences, *Harvard University, USA*

'For decades scholars have produced fine studies of fertility and contraception in modern societies that rely on at most one or two disciplinary perspectives. The limitations of this approach are self-evident: understanding fertility requires precise measurement and an understanding of the way ideas about fertility interacted with medical knowledge, religious notions, and state policy. Violetta Hionidou's *Abortion and Contraception in Modern Greece*, in contrast, is multi-disciplinary study of fertility and its control in modern Greece. Drawing masterfully on the techniques of the demographer, the ethnographer, and the medical and social historian, she has produced both a much-needed, comprehensive account of fertility in modern Greece, she has provided a model for all others to emulate. This work is a triumph of truly inter-disciplinary scholarship.'

—Timothy W. Guinnane, Philip Golden Bartlett Professor of Economic History, *Yale University, USA*

Contents

About the Author

Violetta Hionidou is Senior Lecturer in Modern European History at Newcastle University, UK. She has taught at the University of Southampton and Crete University, Greece. She has recently held the visiting Research Fellowship at Princeton University, Seeger Centre for Hellenic Studies. Her research interests are in all aspects of famines; abortion, contraception and fertility in historical populations; popular and modern medicine in modern Greece; family history; identities and experiences of exile of Pontic Greeks from the former USSR; and experiences of being a famine refugee. Her research is interdisciplinary, transcending the fields of demography, sociology, human geography and history. She has employed oral history, tackling 'difficult' subjects, ranging from abortion, birth control and famine memory in Greece to identity and exile in the Soviet Union. Her research has been published in elite peer-reviewed journals, such as *Medical History*, *Population Studies*, *Journal of Refugee Studies*, *Journal of Contemporary History*, *Journal of the Social History of Medicine*, *Europe-Asia Studies*, *The History of the Family: An International Quarterly*. She is the author of *Famine and Death in Occupied Greece, 1941–1944*, published by Cambridge University Press, and co-winner of the 2007 Edmund Keely Book Prize. She has also recently written *Η κατοχική πείνα μέσα απο προφορικές μαρτυρίες (The Greek Famine of the 1940s Through Oral Histories)* (Athens: Patakis, 2020).

List of Figures

List of Plates

CHAPTER 1

Introduction

The study of fertility decline has seen many hundreds or even thousands of works published in an attempt to answer apparently simple questions such as why, when and how. Answering them is extremely important given the significance of this change, which shaped populations and societies in the nineteenth and twentieth centuries. While the questions are simple, the answers are extremely complicated and definitive ones are yet to be given—if they will ever be given. Moreover, detailed fertility histories of national populations set against a background of that country's social, economic and medical history, all essential in addressing some or all of the above questions, have been scarce outside some Western European and North American examples.[1] Those written as part of the Princeton European Fertility Project (PEFP) were heavily constrained and shaped by the aims of the Project.

The PEFP set the agenda in the 1960s and 1970s and its findings have dominated and shaped much of the research in the decades that followed. However, in the 1990s Timothy Guinnane, B. Okun and J. Trussell were already questioning the claimed 'virtual simultaneity' of the European fertility declines revealed by the project.[2] Subsequently J.C. Brown and T. Guinnane queried the project's statistical methodologies—methodologies that led to uniform conclusions partly because, the authors argue, the same flawed methods were used in all sub-studies.[3] Alongside such criticisms, the Greek results present additional challenges because the conclusions reached about the date of the decline by the PEFP's Greek

V. Hionidou, *Abortion and Contraception in Modern Greece, 1830–1967*, Medicine and Biomedical Sciences in Modern History,
https://doi.org/10.1007/978-3-030-41490-0_1

researchers' own publication and the PEFP itself vary significantly.[4] The lack of *any* actual data during the period of the claimed dates of decline adds significantly to the problem. As the dating of the Greek decline has never been unequivocally resolved, and as new evidence has emerged in the last few decades from family reconstitution studies, it is imperative to re-examine the timing of the fertility decline for Greece.[5]

One of the main findings of the Princeton project—and one that has dominated much of our understanding of fertility change ever since—was the rejection of the adaptation/adjustment hypothesis in favour of the innovation hypothesis. Gösta Carlsson's seminal 1966 paper outlined the implications of these two divergent hypotheses. In the latter case, fertility change is posited as the result of innovation in terms of contraceptive methods, either introduced to or discovered by a population; such knowledge gradually diffuses through and across populations, the direction almost invariably being from higher to lower classes. The adaptation/adjustment hypothesis argues that couples adapt to social and economic changes by adjusting their fertility. This assumes that fertility control methods exist and are understood by the population, or part of the population, whose members choose to use or not use such methods as and when they feel them to be appropriate to their needs. However, Carlsson stressed that, in such a regime, motivation and structural factors are more important than a knowledge of contraception.[6] Nevertheless, in recent years an increasing number of studies of pre-transitional populations have argued that, following crisis situations, the populations studied appear to have quickly controlled their fertility to a significant degree, indicating that individuals could and at times did deliberately control their fertility, even before the fertility transition had occurred.[7] If that was indeed the situation—that is, if populations or groups possessed the relevant knowledge to control their fertility, but chose to do so only in crisis situations—the implication is that adaptation was the mechanism that led to the widespread adoption of fertility control. This also means that populations had knowledge and understanding of how to control their fertility, as, for example, Gigi Santow has argued about coitus interruptus.[8] However, we cannot assume that all couples in any given population were necessarily using the same method.[9] This raises a number of questions, therefore. When and why did couples decide that they would employ the methods of which they were aware to *stringently* control their fertility, rather than just using them occasionally in crises? And was there a time when they were *not* aware of any methods? Greece is an excellent case to address such questions, considering not only the late timing of its fertility decline but also the multiple crises that the country endured in the late nineteenth century and the first half of the twentieth.

Particularly interesting in the discussions outlined above is the terminology employed in referring to the various methods of controlling fertility. While Carlsson explicitly states that he refers to birth control, explaining that this includes abortion, contraception and voluntary abstinence, most authors refer almost exclusively to contraception.[10] Such usage of terms underlines our contemporary understanding of abortion and contraception as separate approaches to fertility control, an understanding that was not necessarily shared by those who controlled their fertility in the past. Some of the most interesting ideas put forward in recent decades in relation to methods of controlling fertility are related to the potential use of emmenagogues and abortifacients before the onset of fertility decline.[11] Angus McLaren, tentatively, and John Riddle, more emphatically, have argued for the importance of early abortion using abortifacients in the Middle Ages and the early modern period in the west, roughly equating emmenagogues with abortifacients.[12] Etienne van de Walle challenged this position, arguing that emmenagogues were used to bring on menstruation when that was delayed, a situation interpreted in the past as pathological.[13] Most recently, Jennifer Evans has persuasively argued that in early modern England women would regulate their menstruation in order to increase their fertility.[14]

Riddle has emphasised the importance of the survival of morsels of knowledge relating to herbal emmenagogues in the west, even in the twentieth century. Considering that the knowledge and use of herbal remedies was widespread in early twentieth-century Greece, it is pertinent, therefore, to ask whether this extended to herbal emmenagogues and abortifacients.[15] If that was indeed the case, who possessed such knowledge and when and in what circumstances did they divulge it to potential users? Did advisors and users differentiate between emmenagogues and abortifacients? And, if so, did such differentiation remain unchanged over time? This monograph will examine the knowledge and use of emmenagogues, including herbal ones, among the Greek population in the nineteenth and twentieth centuries. If emmenagogues were used, what was the purpose of their use? How, if at all, were they linked to abortifacients and how did the latter link to birth control methods? The notable prevalence of abortion in late twentieth-century Greece is very well documented,[16] but why was this the case in a modern society where modern contraception had been accessible for some time? Are there historic pathways to birth control that have determined Greece's extreme reliance on surgical abortion in the second half of the twentieth century?

Much blame for such over-reliance on abortion has been placed on Greek physicians who performed abortions in the post-World War II era. However, beyond that, no attempt has been made to investigate physicians' role in the control of fertility. Then again, this is not specific to the Greek historiography—their potential influence has rarely been considered.[17] Narratives created in individual countries at the time of the decline seem to persist in the absence of research: so, for example, for England Marie Stopes' forceful assertions of ignorant—in terms of contraception—physicians who were unable to provide pertinent advice remain accepted to date. Richard Soloway has offered a thorough account of the negative stance of the British Medical Association towards birth control, and it has been assumed that individual physicians, protective of their reputations, also maintained such a negative stance.[18] For the USA the influential role of Margaret Sanger in bridging the gap between advocates of contraception and the American Medical Association has been acknowledged. Still, the view of individual physicians regarding birth control is again surmised to have been that of their Association, although exceptions existed. In contrast to our limited knowledge of the role of physicians in relation to contraception, much more has been written about them in relation to abortion, where their role has been seen as instrumental, in terms of either providing services to women or their involvement in public rhetoric.[19] This juxtaposition is partly a result of our contemporary understanding of contraception and abortion as separate processes and issues. However, such separation was articulated and promoted by the advocates of contraception in their efforts to legitimise their cause. Considering that traditional, imperfect methods were exclusively used during the fertility decline among historical populations, abortion was their necessary companion for a decline to be achieved, especially so where such a decline was speedy. Therefore, this study will focus on both contraception and abortion, at times referring to them collectively as birth control.[20]

This study will explore the knowledge and use of contraception and abortion in nineteenth- and twentieth-century Greece, examining how and when the population moved from a non-fertility-controlling setting to one where fertility was stringently controlled and attempting to define the ultimate role of physicians, if any, in the shift that occurred. The chronological span of the study covers the period from the creation of the

Greek state in 1832 to 1967—that is, soon after the arrival of the Pill there. The end date has been chosen because there are already a number of—mostly anthropological—studies that have focused on abortion and contraception in Greece in the second half of the twentieth century.[21] While all such studies have significantly contributed to our knowledge and understanding of late-twentieth-century Greek society (most apportioning medicine and physicians a central role), they—understandably so—have not provided the historical background to their findings. This study aims to address this lacuna too.

Chapter 2 outlines what we know about the timing of the start of the fertility decline in Greece. It examines the discrepancies between the dates offered by G.S. Siampos and V.G. Valaoras and the PEFP publication, a gap of 23 years. It utilises all the available data while also incorporating the existing family reconstitution studies. Chapter 3 examines the opposite of fertility—that is, involuntary childlessness—revealing the strong desire for and cultural necessity of procreation on the part of the Greek married couple. A lack of fertility or very low fertility in the past were abhorrent, the absence of children often being interpreted as the result of black magic and a situation that could be cured only by white magic. While physicians made recommendations regarding sterility, their limited effectiveness was understood, leading individuals and their families to turn to religion and magic. This strong desire for procreation was closely linked to the use of emmenagogues, which were employed until the 1920s almost exclusively, but also later on alongside other methods, in order to achieve and sustain fertility. From the 1920s onwards emmenagogues and abortifacients were employed to procure abortion, as is described in Chap. 4. Chapter 5 examines curettage and its history in Greece, revealing its wide use as a cure for both women's ailments and sterility, and as a mechanical emmenagogic method. Since was 1920s the same method was employed to provide early abortions. Chapter 6 considers the abortion law in Greece from the early days of the state to the most recent situation of full liberalisation. It explains why prosecutions hardly ever occurred and outlines the changes in the law that protected the performing physicians. It seems that the law was always liberal in comparison to that of other European states, but was also liberally applied. Chapter 7 examines the ethics of abortion as perceived and practised by physicians, the Church and women. For physicians and the law the mother's life always had precedence over that of the foetus, allowing the physicians to perform abortion in the early twentieth century for mothers whose health was 'under threat', including, for example, cases of pernicious vomiting. The Church had an 'unmoving' position that abortion and contraception should not be practised, but it actually acted—or even reacted—very rarely and only when the political climate was favourable: that is, when the government was distinctly pronatalist. Most low-ranking priests, themselves married and living lives identical to those of their flock, almost certainly did not follow Church's teachings. Many women did have ethical qualms when considering whether to employ emmenagogues/abortifacients or seek surgical abortion, with many—among the early birth controllers—deciding not to do so. However, they linked their unease not to the teachings of the Church or the local priest but to the moral code of the 'elder women'. Chapter 8 describes the natural contraceptive methods widely known and/or used in twentieth-century Greece, as these appear in physicians' publications, oral histories and letters to women's magazines. As much of the fertility change occurred in the 1930s to the 1950s, the analysis is heavily focused on this period. Chapter 9 addresses the same issues but for appliance methods and the Pill. Finally, Chap. 10 examines the role of physicians in facilitating and encouraging couples in employing contraception for, almost exclusively, 'health' reasons. Such encouragement by widely respected physicians, it is argued, enabled couples to adopt contraception much sooner than would otherwise have been the case.

Sources

The sources employed in this study include demographic data, mostly published by the statistical service of Greece; medical publications; the national and local press; women's magazines, especially, the consultation column with the magazine's resident gynaecologist; and oral histories collected by the author.

The medical sources include medical journals addressing either the wider public or the medical profession; monographs published by gynaecologists/obstetricians presenting the essentials of their vocation; and monographs discussing abortion, birth control, contraception, marriage hygiene or marital sexuality. The majority of these have never been used before in a study of this sort.

A source of central importance that enables us to approach the attitudes and understanding of the first users of birth control is oral histories collected by the present author among three island populations between 1994 and 2000. The interviews that I conducted on Mykonos in the spring of 1994 focused on the life histories of those interviewed, addressing issues of migration, family formation, inheritance, living conditions and family limitation.[22] Because of my interest in birth control, I tried to select mainly married or previously married persons. Nevertheless, some persons who had never married were also interviewed, as were couples who were unable to bear children. The initial plan was to interview equal numbers of men and women. However, while all were extremely happy to be interviewed by me, a young Athenian post-doctoral researcher who visited the island during the idle winter months, men were reticent in discussing any aspect of birth control with me. I was rebutted on a number of occasions, eventually leading me to abandon the effort with men, as women did not object to such conversations. When, in 1995, I presented an early version of my subsequently published paper 'The Adoption of Fertility', Simon Szreter commented that the unresponsiveness of Greek men to a female interviewer was, most probably, specific to the Greek culture. Kate Fisher's subsequent attempts to interview elderly British men also encountered failure, and Szreter replaced her as interviewer on some occasions.[23] My lack of access to a male replacement interviewer for the Mykonos interviews meant that the majority of the interviews were conducted with elderly women.

Further interviews were conducted in 1999 and 2000 with survivors of the Greek famine of the early 1940s on Hios and Syros. With the exception of three informants, all were adults at the time of the famine. As these interviews were focused on the famine, the informants addressed issues of birth control only occasionally. Twenty-two interviews were conducted on both Hios and Syros, and 28 on Mykonos. Further interviews were conducted in 2011, mostly in Athens, although one took place on Hios. Seven of these interviews were with retired physicians, exploring their experiences of studying and practising medicine in post-World War II Greece (Nos 1D–7D). The physicians involved, both women and men who had graduated in the 1960s, followed diverse specialisations. One further interview took place in Athens with a non-physician female informant who had lived for most of her life, and all her childbearing years, in a provincial town in northern Greece.

Informants, both men and women, were selected from across all social classes and from both rural and urban environments; and both Orthodox Christians and Catholics were interviewed on Syros.[24] The ages of the Mykonos interviewees ranged from 70 to 101, with the majority being older than 80. The experiences of the informants therefore span as far back as the early decades of the twentieth century. The age range for the Hios interviews was 64–100 and for Syros 68–98. While the initial plan was to interview individuals alone, preferably in the comfort of their own home, this did not always prove possible. In three instances on Mykonos, six on Hios and seven on Syros two people were interviewed together, which changed the dynamics of the interview somewhat. These informants were occasionally cousins or unmarried cohabiting partners, but in most cases they were married couples, and thus something about the intimate relationship of the specific couple was also revealed. In one case on Mykonos, for example, the husband remained present for most of the interview, not interrupting and initially appearing comfortable. When I started asking about birth control, the wife, although continuing to appear comfortable, became less forthcoming, diverting the conversation. The husband, who was becoming increasingly uncomfortable at this stage, left the room, at which point the wife very quickly became vocal, answering all my earlier questions. When the husband returned, the wife returned to neutral topics. When the husband left again, looking increasingly frustrated, she resumed the conversation about birth control and mentioned that the husband was not overly keen on sex.

While a claim to representativeness cannot be made, all the informants were members of the earliest cohorts to control their fertility in Greece, thus providing us with a very rare opportunity to explore their knowledge and thinking at the time. Even more importantly, the interviews allow us to learn about the informants' intentions—as has already been established, for example, breastfeeding was deliberately employed in pre-decline Mykonos in order to postpone the next conception. Such knowledge is invaluable, no matter the criticisms of oral history.

For reasons of anonymity, all interviews conducted by the author are identified by a number. When names are used, these are pseudonyms. While most had no objections to their names being used, the diversity of their wishes on the use of the sources and the level of private information revealed led to the decision not to reveal the identities of any individual.

Notes

1. A notable exception, although it does not directly address fertility decline, is Raúl Necochea López (2014) *A History of Family Planning in Twentieth-century Peru* (Chapel Hill: The University of North Carolina Press). The fertility history of England has been addressed extensively and in depth

(see, for example, Simon Szreter (1996) *Fertility, Class and Gender in Britain, 1860–1940* (Cambridge: Cambridge University Press); Robert Woods (2000) *The Demography of Victorian England and Wales*, Cambridge Population, Economy, and Society in Past Times Series (Cambridge: Cambridge University Press)) and Eilidh Garrett, A. Reid, K. Schürer and S. Szreter (2001) *Changing family size in England and Wales: place, class and demography, 1891–1911* (Cambridge: Cambridge University Press).

2. Timothy Guinnane, B. Okun and J. Trussell (1994) 'What Do We Know About the Timing of Fertility Transitions in Europe?' *Demography*, 31(1), 1.
3. J. Brown and T. Guinnane (2007) 'Regions and Time in the European Fertility Transition: Problems in the Princeton Project's Statistical Methodology', *The Economic History Review*, 60(3), new series, 574–95.
4. G.S. Siampos and V.G. Valaoras (1971) 'Long term fertility trends in Greece', *International Population Conference, London 1969* (Liege: IUSSP), vol. 1, pp. 598–610. Ansley J. Coale and Susan Cotts Watkins (eds) (1986) *The Decline of Fertility in Europe* (Princeton: Princeton University Press).
5. Violetta Hionidou (1993) 'The Demography of a Greek Island, Mykonos 1859–1959: A Family Reconstitution Study' (unpublished PhD thesis: University of Liverpool); Violetta Hionidou (1998) 'The Adoption of Fertility Control on Mykonos, 1879–1959: Stopping, Spacing or Both?' *Population Studies*, 52(1), 67–83; V. S. Gavalas (2001) 'Demographic reconstruction of a Greek island community: Naoussa and Kostos on Paros, 1894–1998' (unpublished PhD thesis: London School of Economics and Political Science, University of London); Ntina Moustani (2014) 'Oi Demografikes Exelixeis s'ena Viomehaniko Kentro: Volos, 1881–1922' (unpublished PhD thesis: University of Thessalia).
6. Gösta Carlsson (1966) 'The Decline of Fertility: Innovation or Adjustment Process', *Population Studies*, 20(2), 150.
7. M. Dribe and F. Scalone (2010) 'Detecting deliberate fertility control in pretransitional populations: Evidence from six German villages, 1766–1863', *European Journal of Population*, 26(4), 411-34; Tommy Bengtsson and M. Dribe (2006) 'Deliberate control in a natural fertility population: Southern Sweden, 1766–1864', *Demography*, 43(4), 727–46; A. Amialchuk and E. Dimitrova (2012) 'Detecting the evolution of deliberate fertility control before the demographic transition in Germany', *Demographic Research*, 27 (article 19), 507–42; Shamma Adeeb Alam and Claus C. Pörtner (2018) 'Income shocks, contraceptive use, and timing of fertility', *Journal of Development Economics*, 131, 96–103.
8. Gigi Santow (1995) 'Coitus Interruptus and the Control of Natural Fertility', *Population Studies*, 49(1), 19–43.

9. See, for example, the situation on Mykonos among the first cohort to control their fertility, where the majority of couples had assumed that all couples were using the same method as them, something that was not true (Hionidou, 'The Adoption', 79).
10. Some use the term contraception almost exclusively and the term birth control only occasionally, without differentiating between the two.
11. According to the Oxford Dictionary online emmenagogues are defined as 'agents which increase or renew the menstrual discharge'. The definition used here for an abortifacient is that of a drug or other agent that causes the expulsion of an embryo or a foetus.
12. Angus McLaren (1984) *Reproductive Rituals: The Perception of Fertility in England from the Sixteenth to the Nineteenth Century* (London: Methuen), pp. 102, 107; John Riddle (1998) *Eve's Herbs: A History of Contraception and Abortion in the West* (London; Cambridge, MA: Harvard University Press), pp. 179–80.
13. Etienne van de Walle (1997) 'Flowers and Fruits: Two Thousand Years of Menstrual Regulation', *The Journal of Interdisciplinary History*, 28(2), 201. Also see Elisha P. Renne and Etienne van de Walle (2001) 'Introduction', in Etienne van de Walle and Elisha P. Renne (eds), *Regulating Menstruation: Beliefs, Practices, Interpretations* (Chicago: The University of Chicago Press), pp. xiii–xxxvii.
14. Evans, Jennifer (2014) *Aphrodisiacs, Fertility and Medicine in Early Modern England* (Woodbridge: The Boydell Press), p. 15.
15. Violetta Hionidou (2016) 'Popular medicine and empirics in Greece, 1900–1950: an oral history approach', *Medical History*, 60(4), 492–513.
16. Eugenia Georges (1996) 'Abortion Policy and Practice in Greece', *Social Science Medicine*, 42(4), 509–19; Heather Paxson (2004) *Making Modern Mothers: Ethics and Family Planning in Urban Greece* (Berkeley: University of California Press); Alexandra Halkias (2004) *The Empty Cradle of Democracy: Sex, Abortion, and Nationalism in Modern Greece* (Durham, NC: Duke University Press); Eugenia Georges (2008) *Bodies of Knowledge: The Medicalisation of Reproduction in Greece* (Nashville: Vanderbilt University Press); Alexandra Barmpouti (2019) *Post-War Eugenics, Reproductive choices and Population Policies in Greece, 1950s–1980s* (London: Palgrave Macmillan)
17. Peel's work is rather exceptional and very valuable. However, Peel was a physician himself and writing at exactly the point when physicians were becoming the main providers of contraception. John Peel (1964) 'Contraception and the Medical Profession', *Population Studies*, 18(2), 133–45.

18. Richard Allen Soloway (1982) *Birth Control and the Population Question in England, 1877–1930* (Chapel Hill: The University of North Carolina Press), chapter 12.
19. Leslie J. Reagan (1997) *When Abortion was a Crime. Women, Medicine and Law in the United States, 1867–1973* (Berkeley: University of California Press), chapter 2; For Greece see Vasilios Valaoras, A. Polychronopoulou and D. Trichopoulos (1965) 'Control of Family Size in Greece (The Results of a Field Survey)', *Population Studies*, 18(3), 265–78; Halkias, *The Empty Cradle*, chapter 5. However, both Georges and Paxson discuss physicians, abortion and contraception, referring mostly to the last decades of the twentieth century (Georges, *Bodies*, chapter 6; Paxson, *Making*, chapter 3). Also, see Barmpouti, who extensively discusses Nikolaos Louros, the most outspoken Greek physician, positioned against abortion (*Post-War Eugenics*).
20. This is not the meaning of the term as it was used prior to 1940. At the time it was used to refer mostly but not exclusively to contraception.
21. Halkias, *The Empty Cradle*; Paxson, *Making*; Georges, *Bodies*; Hara Symeonidou (2006) *Oikogeneia kai gonimoteta sten Ellada. Analyse kata Genees* (Athens: A. Sakkoulas). Also Barmpouti who discusses eugenics and population policies in the same period (*Post-War Eugenics*).
22. Hionidou, 'The adoption', 75.
23. Kate Fisher (2006) *Birth Control, Sex, and Marriage in Britain 1918–1960* (Oxford: Oxford University Press), p. 20; Simon Szreter and K. Fisher (2010) *Sex Before the Sexual Revolution: Intimate Life in England 1918–1963*, Cambridge Social and Cultural Histories 16 (Cambridge: Cambridge University Press).
24. No Catholics lived on Mykonos or Hios.

CHAPTER 2

Fertility Trends, 1870–1967

Introduction

This chapter aims to outline levels of and trends in fertility, and their changes, in Greece over the studied period. Of central importance to the arguments of this book is the establishment of when Greek couples began to control their fertility. One person, Vasileios Valaoras, has shaped much of what we know about Greek historical demography.[1] Valaoras was a trained physician who was already publishing significant works on Greece in the international academic scene of the 1930s. From the 1930s to the 1960s he gained a succession of fellowships, positions and funding, invariably in the US, in prestigious organisations associated with health, demography and reproduction including the Rockefeller Foundation, the United Nations and the International Planned Parenthood Federation (IPPF). In that respect, he was the natural Greek collaborator for the Princeton project. Valaoras had a thorough knowledge of the Greek sources and continued to publish on demographic issues long after his retirement. Not only did his demographic publications carry significant authority but they shaped indelibly how Greeks understand their population history. Few demographic works employing extensive population data had been published even by the end of the twentieth century; most attempted to provide a continuous, in-depth demographic picture of small populations.[2] It should be stressed here that the problems faced when studying the population history of Greece are very significant indeed.[3] First, one has to deal

V. Hionidou, *Abortion and Contraception in Modern Greece, 1830–1967*, Medicine and Biomedical Sciences in Modern History,
https://doi.org/10.1007/978-3-030-41490-0_2

with the frequent boundary (and population) changes that the state of Greece underwent during the first century of its existence. Censuses do exist, but there is a lack of uniformity in terms of the data that were published on each occasion. Worse, for many of the censuses—those before 1861, and those from 1889, 1896 and 1940—the only available data are population figures by sex and administrative unit. For none of the pre-1951 censuses does the original individual-level collected material survive for the whole country. Exceptionally, some census books have been gradually becoming available, but only through the local archives of the area to which they pertain.[4] Furthermore, civil registration suffers from similar problems: intermittent publication of the collected data, with major gaps existing (published material is available for 1861–1884, 1921–1938 and 1956 onwards); and varying quality of the collected data both over time and across space. Thus, Valaoras' work was anything but straightforward. One of his earliest and most fundamental pieces involved 'reconstructing' the demographic history of Greece from 1860 to 1965 utilising the fragmented existing sources, the UN model life tables and extensive assumptions he made based on his in-depth knowledge of the country and the demographic studies he undertook in the US. A number of points are worth identifying here. First, Valaoras states that he employed the 'age–sex composition of the population as found in the censuses of 1861, 1870, 1879, 1889, 1896, 1907, 1928, 1940 and 1951'. As mentioned above, age–sex data do not exist for the 1889, 1896 and 1940 censuses. Second, Valaoras was unable to provide estimates for the period 1910–1919, presumably because of the scant availability of data (both census and civil registration) but also because this was an extremely turbulent period in political, economic and military terms.[5] Third, Valaoras' estimates of Crude Birth Rate (CBR) depict a smoothly declining trend from 1890 onwards.

The Princeton European Fertility Project and Greece

One of Valaoras' main contributions was his collaboration with the Princeton European Fertility Project. In an article co-authored with Siampos they produced Coale's indices for the years 1900, 1928, 1961 and 1971. These same indices were reproduced in the volume *The Decline of Fertility in Europe*.[6] However, Valaoras and Siampos situated the start of the Greek fertility decline in 1890, while the Princeton volume, using the same definition and data, argued for 1913.[7] Beyond the quarter-of-a-century deviation in the start of fertility decline, there are significant issues with the calculation of the indices as well. Valaoras and Siampos explain that, because neither civil registration data nor censuses are available for 1900 or the surrounding years, they used 'interpolation of the two successive censuses of 1896 and 1907'.[8] However, the only available information for 1896 is population figures by sex. The same applies to the preceding census of 1889. The two closest censuses for which an age–sex structure is available are those of 1879 and 1907, and thus an interpolation could only be undertaken for those censuses. These censuses are more than 40 years apart—and, more importantly, 40 years during which major changes took place, such as the start of mortality decline.[9] Moreover, such an interpolation is based on the assumption that the population is stationary, something that the Greek population at the time was certainly not. Such issues pose serious questions relating to both the reliability of their estimates of the 1900 values of the Coale indices and the two suggested dates for the start of fertility decline in Greece.[10] Therefore, a fresh look at the existing sources and studies is necessary in order to establish the timing of the fertility decline.

Fertility Prior to 1920

In assessing fertility changes in the nineteenth and early twentieth centuries, and because of the data problems discussed above, some rather unconventional data must be employed. Thus in the census of 1920 (more accurately, January 1, 1921) each household was asked the number of children born by the head of the household and the number of children that had ever died. The collected data refer to 'Families/Households—in terms of (blood) relatives'—that is, not in terms of co-residence only. The data provided in the census list female heads of households separately from male, and married separately from widowed or divorced. For married couples, the husband was invariably classified as the head of the household and therefore it is the responses of married men that represent the majority of families and their experiences (Fig. 2.1). The data provided in Fig. 2.1 are those for married men who at the date of the 1920 census were heads of their household.[11] Considering that the question cited above referred to 'Children ever born', the answer could potentially have included stillborn children. However, my Mykonos

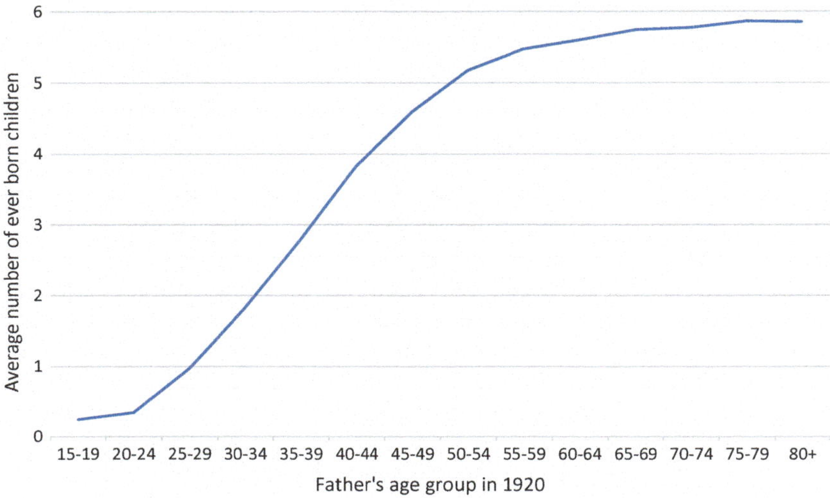

Fig. 2.1 Average number of ever born children by head of household's age group in 1920, male married heads only. (Sources: The data were derived from NSSG (1931) *Statistical yearbook of Greece 1930*, Table 41, pp. 103–4)

informants—particularly the men—when asked about the children they had had, never included any stillborn births. They had to be asked explicitly whether they had experienced any stillbirths and I had to explain why I wanted to include them in my research before they would provide such information. Indeed, to a degree, it was also necessary to ask explicitly about any children who had died in infancy too. Thus, there are clearly issues of accuracy and full reporting of such data in retrospective interviews and potentially also the 1920 census data. However, the large numbers that were available for inclusion in the calculations carried out for this research provide a smooth trend in which the number of children increases along with the age of the father.

Figure 2.1 shows that those aged 65 and over had an almost identical number of ever-born children.[12] That suggests that fertility for those men born prior to 1855 was largely unchanged. Assuming that they got married around the age of 30, this conclusion applies to those reproducing in the years prior to 1885. The 1920 census asked questions not only about children ever born (henceforth CEB) but also about children who died. However, even if one were to assume both that some infants who died were not reported by their fathers and a high infant mortality rate of around 200, an inflation of the reported CEB number by one child would take the figure to 6.8. Such a figure is comparable to that of 7.49 calculated for the 1889–1898 cohort of married women of natural fertility on Mykonos, suggesting that while fertility in Greece was at the time natural, or not controlled in a parity-specific way, it nevertheless reached only moderate levels.

The difference between the levels of fertility achieved in the Cyclades and those of Greece is shown in Fig. 2.2, where the CEB averages are given by the father's duration of marriage for the various regions of the country.[13] For all marriage durations, the average CEB for the Cyclades is higher than that of Greece, ranging from a difference of 0.12 in the first 5 years of marriage to one of 0.79 for those married between 15 and

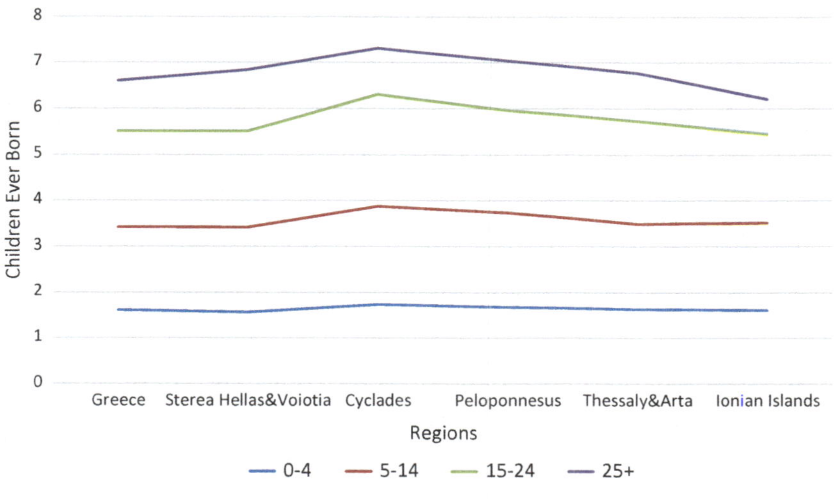

Fig. 2.2 Children ever born by father's marriage duration, 1920. (Sources: NSSG (1928) *Apografe tou Plethysmou tes Ellados. Genika Statistika Apotelesmata* (Athens: National Printers), table IX; NSSG (1927) *Statistika Apotelesmata dia ten Sterea Ellas & Voiotia* (Athens: National Printers), pp. 675–6; NSSG (1929) *Statistika Apotelesmata dia ten Thessalia&Arta* (Athens: National Printers), pp. 488–9; NSSG (1924) *Statistika Apotelesmata dia tas Ionious Nesous* (Athens: National Printers), pp. 378–9; NSSG (1923) *Statistika Apotelesmata dia tas Kykladas Nesous* (Athens: National Printers), pp. 186–7; NSSG (1929) *Statistika Apotelesmata dia ten Peloponneson* (Athens: National Printers), pp. 748–9)

24 years. The values for the Sterea Hellas and Voiotia region, which includes Athens and Piraeus, rest between the two. The average CEB for marriages of more than 25 years' duration in the Ionian Islands is distinctly lower than all the other regions for the same marriage duration.[14] There are many possible explanations for the observed differences, from differences in age at marriage, differences in nutritional status or occupational structure.[15] The significant point is that there *were* regional differences and that these do not seem to have been consistent over time, except for the Cyclades, which consistently exhibited the highest fertility. Moreover, overall levels of surviving children were moderate, the highest being, again, that of the Cyclades, with seven children among those fathers who had been married for more than 25 years in 1920.

Why Were Levels of Fertility Moderate Prior to 1928?

In order to gain an understanding of the situation at the time and in the absence of civil registration data I have resorted to the 1928 population census, which provides population by single year of age up to the age of 30, thus taking the observations back to those born in 1898–1899. These data provide a unique opportunity to observe the changes in childbearing for these pre-1928 years, though keeping in mind the effects of cumulative mortality on the various ages. From the 1928 population census figures issues of 'age heaping' are obvious, particularly for women reporting ages of 25, 22, 20 and 18—all ages associated with the marriage market (Fig. 2.3).[16] Additionally, the 1898–1899, 1916–1917 and 1918–1919 birth cohorts can be identified as abnormally low. The last of these was presumably linked to the Spanish influenza pandemic and its effects, but the involvement of Greece in World War I in 1917–1918 and in the Greco-Turkish War in 1919–1920 would also have had an effect. All these events would have reduced the number of births and increased the number of deaths among the members of this cohort. The shrinkage of the 1916–1917 cohort and possibly that of 1917–1918 were almost certainly associated with the 1915–1917 national schism that almost resulted in a civil war and which included the May 1916–June 1917 blockade imposed on 'Old' Greece by French and British forces,[17] which led to hunger and increased mortality; although it has remained understudied and 'forgotten' among historians, elderly informants did refer to it during my interviews,

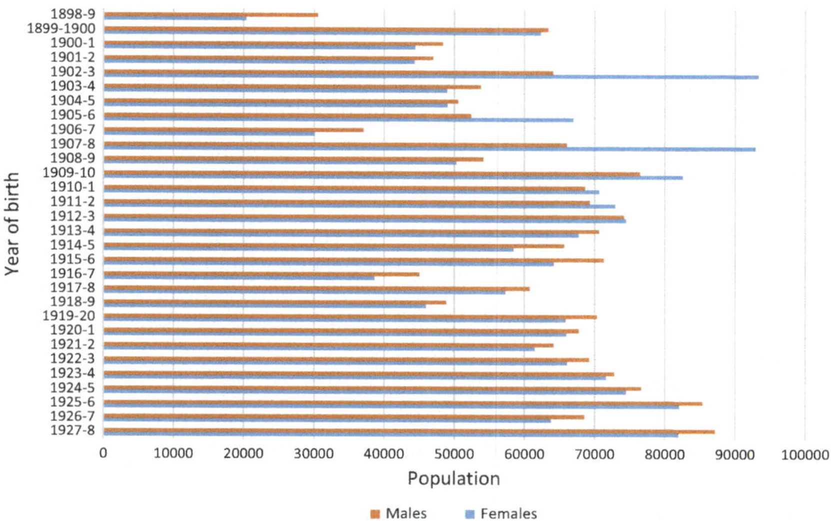

Fig. 2.3 Population pyramid by sex and year of birth, 1928 census. (Sources: NSSG (1935) *Statistika Apotelesmata Apografes Plethysmou tes Ellados 1928* (Athens: National printers), table I, p. 3; refugee data: table II, p. 369)

comparing it to the major famine of 1941–1943.[18] The blockade led to hoarding, increased food prices and an unsettling of the market that continued well beyond its end.[19] For example, according to government sources, the price of cereals increased 3.3 times between 1914 and 1919. By early 1922 the increase was 15 times that of the 1914 prices.[20] However, a further factor may have been a major financial crisis in the early 1920s that led to a 60% increase in the cost of living index in 1922 compared with the previous year[21] and an 86% increase in 1923.[22] The year 1922 also saw the Catastrophe, when the Greek army was defeated in Asia Minor and more than a million destitute refugees arrived in Greece. Inflation rose in the period from 1923 to 1926. The government attributed the increase in food prices to the decline in agricultural production during the war and the extreme inflation.[23] However, A.F. Freris points to the turbulent fiscal situation of the country in the years 1920–1926.[24] Andrianakos, a contemporary practising obstetrician, noted in 1925 that after 1917 births had declined in Athens because of 'worsened living conditions'.[25]

Subsequently, the international financial crisis of 1929 affected Greece in the period 1930–1932, leading to the Greek default of 1932.[26]

Uncertainty and fear regarding the possibility of a full-blown famine almost certainly led to a curtailing of fertility in the years following the 1916–1917 blockade. A similar effect on fertility, associated with an uncertain provisioning situation, was observed in later years on Hios, for example, following the 1941–1943 famine there.[27] While part of the decline may well have been attributable to the physical effects of hunger and malnutrition, in this case much of the decline would have been due to the psychological effects of the possibility of a famine developing.[28] The dire economic situation in 1922–1926 would also have affected levels of fertility.

The 1898–1899 cohort is also exceptionally small, although this may be because of the age heaping of the next birth cohort. On the other hand, it might well be genuinely small, as the 1890s were another decade of insecurity for Greece: the economically important export trade in raisins collapsed in 1893; Greece defaulted the same year; the brief war with the Ottoman Empire in 1897 resulted in a humiliating war indemnity; and Greece was forced to accept the presence of an International Financial Commission (IFC) that ran the Greek economy for a good number of years.[29] There are reports of villages in mainland Greece facing hunger in 1897 and in 1900–1901.[30] The response of their populations was mass emigration to the USA, which led to an estimated annual loss of 25,000 men up to 1924, when restrictions on migration were imposed.[31] These extreme levels of emigration were already evident in 1909, when the commentator on the 1907 census results attributed the halved rate of population increase between 1896 and 1907—compared with that in the period 1889–1896—entirely to 'huge emigration' to the USA.[32] The author added that Greeks at the time also migrated to Latin America, Canada and Australia, as well as Sudan and South Africa.[33] Emigrants were predominantly men, both single and married.[34] In the latter case, families were left behind, only the breadwinner migrating. Single men returned occasionally to Greece to find a bride, or Greek brides were shipped to the USA. During the same period many men remained in the USA while their wives and families stayed in Greece. Children were born to these marriages as a result of rare visits made by the husband to his family.[35] Furthermore, men who were sailors or were employed in Athens or another city for a significant part of the year might also be away for lengthy periods[36]—another factor

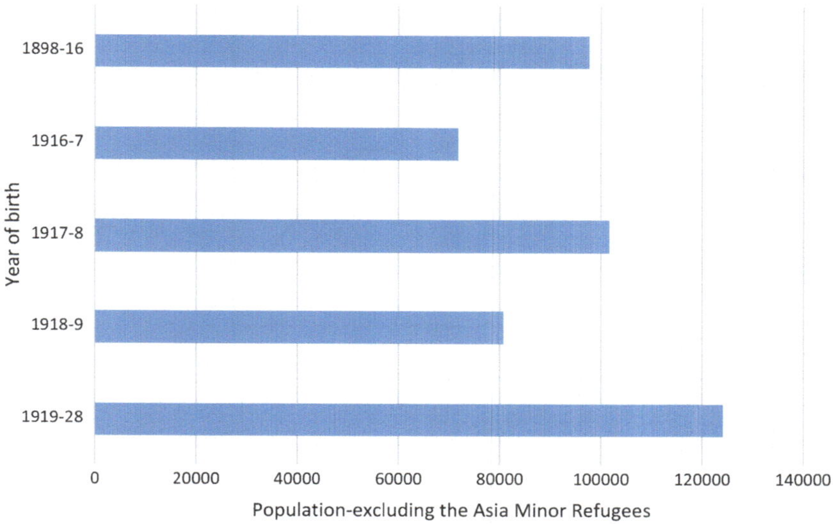

Fig. 2.4 1928 annualised population figures, except for the Asia Minor refugees, by years of birth as reported in the 1928 census. (Sources: NSSG (1935) *Statistika Apotelesmata Apografes Plethysmou tes Ellados 1928* (Athens: National printers), table I, p. 3; refugee data: table II, p. 369)

that kept fertility moderately low in this period, although without couples necessarily intentionally restricting it.[37]

However, when merging various birth cohorts, the annualised 1919–1928 cohort is clearly larger than those of 1898–1916 and 1917–1918 (Fig. 2.4).[38] Here the Asia Minor refugees who were arriving in small numbers in the 1910s and in a massive wave in 1922 have been excluded in order to enable meaningful comparisons over time. While mortality partly explains the difference in the sizes of the various cohorts, the variance is large enough to express a genuine increase of births in the latest period, the years 1919–1928. Moreover, the calculation of the Coale's indices for Greece, including the refugees, gives the index of marital fertility (I_g) as 0.453 in 1879, 0.431 in 1920 and 0.539 in 1928. In comparison, the same index was 0.580 on Mykonos in 1861, when fertility there was certainly natural. Coale's index of overall fertility (I_f) in 1870 was 0.300 for Greece and 0.408 for Mykonos. The 1879 I_f for Greece was a meagre 0.279.[39]

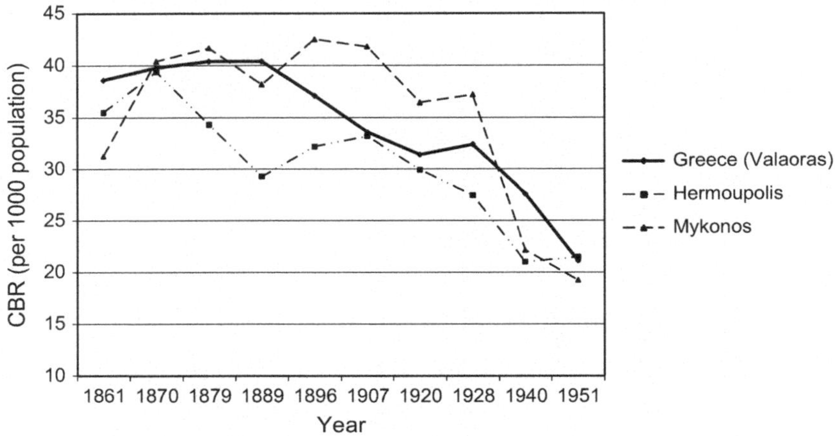

Fig. 2.5 Crude birth rate, Hermoupolis, Mykonos and Greece (Valaoras). (Sources: The Mykonos and Hermoupolis births were obtained from the Mykonos/Hermoupolis Civil Registration books held on Mykonos and Hermoupolis Municipality respectively. The data for Greece are from Valaoras, 'A Reconstruction')

Looking at the CBRs of the two communities for which we have data for over 100 years—that is, Mykonos and Hermoupolis—the disparity is evident and significant (Fig. 2.5).[40] Such a disparity expresses the substantially different socio-economic backgrounds of the two communities, with the merchant town of Hermoupolis attracting large numbers of migrants, many of whom were single. The very different levels of mortality experienced in the two communities—very high in urban Hermoupolis, but much lower on Mykonos—would certainly also have affected fertility levels.[41] For the semi-urban population of Mykonos the effects of the difficult decades of the late 1880s—early 1890s and the 1910s were expressed in the reduced CBR; urban Hermoupolis, which relied on trade, was much more affected, experiencing larger dips in the specific decades but also recovering less well and more slowly than Mykonos. While CBRs in both places declined between 1907 and 1920, those of Mykonos and of Greece recovered to a degree in 1928, before they irrevocably declined.[42] However, that of Hermoupolis did not.

Thus, in the particularly difficult decades from the 1890s to the mid-1920s, financial hardships, wars and emigration, along with the blockade, all had a dampening effect on childbearing. These examples suggest that the condition of the nation had a significant impact on levels of and fluctuations in fertility from year to year; that the effect of such conditions was not uniform across the various localities, but depended also on the local economy and structures; and that the observed changes in fertility in this period were not a result of individual decisions but reflected wider economic and social changes and people's reactions to such conditions. All this is also evident from the findings of the existing family reconstitution studies.

Despite Siampos and Valaoras' assertion that fertility decline started sometime in the late nineteenth century, there is no firm evidence that this was the case. The existing family reconstitution studies show a 'natural fertility' situation for the nineteenth-century marriage cohorts (Fig. 2.6).[43]

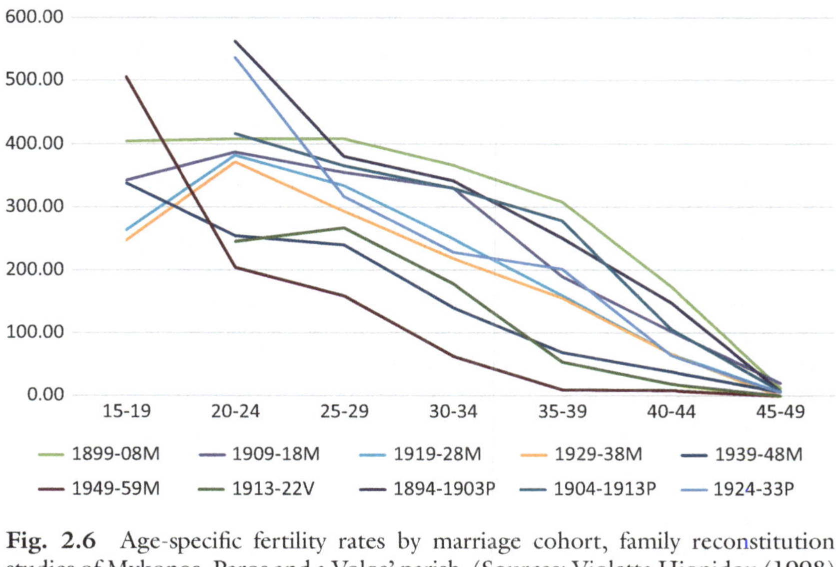

Fig. 2.6 Age-specific fertility rates by marriage cohort, family reconstitution studies of Mykonos, Paros and a Volos' parish. (Sources: Violetta Hionidou (1998) 'The Adoption of Fertility Control on Mykonos, 1879–1959: Stopping, Spacing or Both?', *Population Studies*, 52(1), 67–83; Vasilis S. Gavalas (2002) 'Fertility transition on a Greek island', *Continuity and Change*, 17(2), 133–60; Ntina Moustani (2014) 'Oi Demografikes Exelixeis s'ena Viomehaniko Kentro: Volos, 1881–1922' (unpublished PhD thesis: University of Thessalia))

For Mykonos, I have shown elsewhere that the 1914–1918 marriage cohort was the first to exhibit a different behaviour from the previous ones and only in the later years of its reproductive life, thus situating the start of the decline in the late 1920s at the earliest.[44] Gavalas, in his study of two communities on the neighbouring island of Paros, identified the 1914–1923 marriage cohort as the first cohort to exhibit a slight deviation from natural fertility, but, again, only in the latest years of its childbearing, leading him to situate the start of the decline 'between the late 1920s and early 1930s'.[45] Yet another family reconstitution of one marriage cohort, 1913–1922, of the parish of Agios Konstantinos in the city of Volos, also argues that this cohort controlled its fertility, much more stringently than those of Mykonos or Paros, for that matter.[46] The very low total fertility rate (henceforth TFR) of 3.79 for this cohort suggests that fertility control may well have started earlier in this Volos parish, perhaps indicating earlier fertility control among urban populations.[47] The family reconstitution studies thus support the notion that in rural communities such as those of Paros and semi-urban populations such as that of Mykonos fertility started declining around 1930, whereas for urban populations fertility had already been in decline by that time.

As the interwar period is flagged up as an important one by the family reconstitution studies, it is worth turning our attention to the published national sources on fertility. Demographers, among them Valaoras, have shown that the coverage of vital statistics, which restarted in the early 1920s, became full only later in the decade, with the 1930s data not only having full coverage but also being considered as highly reliable.[48] It is significant that, starting in 1931 and regularly published thereafter, the age of the mother at birth was also recorded on the birth certificate. The availability of the 1928 census thus enables us to calculate the age-specific fertility rates (ASFRs) of the Greek population for the years 1931–1938, the dates for which such data is available (Fig. 2.7).[49]

Two different denominators were used in the calculations: for the years 1931–1933 the 1928 age structure was employed; and for the remaining years the 1935 female age structure, estimated by the National Statistical Service, was used.[50] It is notable that the shape of the age-specific fertility curve for the first three years resembles that of natural fertility, although possibly at lower levels than would be expected for a historical population. Nevertheless, right from the start the values of the 25–29 and 30–34 age range rates decline almost annually, with the younger and older age groups remaining mostly stable. From 1934 onwards the shape of the curve

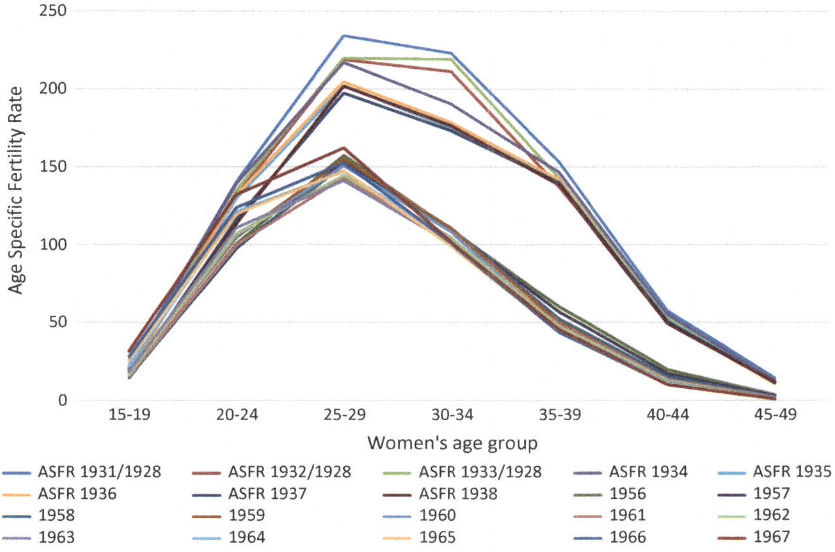

Fig. 2.7 Annual age-specific fertility rates, 1931–1938 and 1956–1967, Greece. Note: The 1931, 1932 and 1933 ASFR figures were calculated using the 1928 census age structure for women. For the rest of the 1930s ASFRs, the NSSG estimated 1935 age structure was employed. (Sources: 1931 births (NSSG [1933] *Statistike tes fysikes kineseos tou Plethysmou tes Ellados kata to etos 1931* [thereafter SKP] [Athens: National Printers], p. ξβ); 1932 births (SKP 1934, p. 62); 1933 and 1934 births (SKP 1936, p. 68); 1935 births (SKP 1937, p. 65); 1936 births (SKP 1938, p. 60); 1937 births (SKP 1939, p. 62); 1938 births (SKP 1940, p. 53); NSSG (1935) *Statistika Apotelesmata tes Apografes tou Plethysmou tes Ellados tes 15–16 Maiou 1928*, vol. 2 (Athens: National Printers), p. μθ, table 17; 1935 estimated female age structure: NSSG (1966) *Demographic Trends and Population Projections of Greece 1960–1985* (Athens: n.p.), p. 29); 1958–62: NSSG (1966) *Demographic Trends and Population Projections of Greece 1960–1985* (Athens: n.p.), p. 33; 1963–1967 ASFRs: Garyfalia Serelea (1979) 'Oi taseis tes gonimotetas tou Ellenikou Plethysmou kata ten periodo 1956–1976 kai oi deiktes metreseos tes', *Greek Review of Social Research*, 36–37, 253)

changes, as the 30–34 group exhibits a downward shift. However, little change seems to exist in the years 1934–1938. It is interesting to note here that post-World War II publications invariably utilise the 1934–1938 rates to illustrate that fertility was controlled in the 1930s, without reference to the earlier rates.

Clearly, the 1930s was a decade of significant and rapid changes in the fertility of the nation. Yet I would argue that the 1931 fertility curve was still very close to that of natural fertility. To determine whether that was the case the indexed values of the age-specific marital fertility rates (ASMFRs) (with the 20–24 group being the index) are depicted in Fig. 2.8, which does indeed depict the natural fertility curve of a population, the curve being almost identical for the years 1931–1933, except for the volatile 15–19 group.[51] Comparing the ASMFRs of the early 1930s for Greece with those of the Mykonos and Paros family reconstitutions shows the 1931 curve for Greece situated between the two marriage cohorts that had

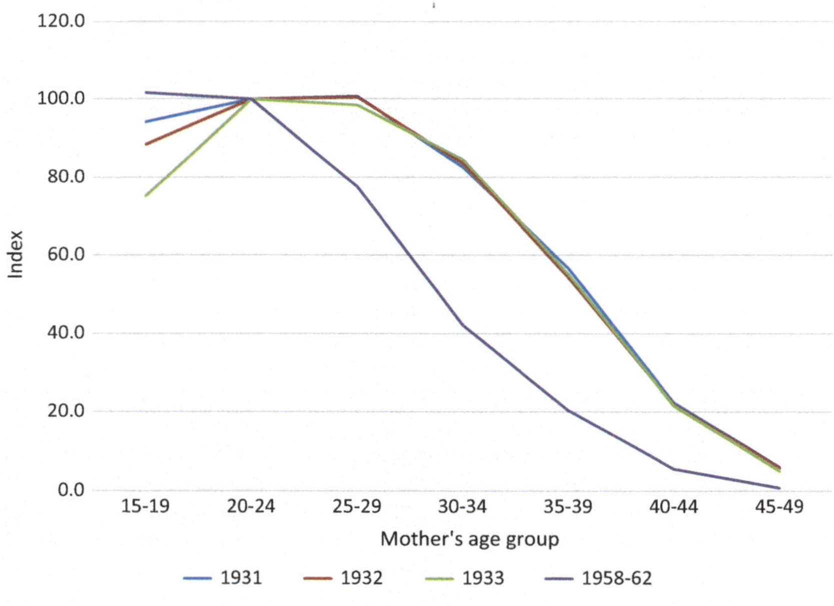

Fig. 2.8 Index of age-specific marital fertility rates (20–24 = 100) for early 1930s and 1958–1962, Greece. (Sources: 1931 births (SKP 1933, p. ξβ); 1932 births (SKP 1934, p. 62); NSSG (1935) *Statistika Apotelesmata tes Apografes tou Plethysmou tes Ellados tes 15–16 Maiou 1928*, vol. 2 (Athens: National Printers), p. μθ, table 17; 1958–1962: NSSG (1966) *Demographic Trends and Population Projections of Greece 1960–1985* (Athens: n.p.), p. 29, Female population by age and marital status from NSSG (1962) *Apotelesmata tes apografes plethysmou-katoikion tes 19 Martiou 1961*, Teuhos 1 (Athens: n.p.), p. 21)

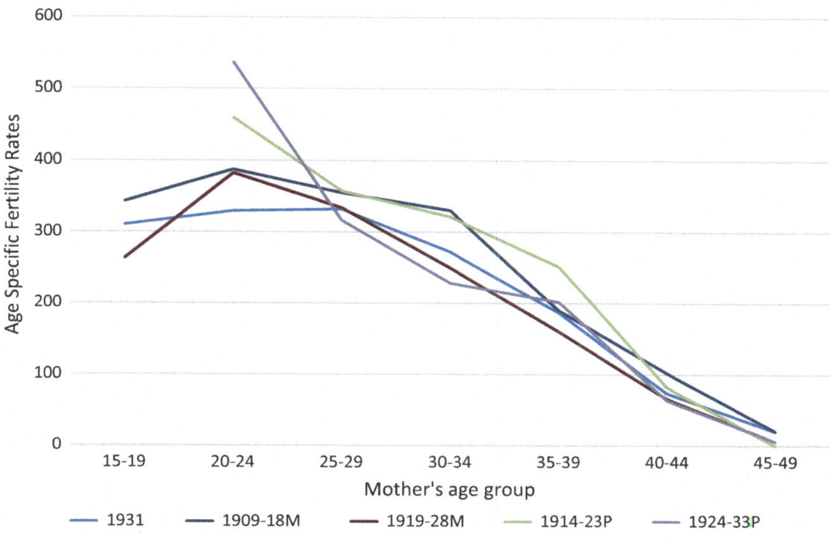

Fig. 2.9 Age-specific marital fertility rates of 1931 Greece and of various marriage cohorts of the Mykonos and Paros family reconstitutions. (Sources: 1931 births (SKP 1933, p. ξβ); Hionidou, 'The Adoption'; Gavalas, 'Fertility')

only just started controlling their fertility (1909–1918 for Mykonos and 1914–1923 for Paros) and the subsequent ones that fully controlled their fertility (Fig. 2.9).[52] Here it should be noted that the 1931 curve is a period measure, whereas the family reconstitution curves represent the experiences of marriage cohorts. Therefore, there is a time gap between the experiences of the latter in comparison to the 1931 marital fertility curve.

Figure 2.7 shows that the ASFRs of the early 1930s were all high. The changing shape and height of the ASFR curves from 1934 onwards indicate the irreversible parity-specific employment of family limitation for the country as a whole.[53] Such quantitative evidence is strongly supported by the qualitative evidence from the last years of the 1930s compiled by E. Averof. Averof focused his research on areas with medium or high levels of fertility, including villages, towns and cities, and determined that between 5 and 34% of couples who got married after 1922 neither controlled their fertility nor wanted to do so. In one of the villages he examined, none of the couples controlled their fertility.[54] Among the urban populations, in contrast, Averof observed an 'intense' control of fertility, even in cities (such as Larissa and Trikala) situated in counties with high levels of fertility.[55] For the three cities he investigated (Larissa, Trikala and Patras), between 53 and 68% of the couples used fertility-control methods of some kind. Among the villages he studied, the same percentage ranged from 17 to 67 (except the one village where no couples restricted their fertility).[56]

Thus, fertility was limited neither in nineteenth-century Greece nor until the late 1920s at the level of the country. After 1934, signs of parity-specific control become evident in the national rates. The effects of repeated wars, maritime blockades, political instability and financial turmoil compressed fertility levels in the 1920s. The affluent sections of urban populations did control their fertility throughout the 1920s. In the early 1930s, and while fertility levels were moderate, with a TFR of 4.2 in 1931, the shape of the fertility curve was still that of natural fertility: that is, a fertility regime where control is not practised in a parity-specific way. This is very much in line with the findings of the family reconstitutions. This combination of a 'natural'-appearing fertility curve with a rather low TFR suggests that any control of fertility that was taking place at the time was not associated with parity but was rather taking place haphazardly, over much of the reproductive life of the woman. This would correspond well to the main reason for controlling fertility in the 1910s and 1920s Greece: that is, a response to the repeated crises experienced by the population. While abortion would have been the reaction of urban women to such crises, for rural women attempts to space or delay the next pregnancy and the inefficient use of rudimentary methods would also lead to the results observed.

Overall, then, Greek fertility experienced significant changes in the 1930s. This is the primary decade of change, although there were places that had experienced significant decline before 1930 (Athens among them most certainly, but probably Hermoupolis too). However, the decline was not fully accomplished during the 1930s. By the next point at which reliable data are available—that is, the mid-1950s—fertility had reached low levels. As had happened earlier in the century, war, occupation, famine, financial dislocation and a civil war had an important effect on the level to which fertility declined but also the speed of the decline, bringing the country's fertility to levels that could be called 'modern' by the mid-1950s.

The 1950s Onwards

Figure 2.7 enables us to imagine the changes that occurred between the 1930s and the 1950s and 1960s. As mentioned above, there are no vital registration data for the years 1939–1954 because the collection of vital statistics by the central statistical service ceased in that period.[57] The figure shows the major decline that occurred in the 25 years from 1939 to 1954: fertility declined for *every* age group, but the decline was most spectacular for the three age groups with the highest fertility rates in 1931, those aged 25–39. The peak of fertility continued to occur within the age group 25–29 in both the late 1950s and the 1960s. The change observed from the 1950s to the 1960s is small, although the 1967 curve suggests further declines for all groups above the age group 25–29 and visible increases for the two youngest groups. This reflects the younger age at marriage in this period and the very close link between marriage and the birth of the first child in Greece. The decline for the older age groups signifies the decline in higher-order births, squeezing childbearing to the lower birth orders. Importantly, it signifies the tight control of fertility by couples who by 1967 were able to control not only the number of their offspring but also the timing of their birth.

Figure 2.8 demonstrates the shape of the ASMFRs curve when indexed for the 20–24 age group. While the curve for the early 1930s shows an essentially identical convex shape for each of the years, by the 1958–1962 period this has become a concave one. As before, most of the decline took place in the most productive post-20s age groups—that is, 25–29, 30–34 and 35–39, especially the middle of these. In subsequent years the indexed curve demonstrated greater control for all age groups, with the older group having almost entirely ceased childbearing by the end of the 1960s, while the 40–44 group had reduced it to very low levels. Thus extremely stringent control was in place for the oldest age groups. The 1970–1972 marriage cohort had further reduced its fertility, in comparison to the 1960–1962 period, in every age group except for the two youngest, which actually increased their fertility. This increase demonstrated that childbearing in Greek society was linked to marriage and that, once marriage had occurred, childbearing was expected to follow soon after. For example, E. Friedl, during her field trip in the village of Vasilika, noted that couples would start considering how many children to have only after they had had 'at least one' child.[58] By the end of the 1960s most married women of childbearing age would have one or two children and the younger age groups were the ones within which most such childbearing was taking place, meaning that childbearing at ages above 30 could essentially be dispensed with.[59] Even during this period of highly controlled fertility, however, demographers pointed to the possible effects of migration on it, arguing that emigration affected fertility negatively.[60]

Friedl was one of the first anthropologists to study life in a Greek village, namely Vasilika, in Voiotia.[61] She explains how, during the second half of the 1950s, regulating family size was not only accepted but seen as 'prudent and sensible', and estimated that those families with children of marriageable age at the time of her fieldwork had around four children, whereas their own parents had had around eight at the same point in their lives.[62] With the age at marriage being between 25 and 30, she situates the start of the decline in the period 1925–1935.[63] Richard and Eva Blum, in their anthropological study of three villages in mainland Greece in the late 1950s and early 1960s, concluded that couples controlled their fertility in all three villages, although in one of them this seemed to have started much earlier than in the other two.[64] Valaoras and his collaborators undertook a fertility survey in 1962–1963, interviewing 3838 families from rural and urban areas.[65] Couples expressed their desire for a small number of children, and 78.7% of rural couples and 87.1% of urban couples said that they used some kind of birth control.[66] For all ages except those 21 or younger (and, curiously, those aged 45), urban women had fewer live children than rural women, indicating that rural–urban differences persisted to the end of our examined period.[67]

It is difficult to examine the rural–urban differences in fertility with the existing sources. However, by employing the CBRs from 1925 onwards it can be seen that the urban rate was lower than the rural one, and that the two rates show a similar trend and parallel fluctuations until 1931 (Fig. 2.10).[68] From 1932 the two diverge: the urban CBR declines from 1932 onwards, whereas the rural CBR decline starts in 1935 but takes place more rapidly than the urban one. Here it should be mentioned that until 1920 the percentage of the urban population residing in cities with populations of more than 100,000 was below 12%; this increased gradually to 19% in 1940 and 37% in 1971.[69] In 1964 the two lines cross and the trend seems to revert thereafter, with the rural CBR becoming lower than the urban one. Considering the problems that are associated with this measurement (for example, increasing reporting of rural births in

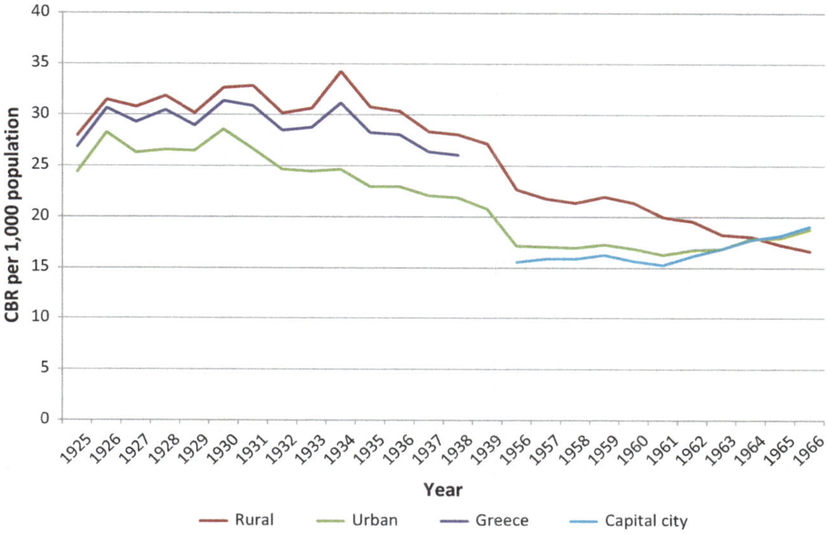

Fig. 2.10 Crude birth rates of rural and urban populations, Athens and Greece, 1925–1966. (Sources: Vas. G. Valaoras (1971) 'Changing Patterns of Fertility Differentials (The Case of Greece)', *International Population Conference, London 1969* (Liege: IUSSP), pp. 2074–80; Gerasimos Alivizatos (1947) *Mnemonion Ygieines* (Athens: n.p.))

urban areas, where births were increasingly taking place) I will not focus on the last three years (1965–1967). Figure 2.2 also offers a glimpse of the rural–urban differences. The 1920 CEB information is plotted there for each county and Greece as a whole, showing that only among the most recently married men (those married for less than five years) Sterea Ellas/Voiotia, which included the capital Athens, the largest urban centre at the time, had experienced a lower CEB value in comparison to the country's value.[70] While the other examined regions did not demonstrate distinctly higher values than those of the country for that specific cohort, nevertheless they were not lower than that of Greece. Beyond the CBR, it is the qualitative information that emphasises the more widespread control of fertility among urbanites in comparison to the rural population in the inter-war period.

Public Discourse on Population Change

The Greek state was created in 1832 following the 1821 revolution, a bloody war against the Ottoman Empire and a civil war. As the Muslim population left the new state over a period of time, the resulting population gaps must have been obvious to see. The loss of the Christian population in the decade of war must have also been noticeable. Much nineteenth-century thinking about population was focused on its natural increase, something that was seen as insurance for the future and prosperity of the new state. This was very much in line with the manner of thinking of other states at the time. As the Greek state was a new one and its main enemy was a sizeable one—the Ottoman Empire—increased population was seen as central and vital to the fledgling state's future. Much public discourse in the nineteenth century moved around the 'unredeemed' Christian populations of the Ottoman Empire, populations that the Greek state claimed and wished to incorporate into its fold. Thus, such people, *the eterochthones*, were welcomed in Greece and were offered equal rights with those born in the Greek state whenever they chose to move within its borders. Ideally, the Greek state aimed to incorporate both those people and the lands they lived on. This was achieved on a number of occasions in the nineteenth and early twentieth centuries. However, on numerous other occasions Greece also received Christian refugees fleeing the Ottoman Empire, the most significant instance of which was in 1922–1923 when, following the Lausanne Treaty, any dreams of territorial expansion were shattered and all Christians living in Turkey had to leave. Thus, the Greek state opened its borders to more than a million refugees, when its own population at the time was around five million. While the Greek population at times contested the presence of refugees in the country, the state has always been supportive. Most historians and politicians, though certainly not all at the time, saw this new 'blood' as a positive addition to the Greek population. Comparison with the burgeoning neighbouring Turkish population has never ceased to occur, even nowadays, encouraging a nationalistic 'obligation' to reproduce for the 'nation'.[71] However, the arrival of refugees in 1922 and the population-centred discussions taking place in interwar Europe more widely led to a population discourse in Greece too.

Despite this, discussions on population had begun some time earlier, although they were mostly restricted to medical publications. For example, the only nineteenth-century reference to population that directly mentions the idea of restricting childbearing appears in a volume authored by a physician focusing on sterility. Antonios Kindynes, in the first page of his introduction, questioned how sterility could be considered as 'beneficial' and described how many people were trying through 'thousands of mysterious precautions' to avoid fertility and, when failing, 'destroy[ing] and exterminat[ing] through the terrible crimes of abortion and infanticide' the pregnancy.[72] Kindynes also referred to Malthus and his 'known theories, in support of which a feverish battle is currently undertaken in his home country among the most prestigious physicians of England', as well as the explosive discussions that 'recently had taken place in the Medical Academy of Paris', where some eminent members supported the 'mostly immoral and destructive for the State principles of Malthus'.[73] When '[neo]Malthusianists' from abroad wrote to an eminent Greek paediatrician to find out whether the Greek population was also employing 'artificial checks', Anastasios Zinnes replied that 'we are busy looking for ways to increase our population'.[74] Kindynes pointed out that philosophers and economists in Greece appeared to be reticent in leading a 'true crusade' against these new principles of restricting the number of children, something that—he noted—is against the Christian spirit. Thus, the onus was on 'medicine—or should I say on physicians—to fight against those destructive principles' of Malthus and his followers. For medicine, Kindynes argued, fertility should always be considered as 'nature's gift'.[75]

Kindynes' assessment was accurate in more than one way. First, it was almost exclusively physicians who spoke publicly about issues of population and birth control.[76] Second, the state and most of the intelligentsia were not keen to hear or publicly discuss, let alone accept, Malthusian or neo-Malthusian ideas. This continued to be the case for the next 30 years. In 1917 Mihael Kaires, within his discussion of eugenics, rearticulated the 'foundational principles of [Greek] society which stands against sterility and the restriction of births, [which if undertaken] repeatedly, [is] against the reduction of the country's population'.[77] In 1922 another physician, M. Moyseides, engaging with eugenics poignantly summarised the essence of his book: 'Marriage, robust motherhood, rich and fertile, that is what our race needs in order to stand back on its feet.'[78] Earlier, Moyseides had pointed out the declining number of marriages that were taking place, attributing this to 'post-war [World War I] ideas and various social reasons', which led to large numbers of single people, 'especially in the cities'.[79] Significantly, Moyseides also mentioned, very briefly, that 'among our most affluent classes, a reduction in the number of births can be observed, something that should not have been the case'.[80] At the same time, the robust expression of the state's desire for an increased population is explicitly supported by the Church in, for example, the writings of an Archimandrite who summarised the Church's guidance with a quote from the bible—'*Be fruitful and multiply*'—and a reprimand for women who 'avoid the familial weight of childbearing'.[81] Interestingly, in his elaborations on this he referred exclusively to abortion rather than to contraception.[82]

It was not until the mid-1920s that questions of overpopulation, mortality, fertility and migration as a whole were addressed for the first time. Gregorios Hatzevasileiou, the head physician of Piraeus, in a lengthy article entitled 'The population problem in Greece', eloquently outlined the rather complicated and unconventional situation at the time. The year 1925 was exceptional in many ways: emigration had been effectively shut down by new laws in the USA; Greece had received more than a million—mostly destitute—refugees just a couple of years earlier; and a decade earlier Greece's northern borders had moved northwards, incorporating areas such as Macedonia and Thrace that had a very different epidemiological profile from that of 'Old' Greece. In addition, this was also a year of extreme increases in prices of food and inflation. Hatzivasileiou emphasised the resulting high mortality levels and destitution of the Greek poor and saw no prospects of improvement in the mortality situation. Fertility, he believed, was high, and contrasted favourably with that of—presumably—western European countries.[83] At the same time, his assessment was that Greece was experiencing an unprecedented 'overpopulation'. However, and even considering the extremely inadequate nutrition of the population, he believed that no attempt should be made to influence fertility; rather, the situation should be allowed to continue as it was—that is, fertility should be unrestricted among the rural population since 'our population has not espoused yet the degenerate tendencies of the so called "individual liberties"'.[84] Nevertheless, he warned, 'in cities the uncontrollable tendency to reduce fertility and the system of one or two children had already begun for some time'.[85]

The rural population was perceived by those writing in the 1920s as one that would not change, that simply had no reason to change: 'Having many children is useful only to the peasant (horiatis), the farmer. For him they are wealth, just like his oxen and his donkeys because as soon as they are 10 years old they will become productive and they will relieve him from his work.'[86] While the rich could afford to have many children and to bring them up properly, 'they are more careful than us [the urban middle/lower class] so that the inheritance will not be shared and the capital reduced'. As for the non-wealthy urbanite, many children represent 'misery and poverty'.[87] A. Sygkelakes demonstrates this with the example of an artisan who marries for love without receiving a dowry and who eventually manages to acquire a house. If he has too many children, these will overspill from the house and he will never be able to provide them with an education or pamper them. They will become the thieves, criminals and prostitutes of tomorrow. But, if, soon after their wedding, a good man[88] said to the artisan and his wife 'do you want to have only two children for your own benefit? This is what you will do', things would be very different.[89] And thus the author proceeded to present the 'necessary' birth control advice in a friendly and approachable manner, unlike most other preceding publications. Sygkelakes put forward new suggestions as to when birth control could be used, moving from the bare necessity of reducing the number of children to recommending the delay of childbearing right at the start of marriage because such a pregnancy 'is a real misfortune as within few days the headaches will start and the vomiting and then [it will be] goodbye sexual games, pleasure and honeymoon'.[90] Other circumstances in which he advocated contraception included women who should not conceive for health reasons. Thus, while Sygkelakes believed that the upper classes, unlike people from other classes, were controlling their fertility while the peasants did not and would not do so in the foreseeable future, he argued that the middle and upper working class, then not controlling their fertility, would do so if they were given the means and were suitably educated.

Sygkelakes was not the only writer to explicitly discuss birth control methods in the 1920s. Other publications also outlined and discussed in detail the various then-existing methods of birth control. One such is a short article appearing in a medical journal, in which the contraceptive information was essentially an acknowledged translation of A. Forel's publication.[91] The author suggests that such methods would be appropriate for young people who wanted to get married but were unable to afford children, presumably referring to the difficult financial situation of the time but also to the situation in which marriages were longpostponed owing to the conflicts in which the country had been involved.[92] In sharp contrast, Moyseides, in his book *The Hygiene of Marriage*, refers to the changing nature of marriage in 'large urban centres', where it had become, as he saw it, a licence to sexual pleasures without motherhood.

He describes how some women, presumably from the upper classes, saw motherhood as the 'nine-month interruption from their high society life', but also pointed to their fear of losing their looks and of giving birth, while men feared the dispersion of the family fortune.[93]

Towards the end of the decade Apostolos Doxiadis, a physician who had also served as Minister of Health (1922–1924) and Deputy Minister of Hygiene (1928–1929) in Liberal governments, wrote a significant piece addressing, as Hatzevasileiou had done three years earlier, the major population questions of Greece.[94] He started by emphasising that, unlike other states, who were aware that their population was not increasing, 'we do not know what is happening in Greece',[95] and went on to outline his own observations:

> The urban population procreates less than those in smaller towns and villages do. But even within the city population, there are differences. The inteligencia, the [white collar] employee, the military officers, the affluent have fewer children than the workers, the artisans, the petit bourgeoisie…the mortality of children is much lower in towns rather than in the provinces.[96] … Among the Athenian families, the number of families with two children is very large and those with only one child is even larger.[97]

Thus, the 1920s ended with a small number of writers making qualitative assessments of fertility in Greece. Although the severe lack of data compelled these authors to utilise their observational and professional skills in judging the situation, they were all among the most qualified people to make such judgements. All came to very similar conclusions: namely, that the rural population did not control their fertility, while urban populations, especially the Athenian upper classes, did so rather stringently. Doxiadis, like others, attributed the decline partly to financial reasons, but also cited psychological ones, especially among the most affluent classes, such as the lack of a feeling of solidarity towards wider society and obligation towards the country.[98]

The 1930s brought both more accurate and plentiful data and many more discussions on the rapidly evolving population situation. Much of the latter took place in the first two years of the decade, 1930–1931, during the Liberal government of E. Venizelos. The open, though short-lived, discussion reflected to a degree events on the international scene. As expected, given the dominance of eugenics in the population discourse of the most advanced states in the 1930s, vocal eugenicists existed in the

Greek scene too (Kaires and Moyseides among those already cited, as well as Drakoulides and Louros, from whom we will hear below), although they achieved little in the inter-war period.[99] For example, Drakoulides lamented in 1933 that when the Civil Code was revised in late 1930 the relevant committee declined to introduce a prohibition to marriage for specific health conditions that affected either the woman or the man, with one of the committee members responding that 'marriage does not mean … childbearing'.[100] Those without a eugenic stance were significantly less vocal. As Eleutheriades pointed out, someone had to be 'bold' to dare to express his innermost thoughts in the 'puritanical atmosphere that we live in'.[101] Very few were 'bold'. Those who were discussed overpopulation, the migration of the excess rural population to cities, the protection of motherhood, the burgeoning orphanage of Athens and the high mortality among urban infants.[102] Some focused on housing and how this had become scarce, partly because of the excessive in-migration of the rural population to cities.[103] Others discussed the changing nature of the urban 'family', which had ceased operating as a single economic unit, unlike the rural one;[104] the high early-age mortality of urban children as a result of the absence of breastfeeding—again, a situation that contrasted with that of their rural counterparts;[105] the burgeoning orphanages of children whose parents had died from 'hunger or other privations'; and begging children, of which there were approximately 6000 in Piraeus alone.[106] Some were convinced that once the financial situation improved the fertility of the urban working class would increase as well.[107] However, others attributed the observed situation to the effects of 'wealth and luxury', but supported the promotion of contraceptive methods in order to avoid the use of abortions and to ensure that women 'have children but do not become childbearing machines'.[108] One of the readers of a journal that repeatedly published on population issues during the 1930s accurately identified the problem of disjuncture between the actions and wishes of the state as opposed to those of private individuals. While the former protected large families 'and provides multiple privileges and facilities', the latter from time to time supported the idea of 'fewer marriages—fewer children'. This, according to the author, was proof that Greece as a whole was 'yet to form a clear understanding of the issue'.[109]

A constant and consistent thread in all writings, mostly explicitly but sometimes implicitly, was the unchanging high fertility of the peasants. Doxiadis offered some numerical guidance on the situation in Greece, emphasising that this was a 'short review and personal examination of a small number of families': the upper class, which included bankers, scientists and so on, had two children; the middle class had three to four; the petit bourgeoisie had four to five and the workers (presumably urban and agricultural ones) and peasants had five to seven.[110] Doxiadis calculates an average family size of 4.5, which, we are told, was close to the one provided by the existing statistics. Elsewhere, Doxiadis explained that '9/10s of parents procreate unconsciously', an observation that one can assume applies to his fourth group, workers and peasants, given that those with lower numbers of children *had* to act consciously to achieve that.[111] In yet another article he refers to the 70–80% of the population making up the group of peasants and workers.[112] Doxiadis was not alone in thinking so. M.R., also writing in *Eleuthero Vema*, argued that for peasants and workers high fertility was not an actual choice but rather an act of desperation. They simply lacked the necessary clarity to realise that high fertility 'is a social misfortune, given the difficulties of today's life'.[113]

Doxiadis' prolific writing in the national press continued throughout 1931 and 1932, reporting from major population events on the international scene and unabashedly discussing all aspects of population change and control, eugenics, abortion and government policy. His position as a physician, politician and member of the government offered him the unique liberty to 'boldly' articulate his thoughts on, many occasions, the first page of the national press. While his position evolved over time, he did not discuss the topic beyond 1932, however.[114] By 1934 M.I. Vastagos, a senior employee of the national statistical service, reported that fertility decline had started in Greece but that the long-term prediction, if the optimistic set of projections was used, was that the population of Greece would double in 65 years.[115] Such a statement pacified those concerned for the future of the country and so dampened all discussions for a few years.

However, in the late 1930s, as discussed above, Averof undertook his excellent research asking physicians to provide him with information about the practices of their patients. His findings indicated that between 5 and 34% of couples who got married after 1922 neither controlled their fertility nor wished to do so,[116] although among urban populations Averof observed an 'intense' control of fertility.[117] Averof was the first to have access to the ASFR that had been collected by the National Statistical Service of Greece (NSSG) since the early 1930s, and so he had the figures showing a decline in the TFR over the decade. The 1933–1934 TFR was found to have been only 3.7 and therefore rather low, creating further concerns about the future of the country.[118] Averof demonstrated for the first time, with the use of both quantitative and qualitative sources, that fertility was declining among *all* social groups in Greece.

By the end of World War II it was an unchallenged truth that fertility had declined to unprecedented levels, following a war, a famine and the country's dislocation during the occupation. This may be why discussions of population control and whether this would be desirable for Greece or not were rare until the end of the 1960s. Topics raised in those uncommon instances in which individuals articulated their stance in this period included the need to avoid demographic decline in the country and the necessity of educating the poor in the use of contraception in order to improve the financial position of their families.[119]

Conclusions

The assertion that fertility decline had started in the 1890s has dominated the understanding of population history and further interpretations of fertility change in Greece. As a result, the dampened levels of—overwhelmingly guesstimated—Greek fertility in the period 1890–1930 were interpreted as volitional fertility decline. The higher levels recorded for the early 1930s were interpreted as a temporary bouncing back of fertility before the irrevocable decline from 1934 onwards. I have offered here an alternative interpretation: levels of fertility in the period from around 1890 to the 1920s were low not because couples were intentionally controlling their fertility but because of the turbulent history of the country in those years and its effects on the lives of the population. This is corroborated by family reconstitution studies and variation in observed levels from locality to locality, since different localities were affected in varying ways by national events. Combining quantitative and qualitative sources, it is safe to conclude that in 1931 national fertility levels represent those of a population that overwhelmingly—and certainly its peasant population—displayed natural/non-parity-specific-controlled fertility. Although affluent urbanites were controlling their fertility from at least the mid-1920s, their small numbers were not sufficient to change the ASFR curve from its 'natural' shape. By 1934, this was no longer the case. Questions regarding how this was achieved will be addressed in subsequent chapters of this book. Nevertheless, the 'natural'-looking fertility levels of 1931 were still rather low, reflecting the use of spacing to some degree. This was, at least, what was detected on Mykonos where intention could be established through the use of oral histories.

However, an important aspect of childbearing in Greece was the cultural 'necessity' to have children, even if few. This will be examined next in an effort to assess its importance and link it to recorded changes in fertility.

Notes

1. Violetta Hionidou (2016) 'Historical demography of Greek populations' in A. Fauve-Chamoux, I. Bolovan, S. Sogner (eds) *A Global History of Historical Demography: Half a Century of Interdisciplinarity* (Bern: Peter Lang), pp. 291–300.
2. Studies that could be included under the category of Population History did appear, mostly in the 1980s, but many of them did not further the discussion on the trends of fertility or mortality. Exceptions are the works of G. Serelea (1978) 'Regards sur la nuptialité et la fécondité en Grèce pendant la seconde moitié du XIXème siècle', *Greek Review of Social Research*, 67(1), 42–50; and, later, E. Kolodny (1992) *Chóra d'Amorgós. Un village Cycladien* (Aix-en-Provence: Publications de l'Université de Provence); Vyron Kotzamanes (1988) 'E anaparagoge ton Ellenon: Mythoi kai pragmatikoteta I. E poreia tes gennetikotetas kai tes olikes gonimotetas ste metapolemike periodo', *Greek Review of Social Research*, 70(70), 136–90; Violetta Hionidou (1993) 'The Demography of a Greek Island, Mykonos 1859–1959: A family reconstitution study' (unpublished PhD thesis: University of Liverpool).
3. For a comprehensive presentation of the existing sources see Vasilios G. Valaoras (1980) 'National primary socio-economic data structures. V: Greece', *International Social Science Journal*, 32(2), 343–63.
4. For example, for Mykonos the 1861 census enumerators' book is available in the local library. Violetta Hionidou (1995) 'Nuptiality patterns and household structure on the Greek island of Mykonos, 1849–1959', *Journal of Family History*, 20(1), 67–102. For Hermoupolis, the 1861, 1870 and 1789 census books are available in the Hermoupolis archives, although the 1870 and 1879 volumes cover only part of the population. Violetta Hionidou (1999) 'Nineteenth-century urban Greek households: the case of Hermoupolis, 1861–1879', *Continuity and Change*, 14(3), 403–27.
5. See also Averof, who adds that during the decade 1912–22 Greek men were nevertheless conscripted in preparation for war even when there was

no war (Evaggelos An. Averof (1939) *Symvole eis ten Ereunan tou Plethysmiakou Provlematos tes Ellados* (Athens: n.p.), p. 85).

6. Ansley J. Coale and Susan Cotts Watkins (eds) (1986) *The Decline of Fertility in Europe* (Princeton: Princeton University Press), p. 166 (the date of the paper is wrongly given as 1960). G.S. Siampos and V.G. Valaoras (1971) 'Long term fertility trends in Greece', in *International Population Conference, London 1969* (Liege: IUSSP), vol. 1, pp. 563–4. The indices of marital fertility for Greece were adjusted for the under-registration of births, which Valaoras had estimated at 35.7 per cent in 1921–24 and 9.6 per cent in 1925–28. V.G. Valaoras (1960) 'A reconstruction of the demographic history of modern Greece', *Milbank Memorial Fund Quarterly*, 38, 135.
7. Siampos and Valaoras, 'Long term fertility trends', p. 565; Coale and Cotts Watkins, *The Decline*, p. 38.
8. Siampos and Valaoras, 'Long term fertility trends', p. 561.
9. For example, childhood mortality started its decline in the 1890s on Mykonos (Hionidou, 'The demography', pp. 139–43).
10. Violetta Hionidou (1997) 'Istorike kritike Anadrome tes gennetikotetas sten Ellada. E periptose tes Mykonou 1859–1959', *Greek Review of Social Research*, 92–3, 39–48; Violetta Hionidou (2006) 'Demografia' in K. Kostas and S. Petmezas (eds) *E Anaptexe tes Ellenikes Oikonomias kata ton 19o aiona (1830–1914)* (Athens: Alexandreia), pp. 81–102. Valaoras' work was ground-breaking at the time and he could safely be named as the creator of the field in Greece. My main objective is to illustrate that some of his results should not be used unquestioningly by contemporary historians and others.
11. During the period examined in this book, illegitimate fertility was extremely low and therefore will not be discussed further.
12. Source for Fig. 2.1: NSSG (1931) *Statistical yearbook of Greece 1930*, Table 41, pp. 103–4.
13. Sources for Fig. 2.2: NSSG (1928) *Apografe tou Plethysmou tes Ellados. Genika Statistika Apotelesmata* (Athens: National Printers), table IX; NSSG (1927) *Statistika Apotelesmata dia ten Sterea Ellas & Voiotia* (Athens: National Printers), pp. 675–6; NSSG (1929) *Statistika Apotelesmata dia ten Thessalia&Arta* (Athens: National Printers), pp. 488–9; NSSG (1924) *Statistika Apotelesmata dia tas Ionious Nesous* (Athens: National Printers), pp. 378–9; NSSG (1923) *Statistika Apotelesmata dia tas Kykladas Nesous* (Athens: National Printers), pp. 186–7; NSSG (1929) *Statistika Apotelesmata dia ten Peloponneson* (Athens: National Printers), pp. 748–9.

14. Serelea pointed out that, in comparison to all other regions, the Ionian islands had the lowest I_m, the highest percentage of single people and the highest mean age at marriage at various points in the second half of the nineteenth century (Serelea, 'Regards', 44–8). The percentages of men and women who never married were also distinctly higher for the Ionian populations compared with those of Greece and the Cyclades both in 1907 and in 1920 (Vasilis S. Gavalas (2008) 'Marriage patterns in Greece during the twentieth century', *Continuity and Change*, 23(3), 517–8). This partly explains the lower CEB for the 25+ marriage duration group.
15. While nuptiality almost certainly played a role in the observed fertility rates, it is currently impossible to ascertain precisely what that role was. According to Gavalas' work, the Singulate Age at Marriage for Greek females in the twentieth century showed a sharp increase of three years to 25 between 1907 and 1920, a decline of one year in 1928, a two-year increase by 1951 and a declining trend after 1951 (Gavalas, 'Marriage', 514). Though these changes strongly reflect war and crisis periods and the reactions of the population to these, it is difficult to link them to fertility owing to the crude nature of the measure.
16. Sources for Fig. 2.3: NSSG (1935) *Statistika Apotelesmata Apografes Plethysmou tes Ellados 1928* (Athens: National Printers), table I, p. 3; refugee data: table II, p. 369.
17. 'Old' Greece refers to the borders of the country prior to 1910.
18. Vaggelis Karamanes (1999–2003) 'Paradosiakes praktikes diaheirises tes elleipses trofimon kata ten anoixiatike metavatike periodo sta Koupatsiarika horia ton Grevenon', *Epeteris Kentrou Laografias*, 29, 138, citing the diary of a local priest in Tsotyli, northern Greece. According to the diary, food prices increased and the villagers 'panicked' when faced with the prospect of a famine. Three of my informants also mentioned the near-famine situation when asked whether they had experienced another 'hunger' situation apart from that of 1941–2 (No. 10 Syros, No. 8 Hios, No. 13 Hios). The first two had had first-hand experiences as children. No. 13 conveyed information she heard from her parents since she was born in 1920. Mortality appeared to have increased, at least in Athens, with deaths recorded there increasing from 402 in November 1916 to 754 in November 1917. Georgios Hristopoulos (ed.) (1970) 'Oikonomia kai koinonia 1914–8', *Istoria tou Ellenikou Ethnous*, 15, 80–1.
19. Hristopoulos (ed.), 'Oikonomia', pp. 80–1.
20. Anonymous (n.d.) *Ypourgeiou Episitismou. Diaheirisis 1920–1923*, vol. 2 (Athens: Denaxas), p. 77.
21. A.F. Freris (1986) *The Greek Economy in the Twentieth Century* (London: Croom Helm), p. 54.
22. Freris, *The Greek Economy*, p. 54.

23. Anonymous, *Ypourgeiou Episitismou*, pp. 79–80.
24. Freris, *The Greek Economy*, pp. 60–1.
25. Tryfon K. Andrianakos (1925) *E Maieutike kai Gynaikologia en Elladi* (Athens: A. Sakellarios), p. 172. Andrianakos stressed that this concerned the affluent more, and that abortion performed by physicians and midwives was the main means of such control.
26. Catherine Brégianni, 'The Gold-Exchange Standard, the Great Depression and Greece; Lessons (?) from the Interwar Greek Default', pp. 2–4, http://www.euro.uni-bayreuth.de/en/research/publications/Euro-Symposium-2012/Catherine_Bregianni/Bregianni_Lessons_from_the_Interwar_Greek_Default.pdf, accessed 16 November 2018.
27. While the famine resulted in the expected fertility reduction, on Hios, because the food situation remained insecure, fertility did not recover in the last year or so of the occupation (1943–44). In contrast, in Athens, where food provisioning was secure by the end of 1942, there was an increase in fertility in the last two years.
28. On the impact on fertility of the psychological effects of hunger—separate from the physiological, and in many cases cumulative, see Violetta Hionidou (2006) *Famine and Death in Occupied Greece, 1941–44*, Cambridge Studies in Population, Economy, and Society in Past Times Series (Cambridge: Cambridge University Press), pp. 178–89.
29. Lefteris Tsoulfidis and Michel Zouboulakis (2016) 'Greek Sovereign Defaults in Retrospect and Prospect', pp. 8–9, https://mpra.ub.uni-muenchen.de/71588/ MPRA Paper No. 71588, accessed 25 Novermber 2018.
30. Demetres Psyhogios (1986) 'Symvole sten melete ton Demografikon fainomenon tou 19ou aiona', *Greek Review of Social Research*, 36, 169.
31. Averof, *Symvole*, p. 87 quoting NSSG, *Statistike Epeteris*, 1937, p. 464.
32. Georgios Homatianos (ed.) (1909) *Statistika Apotelesmata tes Genikes Apografes tou Plethysmou kata ten 27 Oktovriou 1907*, vol. 1 (Athens: National Press), p. νβ.
33. Homatianos, *Statistika*, p. νγ.
34. Psyhogios, 'Symvole', 167, citing K.N. Geragas (1912) *E Metanasteusis ek tou nomou Euvoias* (Halkida: n.p.).
35. Evidence of such a practice is very widespread, and is cited in works ranging from my oral histories on Hios and Mykonos to biographies and to academic works written at the time (see, for example, the following Hios intervews: No. 1, No. 2, No. 3, No. 14, No. 15, No. 22. Of these informants, the last two related the birth intervals between their siblings to the return trips of their fathers). See also the story told by Nicholas Gage, whose married parents lived in the USA and in northern Greece; the author moved to the USA only after his mother's death, towards the end

of the Civil War in 1948 (Nicholas Gage (1989) *Eleni* (London: Harvill), p. 30).

36. Violetta Hionidou (2002) '"They used to go and come". A century of circular migration from a Greek island, Mykonos 1850 to 1950', *Annales de Demographie Historique*, 51–77. Movement between Athens and Mykonos was documented for the 1930s and 1950s, and similar evidence exists for other islands too. Working in ships and thus staying away from home for long periods of time has been documented for Hios, Mykonos and other ports and islands.
37. Nicholas Gage explains in his autobiographical memoir that such marital separation was not unusual: 'The majority of men in Lia were itinerant tinkers and coopers who travelled far from their homes for most of the year, leaving their wives to farm their fields, rear the children, care for their parents and look after things until their husbands returned' (*Eleni*, p. 30). For Mykonos, the oral histories revealed the circular migration of men working as manual labourers in the port of Piraeus in the 1920s and 1930s.
38. Sources for Fig. 2.4: NSSG (1935) *Statistika Apotelesmata Apografes Plethysmou tes Ellados 1928* (Athens: National Printers), table I, p. 3; refugee data: table II, p. 369.
39. Hionidou, 'The Demography', Table 2.10.
40. Sources for Fig. 2.5: The Mykonos and Hermoupolis births were obtained from the Mykonos/Hermoupolis Civil Registration books held on Mykonos and Hermoupolis Municipalities respectively. The data for Greece are from Valaoras, 'A Reconstruction'.
41. On mortality in Hermoupolis see Michalis Raftakis (2019) 'Mortality Change in Hermoupolis, Greece (1859–1940)' (unpublished PhD thesis: Newcastle University); On Mykonos see Hionidou, 'The Demography'.
42. Valaoras' values for the 1930s mirror those published since registration in the 1930s is considered accurate.
43. Sources for Fig. 2.6: Violetta Hionidou (1998) 'The Adoption of Fertility Control on Mykonos, 1879–1959: Stopping, Spacing or Both?', *Population Studies*, 52(1), 67–83; Vasilis S. Gavalas (2002) 'Fertility transition on a Greek island', *Continuity and Change*, 17(2), 133–60; Ntina Moustani (2014) 'Oi Demografikes Exelixeis s'ena Viomehaniko Kentro: Volos, 1881–1922' (unpublished PhD thesis: University of Thessalia). 'Natural fertility' here is taken to represent the absence of parity-specific control of fertility. However, see Chris Wilson, Jim Oeppen and Mike Pardoe (1988) 'What Is Natural Fertility? The Modelling of a Concept', *Population Index*, 54(1), 4–20.
44. Hionidou, 'The Adoption'.
45. Gavalas, 'Fertility', 151.

46. Moustani, 'Oi Demografikes', p. 286.
47. Moustani, 'Oi Demografikes', p. 285.
48. NSSG (1960) *Statistike tes fysikes kineseos tou Plethysmou tes Ellados kata to etos 1956* (Athens: National Printers), pp. xiv–xvi; Averof, *Symvole*, p. 85. According to Valaoras, in the period 1930–34 under-registration of births was at 1.3 per cent—that is, the lowest ever up to 1960 (Valaoras, 'A reconstruction', 135).
49. Sources for Fig. 2.7: 1931 births (NSSG [1933] *Statistike tes fysikes kineseos tou Plethysmou tes Ellados kata to etos 1931* [thereafter SKP] [Athens: National Printers], p. ξβ); 1932 births (SKP 1934, p. 62); 1933 and 1934 births (SKP 1936, p. 68); 1935 births (SKP 1937, p. 65); 1936 births (SKP 1938, p. 60); 1937 births (SKP 1939, p. 62); 1938 births (SKP 1940, p. 53); NSSG (1935) *Statistika Apotelesmata tes Apografes tou Plethysmou tes Ellados tes 15–16 Maiou 1928*, vol. 2 (Athens: National Printers), p. μθ, table 17; 1935 estimated female age structure: NSSG (1966) *Demographic Trends and Population Projections of Greece 1960–1985* (Athens: n.p.), p. 29); 1958–62: NSSG (1966) *Demographic Trends and Population Projections of Greece 1960–1985* (Athens: n.p.), p. 33; 1963–67 ASFRs: Garyfalia Serelea (1979) 'Oi taseis tes gonimotetas tou Ellenikou Plethysmou kata ten periodo 1956–76 kai oi deiktes metreseos tes', *Greek Review of Social Research*, 36–37, 253.
50. The widely quoted figures of ASFRs of Greece in 1934–37 used the 1935 estimated structure. There is no information available relating to how the 1935 structure was estimated.
51. Sources for Fig. 2.8: 1931 births (SKP 1933, p. ξβ); 1932 births (SKP 1934, p. 62); NSSG (1935) *Statistika Apotelesmata tes Apografes tou Plethysmou tes Ellados tes 15–16 Maiou 1928*, vol. 2 (Athens: National Printers), p. μθ, table 17; 1958–62: NSSG (1966) *Demographic Trends and Population Projections of Greece 1960–1985* (Athens: n.p.), p. 29, Female population by age and marital status from NSSG (1962) *Apotelesmata tes apografes plethysmou-katoikion tes 19 Martiou 1961*, Teuhos 1 (Athens: n.p.), p. 21.
52. For Mykonos we know that control started among the couples married in the period 1914–18 rather than among those married earlier (Hionidou, 'The Adoption'). Sources for Fig. 2.9: 1931 births (SKP 1933, p. ξβ); Hionidou, 'The Adoption'; Gavalas, 'Fertility'.
53. The sudden change of shape may well be due to the use of a different female age structure from 1934 onwards. I have chosen to use this since all the published ASFRs of the 1930s use this estimated structure.
54. Averof, *Symvole*, p. 74.
55. Averof, *Symvole*, p. 75.

56. Averof, *Symvole*, p. 74.
57. In most places the vital events continued to be recorded locally and these are available to consult. Mykonos and Hermoupolis are examples, though there are many more.
58. Ernestine Friedl (1964) *Vasilika. A Village in Modern Greece* (New York: Holt, Rinehart and Winston), p. 50.
59. Serelea, 'Oi taseis', p. 260.
60. Serelea, 'Oi taseis', p. 260; Polyzos referred to the 131,000 migrants who left during the 1950s. Nicolas Polyzos (1959) 'Evolution Démographique en Grèce', *IUSPP Conference*, p. 447.
61. John Campbell undertook his fieldwork at the same time as Friedl.
62. Friedl, *Vasilika*, p. 50.
63. Friedl, *Vasilika*, p. 54.
64. Richard Blum and Eva Blum (1965) *Health and Healing in Rural Greece* (Stanford, CA: Stanford University Press), pp. 72–3.
65. Vasilios Valaoras, A. Polychronopoulou and D. Trichopoulos (1965) 'Control of Family Size in Greece (The Results of a Field Survey)', *Population Studies*, 18(3), 265–78.
66. The survey covered women who started their childbearing after 1935 and women who started in the early 1960s. Valaoras et al., 'Control', 271.
67. Valaoras et al., 'Control', 274.
68. Sources for Fig. 2.10: Vas. G. Valaoras (1971) 'Changing Patterns of Fertility Differentials (The Case of Greece)', *International Population Conference, London 1969* (Liege: IUSSP), pp. 2074–80; Gerasimos Alivizatos (1947) *Mnemonion Ygieines* (Athens: n.p.).
69. Lila Leontidou (1989) *Oi Poleis tes Siopes* (Athens: ETVA), p. 301.
70. However, a large part of its population was rural.
71. Tryfon K. Andrianakos (1 May 1930) 'Organosis tes proleptikes iatrikes pros katapolemesin tes tehnetes ektroseos kai prostasian tes teknogonias kai tes metrotetos (anakoinosis en to A Panellenion Synedrion Ygieines)', *Ellenike Iatrike*, 4(10), 1025; Alexandra Halkias (2004) *The Empty Cradle of Democracy: Sex, Abortion, and Nationalism in Modern Greece* (Durham, NC: Duke University Press).
72. Antonios I. Kindynes (1889) *E Steirosis para te Gynaiki kai Therapeia autes* (Athens: Vlastos Varvaregos), pp. 9–10.
73. Kindynes, *E Steirosis*, p. 10.
74. Kindynes, *E Steirosis*, p. 10.
75. Kindynes, *E Steirosis*, p. 11.
76. Thus, unless stated otherwise, the assumption should be that the cited author is a physician.
77. Mihael Nik. Kaires (1917) *E Eugonia. Dialexis genomene en te aithouse tes Sinaias Akademias te 24 Martiou 1917* (Athens: Adelfoi Frantzeskake), p. 12.

78. M. Moyseides (1922) *Eugonismos kai Gamos* (Constantinople: n.p.), p. 22.
79. However, in the preceding paragraph he cited figures showing that marriage rates were the strongest in Athens in 1920–21 (Moyseides, *Eugonismos*, p. 21).
80. Moyseides, *Eugonismos*, p. 21.
81. Athanasios Vettos Danielides archimadrite (1924) *E Zoe ton Neon* (Athens: Paraskeuas Leones), p. 171.
82. Danielides, *E Zoe*, p. 171.
83. Gregorios Hatzevasileiou (1925) 'To provlema tou Plethysmou en Elladi', *Arheion Oikonomikon kai Koinonikon Epistemon*, 5(3), 263.
84. Hatzevasileiou, 'To provlema', 264.
85. Hatzevasileiou, 'To provlema', 264.
86. A. Sygkelakes (1927) *The Secret Hygiene of Woman* (Alexandria: Grammata), p. 53.
87. Sygkelakes, *The Secret*, p. 53.
88. Ironically, the term the author uses is 'a Christian'! Sygkelakes, *The Secret*, p. 52.
89. Sygkelakes, *The Secret*, p. 52.
90. Sygkelakes, *The Secret*, p. 51.
91. Auguste Forel (1931) *The Sexual Question: A Scientific, Psychological, Hygienic and Sociological Study*, translated by C.F. Marshall, 1st edn 1903 (New York: Physicians and Surgeons Book Company).
92. Anonymous (1925) 'Dia ten Praxin. Kathegetes A. Forel. Mesa di on kanonizetai e parakolyetai e syllepsis', *Klinike*, 1(6), 187–9. All three publications refer to eugenic reasons as well. For an extensive discussion of inter-war and post-World War II eugenics see Sevasti Trubeta (2013) *Physical Anthropology, Race and Eugenics in Greece (1880–1970s)* (Leiden: Brill), chapter 8.
93. M. Moyseides (1925) *E Gyne. Ygieine tou Gamou kai tes Eggamou Gynaikos* (Alexandria: A. Katsigone), pp. 60–1.
94. Apostolos Doxiadis (1927) 'Koinonike Viologia, viologike politike', *Ellenika Grammata*, 3(3), (16 July 1928), 95–9. Doxiadis published this piece only after Venizelos' Liberal government was appointed on 4 July 1928.
95. Doxiadis, 'Koinonike Viologia', 95–6.
96. Doxiadis, 'Koinonike Viologia', 95.
97. Doxiadis, 'Koinonike Viologia', 98.
98. Doxiadis, 'Koinonike Viologia', 98.
99. Trubeta, *Physical Anthropology*, pp. 239–46.
100. N.N. Drakoulides (1933) *Ygeia kai Gamos. Me poia mesa prostateuontai? To progamiaio pistopoietiko* (Athens: Hronika), pp. 20–1.

101. Demosthenes Eleutheriades (10 August 1930) 'Liga paidia, kale trofe', *Peitharhia*, 1(43), 7–9.
102. Articles on overpopulation abounded, especially in the early 1930s (I.L. Halkokondyles (12 January 1930), *Peitharhia*, 1(13); Per. D. Rediades (2 March 1930) *Peitharhia*, 1(20); Eleutheriades, 'Liga paidia', 7–9; A. Doxiadis (10 March 1931) 'Yperplethysmos', *Eleutheron Vema*; A. Doxiadis (12 March 1931) 'Mporei e sfaira na threpsei ton auxanomeno plethysmo?', *Eleutheron Vema*).
103. Solon Veras (14 June 1930) 'E prostasia tes teknogonias', *Ergasia*, 1(23), 19–20.
104. Zoe Fragkou (20 July 1930) 'E Oikogeneia kai to mellon tes', part A, *Peitharhia*, 1(40), 9; Zoe Fragkou (27 July 1930) 'E Oikogeneia kai to mellon tes', part B, *Peitharhia*, 1(41), 9–10.
105. Solon Veras (14 June 1930) 'E prostasia tes teknogonias', *Ergasia*, 1(23), 19–20.
106. Eleutheriades, 'Liga paidia', 7–9.
107. N.S. Louros (21 June 1930) 'E prostasia tes teknogonias', *Ergasia*, 1(24), 15–16; M. Yioel (1938) *Steirosis e Egkymosyne kata Voulesin*, 2nd edn, first edn 1936 (Athens: Vasileiou), p. 7.
108. Andrianakos, 'Organosis', 1026–8.
109. Kostas Hatziotes (24 August 1930) 'Allelografia. Ta liga paidia', *Peitharhia*, 1(44).
110. Apostolos Doxiadis (13 September 1930) 'O anaplethysmos tes Ellados', *Eleutheron Vema*. Yoel, writing in 1936, also mentions that the majority of workers and peasants were not restricting their fertility (Yioel, *Steirosis*, p. 79), and adds that, prior to World War I, the majority of urban couples did not control their fertility either.
111. Apostolos Doxiadis (8 March 1931) *Eleutheron Vema*.
112. Apostolos Doxiadis (15 March 1931) *Eleutheron Vema*.
113. M.R. (10 September 1930) 'Polyteknia', *Eleutheron Vema*.
114. In September 1930 Doxiadis was arguing for the improvement of the survival of infants and the 'adjustment' of fertility: that is, more babies among the upper classes and fewer among the lower classes (Apostolos Doxiadis (11 September 1930) 'Periorismos e diarrythmisis ton genneseon?', *Eleutheron Vema*). By March of the following year he had refined his message, arguing that there should be no 'propaganda' encouraging procreation among the lower classes but that the middle and upper classes should be encouraged to have more children (Apostolos Doxiadis (15 March 1931) *Eleutheron Vema*).
115. M.I. Vastagos (30 December 1934) *Eleutheron Vema*, CBR 1928–34: 29.5, rural areas 30.9, towns 25.6.

116. Averof, *Symvole*, p. 74.
117. Averof, *Symvole*, p. 75.
118. V. Katsougiannopoulos and Th. Edipides (1973) *Syghronoi Demografikai Ropai tes Ellados 1951–71* (Thessaloniki: n.p.), p. 496.
119. Demetrios Th. Stefanou (1963) *O Plethysmos tes Ges, o Periorismos ton Genneseon kai to Demografikon mas Provlema* (Athens: n.p.), p. 31; Nikolaos Hr. Settas (1964) *To Demografikon kai to Koinonikooikonomikon Provlema tes Elladas* (Athens: n.p.), pp. 36–8.

CHAPTER 3

Involuntary Childlessness

Introduction

Jennifer Evans, in her examination of eighteenth-century English society, brought attention to the strong desire of couples to procreate, something they put great effort into facilitating. This, for researchers who have been focusing their attention on how couples in the nineteenth and twentieth centuries tried to do the exact opposite, is rather surprising. However, it should be clear that these two aspects of fertility should be addressed together if we are to understand how a population moved from one situation to the other.

As childlessness has been looked at only rarely for the Greek population, it is essential to address this issue before we can determine how the Greek population came to control its fertility. Childlessness is, and has always been, considered a major misfortune for Greek married couples, as the purpose of marriage within Greek culture has been that of procreation.[1] This has been supported and encouraged by the Church and the wider society. Even in the late twentieth century, when fertility declined to well below replacement levels, childlessness was still seen as involuntary, being accepted only as a postponement of the birth of a child.

For much of the twentieth century, childlessness has been tactfully avoided as a topic of research or public discussion in Greece.[2] While there may be many reasons for this, one is the shame and pain that such a condition brings to the subjects of such a study. Moreover, the majority of

V. Hionidou, *Abortion and Contraception in Modern Greece, 1830–1967*, Medicine and Biomedical Sciences in Modern History,
https://doi.org/10.1007/978-3-030-41490-0_3

childless couples would adopt a child once it was clear that procreation was not going to happen. Such 'adoptions' were—again, in the majority of cases—unofficial, especially when the child was not very young. When the adopted was an infant, it would be simply registered as the biological child of the adopting parents. In the former case, legal inheritance documents, usually prepared when the 'parents' reached old age, would ensure the future financial relationship of the parents and the child. In many such cases, although certainly not all, the 'adopted' child was a girl and occupied an ambivalent position in the 'family' which resembled that of servant. Infants registered as the biological children of the adoptive parents were usually—but not exclusively—the children of relatives who had had sufficient children of their own and were willing to 'help' close relatives who were childless. This was not difficult to achieve in a society where the majority of rural births and a large percentage of urban ones were taking place in houses even in the 1960s.[3] For example, among my Mykonos informants, who had been chosen because they were parents, a number of couples had only one child, and most of these proved to have been childless couples who had adopted a child. Some of the informants discussed the adoption and explained that the adopted child was, for example, a niece. Others did not admit that the child was adopted and were unusually reticent about details concerning the child's birth or failed to refer to the child in the interview, even in passing. In one case the provided age of the mother at the time of the birth precluded the possibility of the child being her biological child. It was also common for abandoned infants to be left on the doorstep of childless couples—who were well known in local societies—in the hope that they would adopt such infants,[4] and it seems that this actually happened in some cases.[5]

Childless couples were thus rare because of adoption, and sterility was much more common than any existing statistics may suggest for Greece. The extensive efforts made by couples to adopt hint at an aversion towards childlessness, and the focus in Greek society on procreation is also easy to detect in the fertility-enhancing rituals surrounding the wedding ceremony.[6] Moreover, as anthropologists have emphasised for twentieth-century Greece, the central role of Greek women has been that of motherhood. That role enabled women not only to move into 'adulthood' and assert their position within society but also to become matriarchs in later life.[7] Moreover, for the nineteenth century and possibly to a degree for the twentieth century too, the commemoration of the dead by their children was an important aspect of life and death. This 'duty' was invariably mentioned in eighteenth- and nineteenth-century inheritance notarial contracts, indicating to whom among the children or whoever else inherited part of the estate that duty would fall to and outlining, in some cases, the frequency that such commemorations should have.[8]

'Childlessness as Dishonour'[9] and 'The Passion for Children':[10] The Fear and Undesirability of Childlessness

For much of the nineteenth century—indeed, throughout the reign of the first king, Othon (1832–1862)—Greek society was preoccupied with the first Greek royal couple's lack of descendants. The royal couple's childlessness had significant implications for the future of the young kingdom. However, it seems that the royal couple were not the only ones preoccupied with sterility and, ultimately, fertility.

The paramount importance of fertility is eloquently articulated in popular novels. Palaiologos, for example, in his 1842 novella, describes the lives of three middle-class Athenian sisters whose aim and purpose in life is to marry and have children. He writes of how women 'conceive childlessness as dishonour and in their quest to force nature, they pay with their lives for this irrational desire'.[11] Palaiologos' protagonist consumes 'various and strong medicines' in her attempt to become pregnant, which ultimately leads to her death, 'just as it happens to many other older or even young women'.[12] By that time she had already invoked the help of the Saints, had mineral baths, tried all the 'midwife's herbs' and approached a physician for advice.[13] Palaiologos would have certainly had knowledge of the childlessness of the then queen of Greece, Amalia, who among other therapies had employed natural baths in her efforts to become pregnant.[14]

In the later part of the century Georgios Kyriakides, in a study of the sexuality of married couples, articulates the significance of sterility to nineteenth-century Greek society in no uncertain terms:

> Since she [the barren woman] prevents the realisation of the sacred purpose of marriage—that is, coitus, conception, pregnancy and delivery—this brings the woman to the class of barren women, or, more precisely, makes her useless to society and therefore justly and legitimately [the husband] is obliged to divorce her and remove her to the monastic life.[15]

Kyriakides' understanding of the purpose of marriage as the vehicle for procreation, though crudely put, accurately expressed that of the Church and popular culture. Very similar sentiments were expressed in the 1930s rural north Greece, where childbearing was clearly seen as the 'purpose' of marriage: 'Whoever gets married gets married for that reason [to have children].'[16] Thus, women who were thought to be sterile, even in the 1940s, were expected to become nuns and not to marry.[17] A female informant from Syros, referring to the mid-1940s, mentioned that her future husband fell in love with her but because she had not begun to menstruate, despite being 17 years of age, they could not get married. They had to wait for her period to start.[18] As marriage and procreation were of paramount importance for women, it was a prime responsibility of a mother to trace signs of possible future sterility and to take action that would ensure that her daughter would not suffer from it.[19] In the mid-twentieth century Alexandros Tsakires, a physician, indicated that only in cases of primary amenorrhoea would it be clear, prior to the wedding, that sterility would be a problem, but he added that it was a moral, not a legal, obligation for the bride to let the groom know of such a circumstance.[20] However, in 1928 Nikolaos Vasileiades had argued in an extensive article that cases of primary and secondary amenorrhoea do not 'necessarily result in sterility', thus providing a window of hope.[21] In small communities even the rumour that a single woman was sterile would seriously jeopardise her prospects of marriage, or at least of a good marriage. One informant described how 'a man, richer than me, loved her [his prospective wife]. My wife [to be] could not have children. He found out and backed off. And I got married to her. Despite being unable to have children, I wanted her. She was nice.'[22] Further questioning revealed that the information about his future wife's inability to bear children was a rumour initiated by her relatives, which in fact proved correct.

Folklore accounts of the 1940s and 1960s further support the great importance of childbearing and the corresponding shame, humiliation, 'bad luck' and 'catastrophe' that accompanied childlessness: 'whoever does not have children, people do not respect them'.[23] The pressure to become pregnant and to do so quickly was significant: 'With the first [child], five months had passed [without becoming pregnant] and I thought I would not have any [children] and I was crying.'[24] Even for intellectual women, their journal suggested in 1951, 'life is a silent torture' for the childless.[25] The most popular and progressive sexologist at the time stressed the 'unrestrained longing of people' to procreate.[26] Similarly, the anthropologists Blum and Blum, who studied a small rural population in Central Greece in the period 1957–1962, reported that the 'condition' of childlessness was described as 'shameful' by the villagers.[27] The family members of a childless couple, especially the mother-in-law, are 'tortured and sigh day and night for the major misfortune that befell upon them'.[28] Within the household the treatment of a barren daughter-in-law was far worse than that of one who had children.[29] Moreover, childlessness would be shouted out as an insult, and one that was very painful: 'In our neighbourhood there was a heirless woman and when she quarrelled with her neighbours, they would throw to her that knife; they called her heirless.'[30] The position of childless persons was—even in the 1960s—precarious and highly undesirable: 'Those who do not have children do not enjoy much respect by the society and are considered as fruitless trees. In earlier times they would not be greeted in the street and they would not even be [allowed to] to become priests.'[31] Even in the mid-twentieth century women and men would be called 'heirless (akleroi)', and a common comment in the 1960s was 'what do you expect from a heirless?'[32] At times, 'heirless' and 'godless' would be used together, indicating the extreme negativity of the former term.[33] Childless couples in some communities were not invited to weddings, their bread offering to the Church was declined and women would not accept bread yeast from a childless woman.[34]

The term 'akleros'/heirless refers specifically to the lack of a descendant who will inherit the family property (kleros). In a childless marriage upon the death of the wife her dowry—essentially her parental *inter vivos* inheritance—would revert to her parental family. Having offspring was significant because it solidified the ownership of whatever a couple was given or promised to be given as dowry or gift by their parents at the time of their wedding: if a husband or a wife died without surviving children, all or a significant part of their own inheritance would revert to their parental families.[35] In cases where land or a house was only 'promised' to the couple, usually allowing the couple to make use of it but without actually transferring ownership, such 'promised' land could eventually, if the couple remained childless, be given to another son or daughter who had children.[36] In other cases, in which such promised land remained with the childless son, when the final sharing of the parental estate occurred the childless son might receive less than his fair share:

> When he [the father] made arrangements for me to marry, he gave me the land .... I was working the land [without a legal contract]. Then he prepared the will [15 years after the wedding] .... Then I inherited [from] the [father's] will. And because I did not have children—my wife could not have children—he did not give me as much as I should have got. He loved me a lot.[37]

This informant felt the need to emphasise that he was his father's favourite son, although his mother loved and supported his brother. Despite being his father's favourite son, the fact that he was childless was a major obstacle in giving him his 'fair' share of the inheritance, a decision that the informant did not question.

The importance of property remaining in the family is shown by childless couples' attempts to adopt from within the extended family, so that ultimately the property remained with the family rather than ending up with an 'outsider'.[38] In families where none of the brothers had children the serious issue of the elimination of the family name surfaced, which was even more significant than that of property.[39]

In the 1950s evidence of some change can be detected: pity would be expressed for those who remained childless and the term, in later years, has become synonymous with unhappiness.[40] However, the possibility of facing sterility was disconcerting for women even before they got married.[41] At the same time, and as popular culture seems to have started shifting from 'shame' to pity, the language of some physicians became laden with ethical overtones when addressing sterility and its opposite, fertility. When Tsakires, for example, discussed the benefits of pregnancy in 1954, he pointed out that women who have never had children 'are psychologically less stable than the rest'.[42] This, he argued, was explained by a number of factors: biological, as the absence of pregnancy prevents the fulfilment of the woman's personality; psychological, as the woman feels deficient; and social, owing to the 'shame' of sterility, something that 'is widespread, especially among the popular/lower classes'.[43]

Having a child was also of paramount importance for the care and comfort of aged parents.[44] Though such care did not necessarily mean cohabitation, nevertheless the expectation was that the children would ultimately help their elderly parents if ill or incapacitated. Furthermore, children would play an instrumental role in the commemoration of deceased parents in the church ceremonies that occurred, and still occur, on a number of occasions throughout the year.[45] The importance of these commemorating ceremonies for the aged is clear from eighteenth- and nineteenth-century wills, in which individuals with no surviving children would bequest money to a specific local church on condition that the priest would perform the customary religious memorial services after their death. Alternatively, specific individuals would receive a small inheritance in order to perform such a duty.[46]

Nevertheless, such solutions, along with adoption, were only partial answers to a significant medical, social, religious and cultural problem, and were considered by a couple only after many years of waiting for a child of their own. The significance of childlessness meant that it involved much more than just waiting: in a society so closely focused on procreation a large number of possible means of 'encouraging' procreation were developed, involving popular medicine, religious practices and, ultimately, modern medicine.

Popular Culture

The possible 'solutions' offered to the problem of childlessness by elements of popular culture were varied and apparently endless. In most of these methods folk traditions, popular medicine and religious practices can all be distinguished but rarely separated—and thus no such effort will be made here.[47]

Curing sterility had been one of the central tasks of empirics—that is, those who practised popular medicine—even before the nineteenth century, as a 1745 comedy articulates: 'We can demonstrate our art in curing various illnesses … a sterile woman who cannot bear children we can [help her] have child with a herb.'[48] In the eighteenth century advice in iatrosophic manuscript books on how to cure sterility abounded.[49] For example, one such manuscript contains six different recipes, all aiming to get the woman pregnant.[50] Such manuscripts were widely used in subsequent centuries, being kept and consulted by monks and private individuals.[51] An example is the *Geoponikon*, which was first published in 1634 by Agapios Landos, a Cretan monk at Athos.[52] It is known to have been reprinted in 1686, 1795 and 1796, as well as tens of times in the nineteenth and twentieth centuries.[53] One of its reprints was kept and used as an iatrosophic book in early twentieth-century Hios.[54] Nineteenth- and twentieth-century iatrosophic manuscripts also circulated, similarly replete with recipes to overcome sterility.[55] At times handwritten recipes were added to parts of a manuscript or printed book, or the manuscripts—or extracts only—might be copied from other places or written from scratch (see, e.g., the twentieth-century manuscript studied by Clark).[56] The ownership of such manuscripts was presumably known to the local population, who would seek advice from their keepers.

The popular medicine of the 1930s also offered recipes for childless couples, often rather elaborate. One recommended the use of greens gathered from a church wall, which would thus be sanctified, while a second suggested that the woman should prepare and drink a herbal and use the leaves of a female peony as a pessary.[57] Yet another indicates that the woman who had a child with her first husband but not the second should boil seeds of wild rue with wild roses and drink the herbal, after which she 'with the help of God will have a child'.[58]

Popular and folklore ways of dealing with sterility were thus available in abundance. Euaggelia Fragkake, who collected folklore practices in her native Crete, noted that 'if a woman has the misfortune to be barren or childless' she would employ 'conceptive medicines, fumigation, hot baths and popular religious methods'.[59] A good 'conceptive', we are told, is ground cinnamon, clove and nutmeg, to be put on the belly or the perineum after a warm bath. This 'opens the womb' and helps with conception.[60] Another is fumigation with rose petals from a specific rose tree or washing/douching with chamomile.[61] In mainland Greece fumigation with boiled parsley was employed for the womb to 'close' so that it could conceive and retain the pregnancy.[62] In the Peloponnese, different herbs were used in different locations in order to overcome childlessness.[63] Similarly, various folklore methods existed in early twentieth-century Hios: a pill made from a powder of dried leeches and a mixture of herbs and seeds; or pessaries made from a combination of chamomile, honey, cumin and sheep's wool, or from figs in combination with other materials.[64]

Fragkake adds that white magic or, as the author calls it, 'good magic' was also employed by the childless.[65] She cites three examples. In the first someone would suddenly throw into the childless woman's apron wild baby rabbits and would wish her 'to give birth as the wild rabbit does'. The second involved the use of a piece of mandrake, which the woman needed to carry on her while she engaged in sex. The last dictated that the childless woman had to be the first to eat bread from a newly built oven while wishing 'to have a child, any that God wants'.[66] A similar practice from the town of Eleusis in Gortynia instructed that when a new mill had been constructed the childless woman should sit on top of the millstone during the first grinding of wheat. That flour would then be used by the childless woman to bake bread that she would offer to the church to be blessed by the priest.[67] A folklorist investigating the Cretan community of Kritsa documented a 'traditional'/popular recipe that would, it was hoped, enable the woman to overcome her sterility, one that closely resembled recipes noted in iatrosophic books: the woman would collect leaves from a specific tree (sarantodendro) that would be added to hot water and used for fumigation.[68]

The childless woman could also enlist religion: a physician, writing rather disparagingly in 1880, mentioned that his contemporaries sought help from the Church, performing pilgrimages, promises (taximata) and blessings (euhas). The most popular place for pilgrimage, the author added, was Tenos—which, incidentally, remains so in the early twenty-first century—and it seems to have been the most constant reference in all sources.[69] Fragkake, for example, discussed the widespread knowledge regarding the miraculous powers of Tenos's Virgin Mary in inducing pregnancy in childless couples. She specifically refers to the use of the wick of Mary's oil lamp: women would travel to the island of Tenos, fast, take communion and swallow the wick.[70] Fragkake cites two separate and well-known local cases, one from the 1890s and another in the 1960s/1970s, where this practice resulted in the bearing of children, noting that even very young children were aware of this and thus would be expected to recount the practice in the future when and if necessary.[71] However, the church of Tenos was not the only one to attract childless women in their efforts to enlist the help of a saint or the Virgin Mary. Many childless women would promise (tama) to a specific local church and saint that she would give the child the saint's name and baptise the baby in that same church[72]—a practice that continues unabated to the present.[73] Stauros Semaiakes, researching in Kritsa, on Crete, in 1965, noted that if a woman desired to fall pregnant 'She visits Churches and prays, lights up the oil-lamps [in Church] and vows offerings of bread, candle, golden or silver effigy of the baby, or [a specific] amount of oil matching [the baby's] weight'.[74] Nevertheless, Semaiakes added, this was not all: childless women would also use a drink made of a particular herb, they would seek advice from physicians and they would employ 'all means that someone will recommend to them with the hope that they will have children'.[75]

Considering the abundance of ways of overcoming sterility outlined above, it is appropriate to consider the order of actions taken by affected couples. In one of the folklore reports, prepared in 1940 by a local educated individual for the folklore commission, the author, K. Karapatakes, clearly outlines the sequence of events from the moment of the wedding onwards:

> If it happens for a woman not to give birth within a year from the day she was married and if time passes without signs of pregnancy, then alas! It brings bad luck (grousouzia) and disaster to the house. Promises (tamata), remote Chapels, blessed waters and religious practices [follow]. And if all that does not work out to a miracle, then they start the incantations, the magicians, the fortune-tellers and all those silly [practices] that various people will advise them. The 'sterile' woman is not considered equal to the others [those who procreate]; and the man, he too is considered incapable/impotent (anikanos) and scapegrace. The whole house[hold] and mostly the mothers-in-law are tormented and sigh day and night for the great evil that has befallen on them. They ask the bride, they ask the groom but the cause remains unknown and always secret. Only the [fortune] cards … and maybe a swindler and a charlatan will be able to console them and to blame the 'doing [spell]'. Only one of them can break the spell and perform the miracle. And then the comings and goings of the mother-in-law to the gypsies … start; they [couple] eat the miraculous vine grape, they drink porcupine blood and [do] many silly things, always at the expense of the household and to the benefit of the cunning miracle-makers.[76]

The first steps in avoiding sterility, therefore, involved religion, popular beliefs (such as drinking water from specific wells, or the childless woman rubbing against specific stones widely known to have powers related to fertility[77]) and popular medicine, here disparaged by the educated narrator.

Interestingly, the blame for sterility was apportioned not only to the woman but also to the man.[78] And for men, too, the rumour that they might be impotent was sufficient reason to call off an engagement or even a wedding.[79] Mothers-in-law, when trying to determine the cause of the absence of pregnancy, would ask both the wife and the husband. And while most recipes and guidance offered for sterility addressed the 'woman who does not bear a child', in many cases the advice referred to the husband too.[80] Thus, the man was also seen as a potential cause of the problem, although this was—almost exclusively—thought to be as a result of impotence rather than other physiological reasons. Interestingly, there is little in the written sources concerning popular attitudes and views concerning impotence. Men were, almost exclusively, the creators of these sources, and this may not have been a subject with which they would willingly engage. Almost certainly, everyday exchanges among men would have touched upon such issues, as they did with other, related ones, but these conversations would not necessarily have found their way into the written sources. Therefore, the rarity of references to impotence in writings concerning popular culture does not reflect its frequency or importance, or the engagement of the people with it. However, all engaged with the 'spell'.

The 'Spell': The Binding Curse (Ampodema)

Modern Greek culture is no stranger to magic and witchcraft, performed either for good or for ill.[81] There are ample evidence and discussion of it in the writings of Greek and Western authors. Nevertheless, the binding curse and the spell necessary to counter it are among the most discussed, second only to the 'evil eye'. References to the binding curse abound throughout the nineteenth and twentieth centuries, though earlier references also exist.[82] John Cuthbert Lawson's 1910 description is one of the most thorough ones, perhaps because he was articulating something unfamiliar to his British readers:

> [T]he weapon of witchcraft wherewith a jealous woman takes vengeance upon a man who has forsaken her or who has never returned her affection and takes to himself another for his bride, is truly diabolical. This is known as the spell of 'binding' (desimon or ampodema). Its purpose is to fetter the virility of the husband and so to prevent the consummation of the marriage. The rite itself is simple. Either the jealous girl herself or a witch employed by her attends the wedding, taking with her a piece of thread or string in which three loops have been made. During the reading of the gospel or the pronouncement of the blessing, she pulls the ends of the string, forming thereby three knots in it, and at the same time mutters the brief incantation … 'I bind N. and M. and the Devil betwixt them.' The thread is subsequently buried or hidden, and unless it can be found and either be burnt or have the knots untied, there is small hope for the man to recover from his impotence.[83]

While many variations of the actions and incantations have been recorded, the timing of the spell is consistent among all sources. The witchcraft occurs during the wedding and, as is well known to all, elaborate and varied measures and precautions are taken by the mothers of the bride and groom to prevent such a spell from becoming effective. For example, the bride and groom may be given scissors to carry under their clothing so that they can 'cut' the spell and prevent it from taking hold. When the wedding takes place at home, which was the most common practice in pre-1950s rural Greece, the couple would lock and unlock a door so that the spell would not become effective.[84] It was believed, however, that if the binding spell takes effect the groom would become impotent and the marriage could not be consummated, resulting in the couple's sterility.[85] The only hope remaining, therefore, was to 'untie' the binding spell. Since untying the binding spell is considered 'good' magic, recipes for untying spells are mentioned in iatrosophic manuscripts, and either a witch or a priest could perform them.[86] In contrast, performing the binding spell is considered to be black magic, and thus priests are never involved in performing it.[87] Lawson cites specific cases of couples who were 'cured', either those mentioned to him or couples he met in person, and he remarks that one couple explained to him how they had the curse removed and how the peasants 'thought no shame to confess it'.[88] The lack of embarrassment in admitting the use of magic in order to remove the binding curse demonstrates how strong and pervasive the belief surrounding this curse has been in Greece throughout the period of study. The enormous number of references to it in the sources spanning the nineteenth and twentieth centuries is a further indication of its survival and significance.[89] Even in Perth, Australian Greek migrants—some second or older generation—maintained such beliefs in the late twentieth century.[90]

The strong belief in and the fear of the effects of the binding spell are present in literature, too. For example, in Kondylakes' 1892 novella *O Patouhas*, when the spell is mentioned to the naïve young protagonist by both his mother and a third person fear is expressed, as both are aware of its effects.[91] For those affected by the spell, the feeling conveyed was that of desperation. In contrast, some rational, educated authors rejected such 'irrational' beliefs, while others who met affected couples attempted to explain rationally the 'real' reasons that lay behind the couples' stories.[92]

The impotence of the husband was devastating for couples and their families, not just for the individual man, and efforts to resolve impotence were thus of central importance to the families of the husband and wife. For the couple, it seriously undermined the success and happiness of the marriage because, for the Greek Orthodox Church and wider society, sex was central in the fulfilment of the marriage, and an inability to perform marital duties was a reason for the annulment of marriages.[93] Equally important was the guaranteed childlessness that resulted from impotence. However, impotence was not seen as a direct challenge to a man's masculinity, but rather as a temporary phenomenon that was beyond his control;[94] the only solution was performing the untying of the binding curse.

Almost all such recipes cited in iatrosophic manuscripts are titled 'to untie a bound couple' and only rarely 'to untie a bound man/woman' (the gender-neutral term *Anthropos* is used).[95] While, in discussions of the binding curse, the man and his inability to perform are central—as the woman is central when sterility is discussed—in the same texts it is indicated that it is the *couple* that is 'bound': that is, the magic concerns the couple specifically.[96] In cases where the marriage was annulled and the man married someone else, the expectation was that he would be able to perform.

Thus in popular culture sterility was an affliction of the couple and their families of origin; it could be the responsibility of either the woman or the man, in the latter case exclusively through impotence rather than less immediately visible physiological reasons; and an array of methods was employed to overcome the problem, whatever its cause, in order that the purpose of Greek marriage, procreation, should be fulfilled.[97] For that reason, it was not sufficient for the couple to prove that conception had taken place; subsequently, significant time and effort were invested in ensuring that the pregnancy came to term. Again, popular medicine, popular culture and religious and magical practices contain numerous recipes, pieces of advice and amulets that would help to sustain the pregnancy and avoid an early miscarriage.[98]

The Physician's Perspective on Men's Sterility and Impotence

The few medical writings that do refer to men cover both the nineteenth and the twentieth centuries. Pyrros, an Italian-educated priest and physician, writing in 1836, attributed the responsibility for sterility to both women and men since, he explained, women's eggs cannot be enlivened without men's 'spermiogenic worms'. As these 'worms' could be damaged by diseases, syphilis or mercury, men could be the source of sterility too.[99] However, Pyrros focused almost exclusively on impotence, which he attributed to the 'passions' of the young men, presumably referring to onanism, and to their shyness, which prevented them from approaching their wives and/or fulfilling their 'duty'.[100] Pyrros recommended cantharides (Spanish fly), a well-known aphrodisiac,[101] as well as preparations that would improve the general well-being of the afflicted man, including opium, aromatic oils, cold sea swims, 'good life' and 'joy'.[102]

Two subsequent publications engaging with male sterility either relied heavily on or were straightforward translations of western writings. So, Meliareses' 1875 volume was published outside Greece and translated Frederick Hollick's writings.[103] Meliareses, following Hollick, attributed impotence to spermatorrhoea, which, he states, was caused by 'excesses and onanism'—a view that was echoed in the following 75 years.[104] He discussed in detail possible remedies for impotence, rejecting old substances such as cantharides and potassium nitrate but recommending phosphorus and ergotine, the latter—albeit only in combination with other substances—a 'valuable medicine for impotence and spermatorrhoea'.[105] He emphasised the very high demand worldwide for aphrodisiac preparations, noting that these 'are not used with care'.[106] Oikonomopoulos, in his two-page discussion of male sterility and impotence, followed Debay verbatim in attributing sterility to a range of physical causes, such as hydrocele or obstruction of the penis, but also to spermatorrhoea, whose cause was identified once again as onanism.[107]

Similarly, Panas, in his 1915 study, identifies analogous causes of male sterility: that is, physiological reasons and impotence consequent to masturbation, but also syphilis and its detrimental therapy with mercury.[108] Interestingly, he also introduced into the discussion the 'psychological' dimension, citing as examples forced marriage under the threat of violence or rumours concerning the bodily—that is, the hidden—imperfections of the bride.[109] He discussed possible cures, though he declared that where physiological reasons were the cause these could not be cured.[110] For impotence he recommended a number of preparations, one of which contained ergotine, as well as electrotherapy and the use of a device he had invented. This, he suggested, would produce well-sustained erections.[111] Panas' most focused and lengthy discussion concerned masturbation and, among its wide and diverse effects, impotence.[112] Later publications presented similar positions with a slightly modified message, and usually forgoing Panas' authoritarian tone, for example.[113] Psychological reasons were given more prominence in the literature and a wider range of therapies was proposed, including hormone therapy, electrotherapy and psychotherapy.[114] Authors continued to emphasise the link between onanism and impotence through spermatorrhoea, although by the late 1940s masturbation was directly linked to impotence.[115] From the 1920s onwards authors also mentioned continence (egkrateia) and abstinence as well as coitus interruptus as causes of impotence.[116]

That this was a topic that physicians engaged with in their practice much more than the meagre publications suggest is evidenced by the explicit mentions of impotence in the abundant advertisements of physicians in the national or Athenian press published from 1898 to the 1950s. One of the most prominent advertisers was Socrates Louizidis, who invariably referred to his five-year studies in Paris. In an early advertisement we read that he guaranteed a 'cure of impotence spermatorrhoea sterility'.[117] In the 1940s his description of his expertise read: 'Venereologist, Syphilis-expert, Gynaecologist, SEXOLOGIST (impotence)', indicating both the emergence of the field of sexology and the changes in the treatment and understanding of impotence.[118] An earlier physician's advert, for example, had referred to the use of tonics, serums, injections and mechanical methods in order to cure impotence.[119] Tonics were also advertised in the press, though the word 'impotence' was never explicitly mentioned. Instead the sketch of a virile centaur was the centre of the advertisement with the text focusing on how the tonic 'enriches the genital glands' and 'restores the natural potency' (Plate 3.1).[120] Moreover, the word 'tablets' was discreetly embedded into the sketch, emphasising that the use of this tonic did not necessitate the involvement of a third person, thus protecting the anonymity of the user. A couple of decades later a cartoon in a popular medical magazine was also referring to such a tonic but in a more light-hearted manner. The cartoon showed a husband, who after having taken a tonic prescribed by the sexologist physician, was chasing the physician's receptionist—a rather plain woman—while the wife—a young, well dressed and modern woman—was complaining that the effects of the tonic were too strong (Plate 3.2).[121] The wife's body image is discreetly over-sexualised suggesting her high demands on that sphere. A 1951 article authored by a psychiatrist and entitled 'Sexual inadequacy of man' outlined the modern interpretation of impotence, which included both physiological and psychological causes. Appropriately for a time following significant societal dislocation and disruption, the article stated that only once all other health and food issues are resolved was impotence acknowledged as a problem,[122] and went on to suggest that, as the problem was complex, different therapies would be recommended to different patients, depending on the specific case. However, it concluded with the recommendation of a 'very strong and effective' new tonic. In the same period, short entertaining stories outlining the plight of the impotent husband were published in a physician's magazine under the title 'From the profession's secrets'.[123]

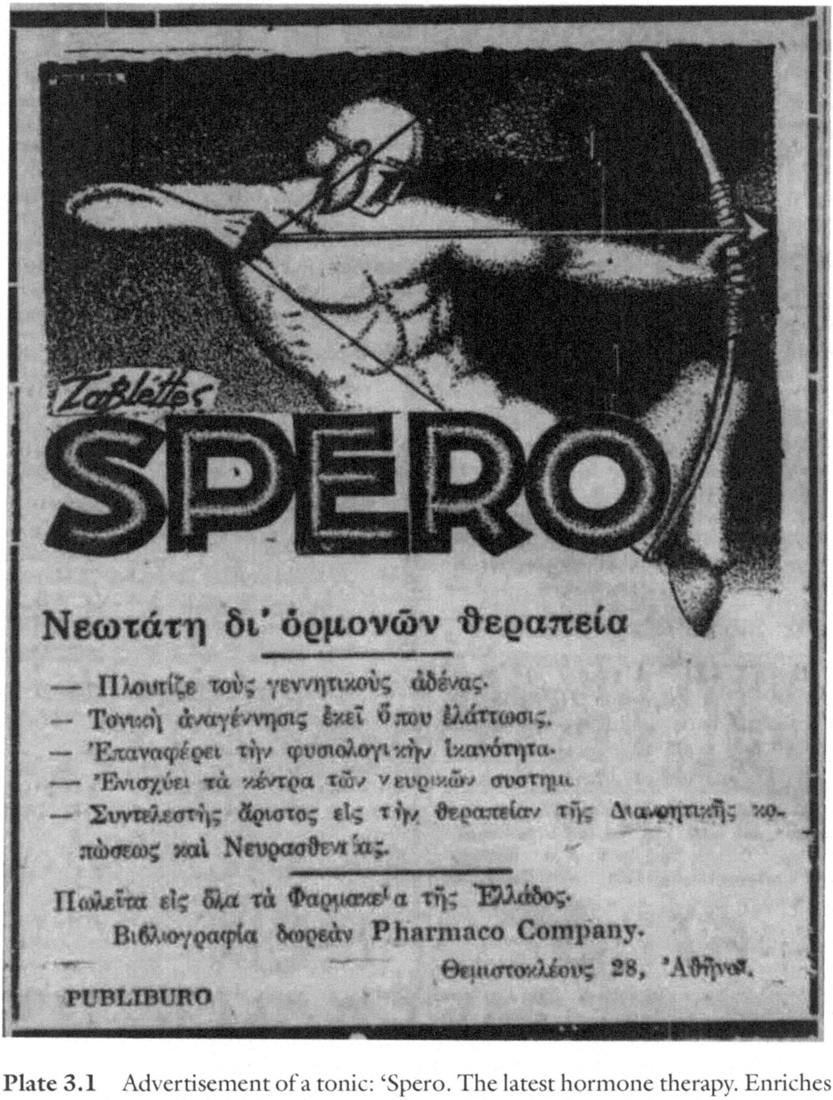

Plate 3.1 Advertisement of a tonic: 'Spero. The latest hormone therapy. Enriches the reproductive glands. Tonic regeneration where there is reduction. Restores the natural ability. Reinforces the centres of the nervous system[s] [sic]. Excellent contributor to the therapy of Mental fatigue and Neurasthenia. Sold in all pharmacies in Greece. Free bibliography *Pharmaco Company* Themistokleous 28, Athens.' (Source: Anonymous (23 September 1930) 'Spero. Neotate di'Ormonon Therapeia', *Akropolis*, 2(594), p. 3)

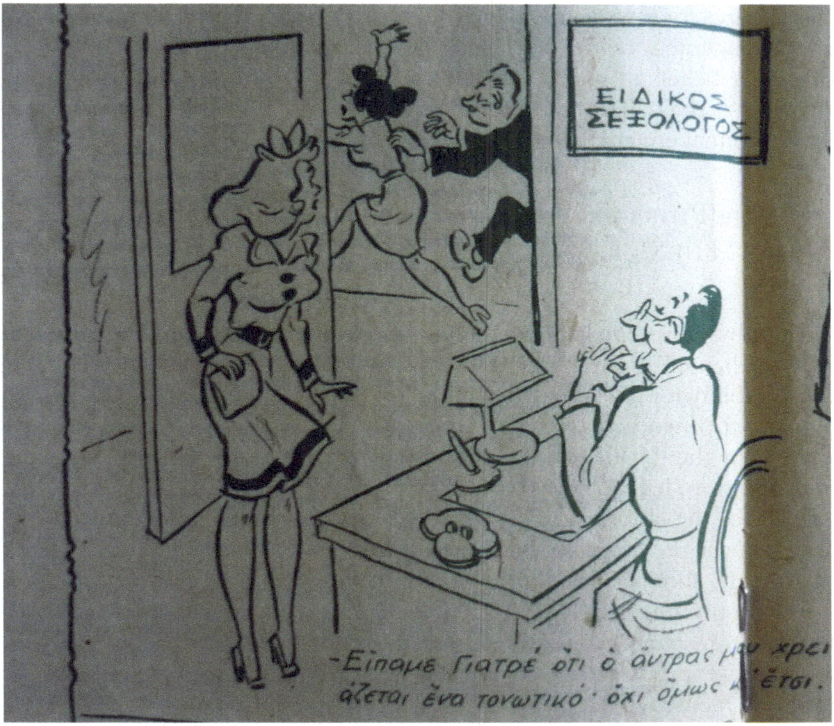

Plate 3.2 'We said Doctor [Sexologist] that my husband needs a tonic. But not like that!'. (Source: Anonymous (June 1949) 'Eipame Giatre', *To Saloni tou Giatrou*, 15(3), p. 13)

The lack of many direct references to impotence in the medical writings should not be taken as an indication of the absence of a problem but rather as evidence of the lack of an open discussion of an issue that was, for many, significant and troubling. Just as in popular culture, this was not an issue frequently discussed between patient and physician and neither was it frequently addressed in medical writings. Patients, especially in rural areas, were in fear of being identified by their fellow islanders on visiting, for example, a venereologist, and adverts promised secrecy to patients from the provinces and abroad who wished to consult the physician by letter.[124] However, the few existing works make it clear that there were no actual cures for impotence, which explains not only the absence of significant engagement by the physicians but also the prevalence and endurance of strong beliefs in magic. As Kyriakides declared in the mid-nineteenth century, 'if the hand of a beautiful woman cannot enliven it … all the rest have minimal effect'.[125]

The Physician's Perspective on Women's Sterility: 'The Purely Medical Therapy Is Completely Powerless Against Sterility'[126]

Greek physicians engaged with much more vigour with women's sterility than with men's, partly because women were apportioned most of the responsibility for infertility. Multiple possible causes are cited in the medical discussion of women's sterility, although these change over time. Pyrros, writing in the 1830s, attributed women's sterility to 'the suspension of menstruation, leucorrhoea, cachexia, fatness, [?] of the utero, syphilis, [?], the size of the clitoris, great weakness and the obstruction or blocking of the utero or the 'so called' fallopian tubes'.[127] He recommended internal treatments, fumigation, douching and putting menstruation in order, as well as rosewater mixed with *kastorhion* (literally a preparation based on beaver's testes; most probably using castoreum sacs), warm baths (plain or aromatic), tonics and 'sweets' internally (that is, pessaries).[128] He discussed blocked menses—which, he advised, could lead to sterility and even death—in a different section of the same book and offered a much longer list of recommended medicines for it than for sterility. Pyrros argued that if the woman had followed all his recommendations and did not conceive 'the damage is with the man and not with the woman'.[129] Almost half a century later Vitsares attributed sterility primarily to the physical construction of the vagina or the uterus, and problems might include stenosis, which would be treated with sea-baths, hydrotherapy, ergot or cleansing, or a twist of the uterus, which could be treated with the continuous and repeated use of laminaria, a type of seaweed; other cases could be treated with pessaries during coitus.[130] However, he also attributed sterility to the long-term suspension of menstruation.[131] For Kindynes, writing in the 1880s, dysmenorrhoea, stenosis, obstruction and metritis were all conditions associated with sterility.[132] By 1886 sterility was linked to conjugal onanism—that is, coitus interruptus—while the rest of the consequences of withdrawal (metritis, leucorrhoea, metrorrhagia, menorrhagia, haematocele, polypus and women's ailments) were also subsequently considered to lead to sterility.[133] Oikonomopoulos, writing at the start of the twentieth century, argues for a position combining the ideas of Vitsares and Pyrros, discussing the physical imperfections of the women's reproductive system and recommending good and 'stimulant' food, sea-baths, douching and warm sitz baths, but also the use of 'the so called aphrodisiac medicines'.[134] As earlier, stenosis was seen as a significant cause of sterility and, while he did not recommend laminaria (as most others did), his suggestions were the equally commonly employed pessaries, 'gradually larger in volume, the best of which are those made of sponge'.[135] Furthermore, he made the explicit link between menorrhagia, dysmenorrhoea, amenorrhoea and sterility, with the former conditions being either the preceding cause or the resulting consequence of sterility.[136] When discussing menstrual irregularities, his discussion was framed almost exclusively around the general health of the woman and only once did he suggest that menstrual irregularity could impair conception.[137] Others linked amenorrhoea with sterility and recommended dilation with candles as therapy.[138] It should be noted that this was an article originally written by Prof. Herman of London, translated, and published in Greek. It is rather telling that at this point in time Oikonomopoulos declared physicians unable to actually deal with women's sterility. In the same decade curettage was advocated, rapidly introduced and widely utilised by Greek gynaecologists for the subsequent 50 or so years in order to treat those women's ailments that were linked to sterility, namely metritis and endometritis.

Antonopoulos' 1926 book focused exclusively on women's sterility. His ideas, which appear to be heavily based on those of Vitsares and Oikonomopoulos, identify a number of female physical pathologies, such as atresia, stenosis and tilted uterus, as causes of sterility. Suggestions for their treatment included, for example, the dilation of the cervix with laminaria or Helger candles for stenosis.[139] Interestingly, Antonopoulos cautioned women who *wanted* to become pregnant not to use douches for reasons of cleanliness and certainly not ones with an antiseptic solution.[140] On the same issue, Drakoulides, writing probably in the 1930s, strongly recommended 'cleanliness' to all women and suggested douching twice a day, although, like Antonopoulos, he advised that those who wanted to become pregnant should wash themselves only externally. A lack of cleanliness, he warned, led to sterility.[141] Elsewhere, Drakoulides argued strongly that gonorrhoea was the main reason for sterility and Zouraris also articulated similar ideas in the 1940s.[142] However, most works from the mid-1920s to the early 1960s yet again put forward different sets of 'causes', now focusing on the use of contraceptives and their side effects, which included inflammation, ulceration, metritis and 'women's ailments', all of which, according to the authors, led to sterility.[143] Virtually all contraceptive methods known at the time were directly linked to sterility, as was curettage by some writers. For the first time, there is also a reference to female onanism, which, we are told, led to sterility, even after marriage.[144]

Discussion and Conclusions

Procreation was central to and essential for Greek society and families, and its absence or inadequacy was seen as a considerable problem. The problem was primarily a social rather than a religious one, as is made clear by eighteenth-century religious teachings that attempted to comfort couples who found themselves in such an unfortunate position.[145] The Church also 'helped' such couples by ignoring the performance of 'good' magic by priests. However, the social status of a childless couple was compromised and they were widely pitied, hence the efforts they would make to remedy the problem. While primary sterility was life-shattering, secondary sterility was problematic too if the couple had only a small number of children.

Unfortunately, neither traditional healers nor physicians were able to offer an effective 'cure', whether this was aimed at addressing women's sterility or men's impotence. Such a lack of successful strategies from popular healing and medicine amplified not only the importance of religious and 'good' magical practices but also the strong belief in 'evil' practices. All in all, a myriad of suggested solutions existed for newly married couples, and trialling many of them discreetly could occupy decades before the couple came to consider some form of adoption.

In explaining and offering therapies for sterility and impotence, Greek physicians were heavily influenced by western European physicians, their publications either being translated or incorporated into Greek publications. For impotence, aphrodisiacs—especially cantharides—were seen as the answer, mirroring the advice Jennifer Evans cites for early modern England.[146] Physicians' attributed causes of sterility varied over time: male masturbation was implicated for the entire nineteenth century and the first half of the twentieth, gonorrhoea and syphilis in the 1930s and 1940s, contraception in the period from the 1920 to the 1970s and curettage in the second half of the twentieth century. Menstrual disorders were also constantly referred to, partly as a remnant of earlier times, partly because of popular beliefs. The therapies proposed are intriguing—a combination of medical modernity, popular remedies and the adaptation of the latter into the former: douching with added chemicals, pessaries and dilation were commonly advocated in the nineteenth and early twentieth centuries and curettage in the first half of the twentieth century. As emmenagogues were also associated—in theory at least—with efforts to overcome sterility and enhance fertility, we turn now to their examination.

Notes

1. See, for example, Richard Blum and Eva Blum (1965) *Health and Healing in Rural Greece* (Stanford, CA: Stanford University Press), p. 75; in addition, a 1950 article in a popular Greek women's magazine emphasises to its middle-class readers that the purpose of marriage is not sexual gratification but procreation (Anonymous (4 October 1950) 'Syzygike Zoe', *Gynaika*, 1(18), p. 12); and for the position of the Church see Anna Matthaiou (2006) 'Syzygikes Sheseis kai Sexoualikoteta sta Hronia tes Othomanikes Kyriarhias: Kanones, Protypa, Sympsefismoi', *Ta Istorika*, 23(44), 147–60.
2. The one article that explicitly deals with childlessness focuses on the waning custom of taking a second 'wife' when the first was not fruitful. Dem. A. Petropoulou (1952) 'E Akleria eis ta Ethima tou Ellenikou Laou', *Epeteris tou Laografikou Arheiou*, 7, 28–44.
3. In 1893 all births occurred in houses, except those of destitute women, who would seek help in the Athens State Maternity Hospital: K. Alexandropoulos (1954) 'Ioannes Anton. Poumpouras 1870–1954. O Vios kai to Ergon Autou', *Arheia Maieutikes kai Gynaikologias en Elladi* 23(1), 5. *Movement Naturel de la Population de la Grèce en 1961* (1963) (Athens: National Printers), p. xv; *Movement Naturel de la Population de la Grèce en 1969* (1971) (Athens: National Printers), p. xv.
4. Despoina Damianou (2005) *Laikes Afegeseis. Mythoi kai Paramythia ton Kytheron* (Athena: Etaireia Kytheraikon Meleton), p. 175, citing G.H. Papaharalampous (1965) *Kypriaka Ethe kai Ethima* (Nicosia: Etaireia Kypriakon Spoudon), p. 83. Alternatively, they would be left in a church and the parish priest might have passed them on to a couple (No. 9, Syros, referring to the Catholic community of Ano Syros).
5. Kyriakos Ntelopoulos (ed.) (2006) *Minos Dounias. Tha Nikesoume alla Yper ten Niken Doxa. To «Saranta» mesa apo tis Epistoles ton Polemiston kai ton Amahon* (Athens: Agra), p. 57, referring to the period November 1940–April 1941.

6. As the Great Greek Encyclopaedia outlines for rural weddings, on wedded couples' return to the home after the ceremony a number of 'magical acts' were performed before entering the home, intended to 'protect the couple from any bad influences and to offer the couple fertility, happiness, peace, male descendants and every good' (Paulos Drandakes (ed.) (1956) *Megale Ellenike Egkyklopaideia*, 2nd edn, vol. 8 (Athens: Phoenix), p. 131). Vassiliki Chryssanthopoulou (2008) 'The evil eye among the Greeks of Australia: Identity, continuity and modernization' in John Petropoulos (ed.) *Greek Magic: Ancient, Medieval and Modern* (London: Routledge), p. 114; Theodore Paradellis, 'Erotic and fertility magic in the folk culture of modern Greece' in John Petropoulos (ed.) *Greek Magic: Ancient, Medieval and Modern* (London: Routledge), pp. 128–9; On Leros mandrake was placed under the pillow of newlyweds for procreation and protection from magic: Pan. Kretikos (1961) 'O Mandragoras', *Laografia*, 19, 38.
7. See, for example, J.K. Campbell (1979) *Honour, Family, and Patronage*, 1st edn 1964 (New York: Oxford University Press), p. 150.
8. The commemoration of the dead is still a significant religious practice today, although it is not necessarily or exclusively performed by the children of the deceased.
9. Gregorios Palaiologos (1989) *O Zografos*, first edition 1842 (Athens: Nefele), p. 327.
10. Folklore Archives of the Academy of Athens (henceforth FAAA) 1426, Asterios Zampouras, Krousevo (NW Macedonia), 1939.
11. Palaiologos, *O Zografos*, p. 327.
12. Palaiologos, *O Zografos*, p. 327.
13. Palaiologos, *O Zografos*, pp. 283, 289. FAAA 1631, Panagiotes Fragkeles, Lesvos, 1950.
14. Vana Bouse and Michael Bouse (eds), *Anekdotes Epistoles tes Vasilissas Amalias ston patera tes*, vol. 1 (Athens: Estia), pp. 278, 290, 572–3. In her case, the advice came from her Bavarian physician.
15. Georgios N. Kyriakides (1882) *Ta Mysteria tou Syzygikou Erotos etoi Fysiologia kai Ygieine kata tas Axiologous tes Zoes Epohas ton Syzygon*, 1st edn 1865 (Athens: Io. Kostopoulos), p. 170.
16. Kyriakides, *Ta Mysteria*, p. 176. See also FAAA 1426, p. 1, Asterios Zampouras, Krousevo (NW Macedonia), 1939; Damianou, *Laikes Afegeseis*, p. 171 citing Euaggelos Audikos (1996) *To Paidi sten Paradosiake kai te Syghrone Koinonia* (Athens: Ellenika Grammata), p. 52.
17. Sevaste Haviara-Karahaliou (1993) *E Laike Iatrike tes Hiou* (Athens: GasciHellas), p. 47, where a Chian informant referred to amenorrhoeal women, perceiving them to be sterile.
18. No. 22 Syros.

19. Euaggelia K. Fragkake (1978) *E Demodes Iatrike tes Kretes* (Athens: n.p.), pp. 33–4.
20. Alexandros Tsakires (1954) *Megale Sexologia. Anikanotes, Steirosis kai e Syghrone Therapeia ton*, 3rd edn, first published 1947 (Athens: n.p.), p. 534.
21. Nikolaos Vasileiades (August 1928) 'Peri Amenorroias', *O Praktikos Iatros*, 6(8), 353.
22. No. 11 Mykonos.
23. Folklore collection of Athens University (henceforth FCAU), 262, p. 9, Maria Memou Emmanouel, Anogeia Mylopotamou Rethymno, Crete, 1967–8, https://pergamos.lib.uoa.gr/uoa/dl/object/3398, accessed 17 September 2018; FAAA 1427, p. 1, K. Karapatakes, Grevena, 1940.
24. No. 21 Mykonos.
25. Pope Speliotou-Mpazina (1951) 'Steirosis', *Alkyonides. Deltio tes Panelleniou Enoseos Dianooumenon Gynaikon*, 2(7), p. 10.
26. Georgios K. Zouraris (1947) *E Steirosis eis tous Andras kai tas Gynaikes kai to Thauma tes Syllepseos*, 2nd edn (Athens: n.p.), p. 14.
27. Blum and Blum, *Health and Healing*, p. 57.
28. FAAA 1427, p. 1, K. Karapatakes, Grevena, 1940.
29. FAAA 1426, p. 2, Asterios Zampouras, Krousevo (NW Macedonia), 1939.
30. FCAU, 262, p. 9, Maria Memou Emmanouel, Anogeia Mylopotamou Rethymno, Crete, 1967–8, https://pergamos.lib.uoa.gr/uoa/dl/object/3398, accessed 17 September 2018.
31. FCAU, 17, p. 2, Stauros Semaiakes, Kritsa Lasithi, Crete, 1965, https://pergamos.lib.uoa.gr/uoa/dl/object/308, accessed 17 September 2018.
32. Fragkake, *E Demodes*, p. 31; FAAA, 1566, Informant Katsoulena, Maniaki, 1944; Blum and Blum, *Health and Healing*, p. 65; Nikiou N. Konsola (1965) 'Laografika Olympou Karpathou', *Laografia*, ΚΔ, 228 (the author and interviewer was a teacher).
33. FAAA, 1628, Maria I. Kokkine, Patra, 1950. Also see T.I. Athanasopoulos (1915) 'Magikai teletai pros teknopoiesin', *Laografia* E, 408. See also Damianou, *Laikes Afegeseis*, p. 170, referring to sterility as a 'curse'.
34. Konsola, 'Laografika Olympou Karpathou', 228.
35. If the widow remained unmarried, in many cases she would enjoy the usufruct of whatever her late husband owned. Upon her death, his relatives would become the owners. G.L. Maurer (1976) *O Ellenikos Laos: Dimosio, Idiotiko kai Ekklisiastiko Dikaio apo ten Enarxi tou Agona gia ten Aneksartisia os tin 31 Iouliou 1834*, translated by O. Rompaki, original edn 1835 (Athens: Tolidi Bros), pp. 706–9; Aglaia E. Kasdagli (2004) 'Family and inheritance in the Cyclades, 1500–1800: Present knowledge and unanswered questions', *The History of the Family*, 9, 266.
36. Violetta Hionidou (2012) 'Marriage, inheritance and household formation on a Greek island, Mykonos (mid-nineteenth to mid-twentieth

century)' in A.L. Head-König (ed.) in collaboration with P. Pozsgai *Inheritance practices, marriage strategies and household formation in European rural societies* (Turnhout: Brepols), pp. 261–82.
37. No. 11 Mykonos, married in 1946.
38. See Hamish Forbes on adopting within the kinship group: (2007) *Meaning and Identity in a Greek Landscape* (Cambridge: Cambridge University Press), p. 170. This was also the case for one of my Mykonos informants.
39. FAAA, 1631, Panagiotes Fragkeles, Lesvos, 1950.
40. FAAA, 1631, Panagiotes Fragkeles, Lesvos, 1950; Vaios F. Kaminiotes (2016) *Magisses kai Mageirisses. Diatrofe, Mageia kai Gynaikeia Exousia stous Karagkounedes tes Dytikes Thessalias* (Athens: Erodotos), p. 454, citing FAAA, 306, informant Vassiliki, born 1896; Demetrios Petropoulos (1956) 'Le rôle des femmes et de la terre dans quelques pratiques magiques' in O. Merlier and M. Merlier, *Melanges offerts a Octave et Melpo Merlier a l'occasion du 25e anniversaire de leur Arrivée en Grèce* (Athens: n.p.), p. 276.
41. Anonymous (20 November 1950) 'O Gynaikologos Apanta: Reply to Polyvasanismene', *E Gynaika* 1(20), p. 31; Anonymous (20 November 1950) 'O Gynaikologos Apanta: Reply to Hamena Oneira', *E Gynaika* 1(20), p. 31.
42. Tsakires, *Megale Sexologia*, pp. 542, 546.
43. Tsakires, *Megale Sexologia*, pp. 542–8.
44. FAAA 1426, p. 2, Asterios Zampouras, Krousevo (NW Macedonia), 1939.
45. Forbes, *Meaning and Identity*, p. 170.
46. See, for example, Emm. G. Drakakes (1999) *Emmanouel Kasimates notarios Kytheron (1560–1582)* (Athens: Etaireia Kytheraikon Meleton).
47. The close link between magic and Orthodoxy is eloquently outlined in Charles Stewart (2008) 'Magic and Orthodoxy' in John Petropoulos (ed.) *Greek Magic: Ancient, Medieval and Modern* (London: Routledge), pp. 87–94. Also see Violetta Hionidou (2016) 'Popular medicine and empirics in Greece, 1900–1950: an oral history approach', *Medical History*, 60(4), 492–513.
48. Gerasimos Regatos (2003) 'Oi Empeirikoi Therapeutes os Antikeimeno Satyras: E Periptose tes Komodias ton Pseutogiatron tou Savogia Rousmele', *Deltos*, 25, 26.
49. These were hand-written healing manuscripts listing diseases and their therapies, including incantations. The language was always vernacular Greek. See also Hionidou, 'Popular medicine', 498.
50. University of Athens, Greece, Library of Byzantine and Modern Greek Philology, *Iatrosofion* 46, pp. 6–7, eighteenth century, https://pergamos.lib.uoa.gr/uoa/dl/object/183213, accessed 3 July 2019. In a

Cypriot medical recipe of 1842 the recommended cure involves the use of a herbal pessary based on rue: Kypros Hrysanthes (1951) 'Ena Kypriako giatrosofi', *Kypriakes Spoudes* 15, η.

51. On the definitions of such medical recipes and the creation and use of such manuscripts see under 'iatrosophion': Paulos Drandakes (1929) *Megale Ellenike Egkyklopaideia* vol. 12 (Athens: Pyrsos), p. 828. Also Hionidou, 'Popular medicine'.
52. Agapios Monahos o Kres (2002) *Geoponikon. Giatrosophia kai Palies Syntages*, digital reprint from the 1850 publication (Athens: Koultoura).
53. For the first edition see Dionysios Stathakopoulos (2007) 'Between the field and the plate: how agricultural products were processed into food' in Leslie Brubaker and Kallirroe Linardou (eds) *Eat, Drink, and be Merry (Luke 12:19): Food and Wine in Byzantium*, Papers in honour of Professor A.A.M. Bryer (Aldershot: Ashgate), p. 29. For subsequent editions, see the catalogue of the National Library of Greece under 'Geoponikon' (https://catalogue.nlg.gr/).
54. Haviara-Karahaliou, *E Laike*, p. 384.
55. Emmanouel I. Emmanouel (1938) *Iatrosofia kai Tsarlatanoi* (Athens: n.p.), p. 13, referring to a herbal (Kodikas Leipsias, published 1873–4); Argenti and Rose mention a recipe for curing sterility originating from a privately written and owned manuscript dated 22 February 1873: Philip P. Argenti and H.J. Rose, *The Folk-Lore of Chios* (Cambridge: Cambridge University Press, 1949); Hrysanthes, 'Ena Kypriako', θ–ιδ, who discusses an iatrosophic manuscript bound to the printed book Γ.Φ.Β. (1835) *Greek Pharmacopoeia* (Smyrna: n.p.). Hrysanthes argues that this is not a Cypriot iatrosophic but rather that at some point it was transcribed by a Cypriot (στ). Evidence abounds for the seventeenth and eighteenth centuries too: see, for example, V. Skouvara (1967) 'Magika kai Iatrosofika Eranismata ek Thessalikou Kodikos', *Epeterida Kentrou Ereunes Ellenikes Laografias* ΙΗ-ΙΘ, 79–80, 89 (utilising a mid-eighteenth-century manuscript). For a sixteenth-century manuscript offering such recipes see Labrini Manou (2008) *Giatrosofia 16ou aiona* (Thessaloniki: Kyriakides), p. 26 citing manuscript 181, Iveron Monastery.
56. Patricia Ann Clark (2011) *A Cretan Healer's Handbook in the Byzantine Tradition: Text, Translation, and Commentary* (Farnham: Ashgate).
57. Clark, p. 52, 114; FAAA, 1628, Maria I. Kokkine, Patra, 1950; FAAA 1631, Panagiotes Fragkeles, Lesvos, 1950; Xen. G. Anagnostopoulos (1961) *Ta Votana. Laike Farmakologia kai Therapeutike* (Athens: n.p.), p. 118; Konsola, 'Laografika Olympou Karpathou', p. 228.
58. Haviara-Karahaliou, *E Laike*, pp. 168–9.

59. Fragkake, *E Demodes*, p. 31. The terms the author uses are 'sulleptika farmaka, ahnismata, hamamia, agiotika'. Religious methods and herbals are mentioned also by Konsola, 'Laografika', 228.
60. Fragkake, *E Demodes*, p. 31.
61. Fragkake, *E Demodes*, p. 31. Fumigation, though with different ingredients, is also described as a cure for sterility in other Cretan localities. Again, the aim was to 'open up' the womb, which was 'closed up', resulting in sterility. Kostas D. Moutzoures (2003) 'Laike iatrike sto Akroteri Hanion', *Laike Iatrike, Diethnes Epistemoniko Synedrio Rethymno 8–10 Dekemvriou 2000, Praktika* (Rethymno), p. 288.
62. Kaminiotes, *Magisses*, p. 455, citing FAAA, 306, informant Vasiliki born 1896. Kaminiotes cites other folklore methods as well.
63. Aglaia Mpimpe-Papaspyropoulou (1985) 'Paradosiake iatrike sten Peloponneso' (PhD thesis, Athens: Ethniko kai Kapodistriako Panepistemio Athenon), p. 323.
64. Argenti and Rose, *The Folk-lore of Chios*, p. 410.
65. Fragkake, *E Demodes*, p. 31.
66. Fragkake, *E Demodes*, pp. 31–2.
67. Athanasopoulos, 'Magikai teletai pros teknopoiesin', p. 408–9.
68. FAAA 1426, p. 2, Asterios Zampouras, Krousevo (NW Macedonia), 1939. Also FAAA 1631, Panagiotes Fragkeles, Lesvos, 1950.
69. Antonios N. Kindynes (1880) *E Steirosis para te Gynaiki kai Therapeia Aytes* (Athens: Vlastos Varvarregos); Evy Johanne Håland (2009) '15 August on the Aegean Island of Tinos', *Bulletin of the Institute of Ethnography*, SASA, LVI I (2), 95–110.
70. Prior arrangements would have been made with the church so that the specific wick used on the day was made of cotton (Fragkake, *E Demodes*, p. 32). Similar practices are mentioned in FAAA, 1628, Maria I. Kokkine, Patra, 1950.
71. Fragkake, *E Demodes*, p. 32.
72. FCAU, 17, p. 2, Stauros Semaiakes, Kritsa Lasithi, Crete, 1965, https://pergamos.lib.uoa.gr/uoa/dl/object/3083, accessed 17 September 2018; FAAA 1631, Panagiotes Fragkeles, Lesvos, 1950; on Hios the Monastery of Nea Mone was the one where the childless promised their children to the church: Mikes Paidouses (1964) 'E Iatrike eis ten Hion. Sympleroseis kai Diorthoseis', *Periodikon tou en Hio Syllogou Argente*, 6, 103–8, cited in Haviara-Karahaliou, *E Laike*, p. 375.
73. Jill Dubisch (1995) *In a Different Place: Pilgrimage, Gender, and Politics at a Greek Island Shrine* (Princeton, NJ: Princeton University Press).
74. FCAU, 17, p. 2, Stauros Semaiakes, Kritsa, Lasithi, Crete, 1965, https://pergamos.lib.uoa.gr/uoa/dl/object/3083, accessed 17 September 2018; FAAA 1426, p. 2, Asterios Zampouras, Krousevo (NW Macedonia), 1939.

75. FCAU, 17, p. 3, Stauros Semaiakes, Kritsa, Lasithi, Crete, 1965, https://pergamos.lib.uoa.gr/uoa/dl/object/3083, accessed 17 September 2018.
76. FAAA 1427, K. Karapatakes, Grevena, 1940. For a very similar account from Eleia a different area in 1951 see Ntinos D. Psyhogios (1951) 'Eleiotika Paidokomia', *Laografia*, 13, 341–2.
77. N.G. Polites (1975) 'Okytokia', *Laografika Symeikta* B, originally published in 1918, 345–6, 354, citing sources referring to the first half of the nineteenth century. Similar practices were observed in the late twentieth century on the island of Tinos at the Church of Virgin Mary (Håland, '15 August', p. 99). Also M. Meliareses (1875) *O Odegos ton Eggamon*. By Frederick Hollick M.D. part b, translated by M. Meliareses (Vraila: M. Pestemaltziogou), p. 69.
78. Pyrros articulates clearly that both men and women can be responsible for sterility: Dionysios Pyrros o Thettalos (1840) *Egkolpion ton Iatron etoi Praktike Iatrike*, 1st edn 1831 (Athens: Aggelou Aggelidou), pp. 192, 196.
79. Psyhogios, 'Eleiotika', 341. When there was evidence 'that there was some deficiency that would prevent the great task of procreation', calling off the engagement was legal (Kyriakides, *Ta Mysteria*, p. 158).
80. Anagnostopoulos, for example, provides popular/magical recipes for childless couples that involve both man and woman (Anagnostopoulos, *Ta Votana*, p. 118). He also provides a couple of popular recipe for curing impotence (powdered cockerel comb, spurge) (Anagnostopoulos, *Ta Votana*, pp. 99–100, 32). Oikonomopoulos emphasises that 'sterility is very rare [in] men' but 'extremely common' in women: Elias I. Oikonomopoulos (1902) *O Gamos* (Athens: O Kadmos), p. 65.
81. Stewart's book is the best text in English introducing such concepts from the Greek culture: Charles Stewart (1991) *Demons and the Devil. Moral Imagination in the Modern Greek Culture* (Princeton, NJ: Princeton University Press). On spells, see chapter 9. Also Richard Blum and Eva Blum (1970) *The Dangerous Hour: The Lore of Crisis and Mystery in Rural Greece* (London: Chatto & Windus), pp. 127–9, 173–5, 192–5; Hionidou, 'Popular medicine'.
82. See Stewart, for example, who cites eight nineteenth- and twentieth-century authors discussing the spell, only one of whom is cited in this publication (*Demons*, p. 289); Pyrros when discussing impotence refers to that 'some [people] think, is caused by magic' (Pyrros, *Egkolpion*, p. 23); Blum and Blum, *Health and Healing*, pp. 128, 195; manuscript notebook of priest Georgios Saramantioudhis, written around the 1890s (Argenti and Rose, *The Folk-Lore of Chios*, p. 387; from the mastic growing area of Hios Argenti and Rose recorded a different 'remedy' to the binding spell (*The Folk-Lore of Chios*, p. 412). See also Paradellis, 'Erotic', for an excellent introduction to the binding spell.

83. John Cuthbert Lawson (1910) *Modern Greek Folklore and Ancient Greek Religion. A Study in Survivals* (Cambridge: Cambridge University Press), p. 19. Though the author here refers to the witch as a female, in Greece bewitchers were equally common (see, for example, Blum and Blum, *The Dangerous Hour*, pp. 195–8; also Ioannes Kondylakes (2005) *O Patouhas*, 1st edn 1892 (Athens: Pelekanos), pp. 62, 114–15).
84. FAAA, 1636, p. 21, Mary Tounta, Aharnai Athens, 1948.
85. FAAA, 1620, p. 5, Themelis, Leukada, [1940s]. Kaminiotes, *Magisses*, pp. 466–7, 469. In the village of Gelanthe the first sexual intercourse of the couple took place the night before the wedding, in order to ensure that any magic during the wedding could not have an effect, as the groom would have already proved his sexual ability (Kaminiotes, *Magisses*, p. 471).
86. Lawson, *Modern Greek Folklore*, pp. 19–21.
87. A sixteenth-century Church canon banned those 'practicing binding spells on married couples' (Stewart, *Demons*, p. 231, citing W.H.D. Rouse (1899), 'Folklore from the Southern Sporades', *Folklore*, 10, 153).
88. Lawson, *Modern Greek Folklore*, p. 20.
89. Clark, *A Cretan*, p. 56, p. 108; Agapios, *Geoponikon*, p. 140; Skouvara, 'Magika', 71–113.
90. Chryssanthopoulou, 'The evil eye', p. 111.
91. Kondylakes, *O Patouhas*, pp. 114–16.
92. Vounas, after presenting the popular beliefs about the 'spell', attributes the impotence of the groom to excessive consumption of wine and the prolonged celebration of the wedding: Christos Vounas (1968) *Laografika tes Kefalonias* (Patra: n.p.), p. 18. Kyriakides explains that the threat of the spell had a psychological effect as a result of the fear that it engendered (*Ta Mysteria*, pp. 178–9).
93. Tsakires emphasised that 'impotence is a legal impediment to marriage and a strong reason for divorce' (*Megale Sexologia*, p. 533).
94. Stewart mentions that men who slept with a nereid also become impotent (*Demons*, p. 175, citing Nikolaos Polites (1904) *Paradoseis*, vol. 2 (Athens: Gregorios Marasles), p. 389). Again, the individual is not responsible for the impotence; rather, it is the fault of supernatural creatures. This seems to refer to non-irreversible situations.
95. Skouvara, 'Magika', 90, 105, 108 (One refers to anthropos [i.e., it is not gender specific] and three to a couple); Argenti and Rose, *The Folk-lore of Chios*, p. 387.
96. Magic in most cases targeted the groom, but it could also be used to render the virgin bride unable to lose her virginity or, later, to make the woman sterile (by throwing a snake to the entrance of her house) (Kyriakides, *Ta Mysteria*, pp. 176–85).

97. The most unusual situation, and one rather specific to the area of Mani, was the unofficial co-habitation of the childless couple with a second woman, who would bear children for the family. The custom survived well into the twentieth century (Petropoulou, 'E Akleria', pp. 28–44).
98. Agapios advises that an amulet should be used, but also that the pregnant woman should avoid particularly heavy jobs (Agapios, *Geoponikon*, p. 146). Argenti and Rose list a variety of protective methods, ranging from an amulet—seeking the protection of a specific saint, Saint Stylianos—to various herbals (Argenti and Rose, *The Folk-lore of Chios*, pp. 374, 427, 524, 528, 540, 545). FAAA 1427, p. 2, K. Karapatakes, Grevena, 1940. FCAU, 17, p. 3, Stauros Semaiakes, Kritsa, Lasithi, Crete, 1965, https://pergamos.lib.uoa.gr/uoa/dl/object/3083, accessed 17 September 2018. Vivliotheke Vyzantines kai Neoellenikes Filologias, Iatrosofion IΘ, 46, https://pergamos.lib.uoa.gr/uoa/dl/object/183213, pp. 6–7, 'For the child not to be killed'. Psyhogios, 'Eleiotika', p. 343. Konsola, 'Laografika', 231. Damianou, *Laikes Afegeseis*, p. 171.
99. Pyrros, *Egkolpion*, p. 192.
100. Pyrros, *Egkolpion*, p. 23.
101. Kyriakides, though not a physician, also recommended cantharides as an aphrodisiac in order 'to make him more amorous'. He also listed celery, artichoke, asparagus and crocus as additional aphrodisiacs (Kyriakides, *Ta Mysteria*, pp. 245, 248).
102. Pyrros, *Egkolpion*, p. 23.
103. Meliareses, *O Odegos*.
104. Meliareses, *O Odegos*, p. 69; M. Moyseides (1927) *Ygieine tes Egkyou, Epitokou, Lehoidos, kai tes Galouhouses* (Alexandreia: Kasigone); Antonios Gregoriades (1949) *Afrodisia Nosemata kai Anikanotes. Ygieina paraggelmata kai profylaxis ton neon* (Athens: n.p.).
105. Meliareses, *O Odegos*, pp. 74–9.
106. Meliareses, *O Odegos*, p. 82. Interestingly, the next reference to 'stimulants and aphrodisiacs' appears when masturbation is addressed, with the advice to avoid both sets of medicines: M. Moyseides (1927) *Aunanismos kindynoi-profylaxis-therapy* (Athens: Gerardon Bros), p. 19.
107. Oikonomopoulos, *O Gamos*, pp. 65–7.
108. A.V. Panas (1912) *Tria Themata Iatrokoinonika Ypsistes Meletes* (Athens: Estia), pp. 25–30.
109. Panas, *Tria Themata*, pp. 32–3. The author calls this the 'moral' dimension.
110. Panas, *Tria Themata*, p. 44.
111. Panas, *Tria Themata*, pp. 41–51.
112. Panas, *Tria Themata*, pp. 55–120.

113. Gregoriades, *Afrodisia Nosemata*, pp. 53–61.
114. Gregoriades, *Afrodisia Nosemata*, p. 61.
115. Gregoriades, *Afrodisia Nosemata*, pp. 20–1, 56–8; Tsakires, *Megale Sexologia*, pp. 666–7. In Britain the preoccupation with spermatorrhoea died out in the 1860s. Elizabeth Stephens (2009) 'Coining Spermatorrhoea: Medicine and Male Body Fluids, 1836–1866', *Sexualities*, 12(4), 480.
116. Moyseides, *Aunanismos*; Tsakires, *Megale Sexologia*, pp. 667–73; Gregoriades, *Afrodisia Nosemata*, pp. 20–1, 56–8; Georgios K. Zouraris (1947) *Sexoualike Zoe: Apohe, Egkrateia, Akolasia kai e Exasthenisis tes Ormes*, 3rd edn (Athens: n.p.), pp. 54–5. However, that *egkrateia* could lead to impotence had already been suggested by Kyriakides in 1882: *Ta Mysteria*, p. 159.
117. Anonymous (13 December 1924) 'SOKRATES I. LOUIZIDIS, EIDIKOS IATROS', *Skrip*, 29(1877), p. 4.
118. Anonymous (10 June 1947) 'SOKRATES I. LOUIZIDIS, EIDIKOS IATROS', *Rizospastes*, 30(10088), p. 2.
119. Anonymous (1 April 1900) 'SYFILIDIKA-GYNAIKEIA. O IATROS ANASTASIOS TH. DOUSES', *Skrip*, 5(1658), p. 6.
120. Anonymous (23 September 1930) 'Spero. Neotate di'Ormonon Therapeia', *Akropolis*, 2(594), p. 3.
121. Anonymous (June 1949) 'Eipame Giatre', *To Saloni tou Giatrou*, 15(3), p. 13.
122. Ioannes Ch. Nikoletsopoulos (30 December 1951) 'Sexoualike Aneparkeia ston Andra', *E Gynaika*, 3(51), p. 61.
123. Staurou I. Vosyniote (November–December 1950) 'Apo ta Mystika tou Epaggelmatos. Otan e sarx … aperge', *To Saloni tou Giatrou*, 16(17), p. 12, 14.
124. Informant No. 7d Hios discussed the fear of patients visiting venereologists for treatment at length: if their visit were to become known, their reputation would be destroyed. Even those who dared to confide to a physician subsequently had an ambivalent relationship with them, fearing that their secret might become widely known. Adverts in the daily press promised 'utter secrecy' to clients from the 'provinces or abroad', who could consult the physician through correspondence: Anonymous (1 April 1900) 'SYFILIDIKA-GYNAIKEIA. O IATROS ANASTASIOS TH. DOUSES', *Skrip*, 5(1658), p. 6.
125. Kyriakides, *Ta Mysteria*, p. 160.
126. Oikonomopoulos, *O Gamos*, p. 74.
127. Pyrros, *Egkolpion*, pp. 191–3.
128. In a different publication, Pyrros explains that Kastorhion is an emmenagogue. Dionysios Pyrros o Thettalos (1838) *Votanike Praktike*

Prosarmosmene eis ten Iatriken & Oikonomia (Athens: Aggelou Aggelidou), p. 168. Such 'sweets' were heavily based on sugar.

129. Pyrros, *Egkolpion*, p. 192.
130. A. Vitsares (1874) *Nosoi ton Gynaikon*, vol. 1 (Athens: Ermou), pp. 132–3, 138.
131. Vitsares, *Nosoi ton Gynaikon*, pp. 138, 155.
132. Kindynes, *E Steirosis*, pp. 85, 110, 124, 138, 145. He cites and quotes only British and French authors.
133. K.P. Kardamates (1886) *Peri Aunanismou, ton Apotelesmaton kai Therapeias Autou* (Athens: n.p.), pp. 101–10. Interestingly, all the case histories provided by Kardamates are from Bergeret's publications, unlike in the earlier part of the book, where he provides Greek cases too.
134. Oikonomopoulos, *O Gamos*, p. 68. See also Jennifer Evans (2014) *Aphrodisiacs, Fertility and Medicine in Early Modern England* (Woodbridge: The Boydell Press).
135. Oikonomopoulos, *O Gamos*, p. 68.
136. Oikonomopoulos, *O Gamos*, p. 67.
137. Oikonomopoulos, *O Gamos*, pp. 31–2. An interesting and unusual case presented by Oikonomopoulos is his reference to women who preferred female sexual partners; he suggested that a cutting of the clitoris would resolve the problem. No further references to this have been traced (p. 67).
138. Prof. Herman (1906) 'Peri Dysmoinoroias', *Iatrike Proodos*, 11(11), 118–22.
139. Dem. Antonopoulos (1926) *E Steirosis para te Gynaiki* (Athens: Koronaiou, Denaxa and Co), pp. 20, 36–8.
140. Antonopoulos, *E Steirosis*, p. 32.
141. N.N. Drakoulides (1956) 'Ygieine Genetesiou Omilias' in Paulos Drandakes (ed.) *Megale Ellenike Egkyklopaideia*, vol. 8, 2nd edn (Athens: Phoenix), p. 187.
142. N.N. Drakoulides (1933) *E Vlennoroia. Ston Andra kai ste Gynaika. Synepeies-profylaxis-Therapeia* (Athens: K. Papadogiannes), pp. 6–11; Zouraris, *E Steirosis*, pp. 80–1.
143. M. Moyseides (1925) *E Gyne. Ygieine tou Gamou kai tes Eggamou Gynaikos* (Alexandreia: A. Kasigone), p. 72 (Moyseides advised that in women intellectual work can lead to sterility as well: p. 71); M. Yioel (1938) *Steirosis e Egkymosyne kata Voulesi*, 2nd edn, 1st edn 1936 (Athens: Vasileiou), pp. 13, 20, 22; N.N. Drakoulides (1936) *E Sexoualike Leitourgia* (Athens: n.p.), p. 11; Anonymous (1954) *Egkyklopaideia tes Ellenidos. Iatrike ton Oikogeneion, Diaitetike, Gynaikeia Provlemata, Kallone, Symperifora* (Athens: Papademetriou); Konstantinos

Metropoulos (1954) *Ygieine tes Egkyou. Enas Polytimos Odegos gia ten Ygieine Diaviose tes Egkyou* (Athens: Papademetriou), p. 306; Tsakires, *Megale Sexologia*, pp. 536, 539.

144. Alkaios Vyzantinos (1946) *O Sexoualismos sten Ellada* (Athens: H. Symeonides), p. 30.
145. In contrast to the findings of Daphna Oren-Magidor for early modern England ((2017) *Infertility in early modern England* (London: Palgrave Macmillan)), the teachings of Kosmas o Aitolos urged the people not to divorce their wives because of childlessness (Matthaiou, 'Syzygikes Sheseis', pp. 152–3).
146. Evans, *Aphrodisiacs.*

CHAPTER 4

Emmenagogues and Abortifacients

Introduction

In the 1980s and 1990s, as noted in the Introduction, Angus McLaren and John Riddle argued for the importance of abortion in the early stages of pregnancy in medieval and early modern England and in the west, respectively. These abortions, they argued, were carried out with the use of abortifacients, with which they roughly equated emmenagogues. As Riddle noted, what was called an emmenagogic herb in one place was termed an abortifacient somewhere else, making the naming of a substance a matter of the user's intention.[1] In his work Riddle also examined the significance of emmenagogic herbs and women's knowledge and use of them over time; he argued that such knowledge, which was primarily possessed by women, although largely forgotten after the Middle Ages, survived to the twentieth century in some small measure.[2] Moreover, Riddle equated western women's desire to make 'themselves regular' with inducing abortion, a process undertaken by women who wanted to avoid childbearing.[3]

In contrast with the views of McLaren and Riddle, Van de Walle provided evidence that emmenagogues were not equated with abortifacients and that the aim in using the former was not to be equated with the desire to achieve an abortion. Rather, emmenagogues were used to bring on menstruation when it was delayed, as deviations from the perceived 'norm' of menstruation—that is, excessive, insufficient or absent menses—were

V. Hionidou, *Abortion and Contraception in Modern Greece, 1830–1967*, Medicine and Biomedical Sciences in Modern History,
https://doi.org/10.1007/978-3-030-41490-0_4

viewed as pathology.[4] Van de Walle strongly argued that there was a 'genuine market for emmenagogues', rather than a covert one that catered for those seeking abortion.[5] Though Van de Walle and others made it clear that irregular menses were treated as pathology, Cadden's linking of menstruation with conception ('no menses, no conception') has passed largely unnoticed for quite some time.[6] Porter's repeated comments on quacks trying to make sales by targeting women 'wishing to conceive and be fruitful' in eighteenth-century England have also been largely ignored.[7] Van de Walle and Renne's edited volume, in which the regulation of menstruation is examined from ancient Greece to contemporary populations, provides a very rich range of evidence on how the regulation of menstruation was and is perceived and achieved in past and contemporary populations. The combination of historical, demographic and anthropological evidence which they offer allows a much more in-depth understanding of the reasoning behind the regulation of menses and the ways women tried to achieve that, and also highlights the ambiguity of the intentions behind such actions. More recently, Jennifer Evans has argued that for early modern England regular menstruation was linked to the promotion of conception: that is, women would regulate their menstruation in order to increase their fertility.[8] Similar arguments have been put forward for eighteenth-century American and contemporary African populations.[9]

This brings us to the question of the significance of herbal preparations as emmenagogues or abortifacients among Greek populations. Greek women have always had a very good knowledge of herbs and wild vegetables, and abortion has been a prime birth control method among those contributing to Greek fertility decline from the first half of the twentieth century onwards. If such herbs were used, what was their relationship with fertility and what were the intentions of their users? Were Greek women practising abortion even before the onset of the fertility decline? Certainly, the use of the term 'emmenagogue' continued well into the twentieth century among Greek physicians, unlike in Western Europe and the USA, where gynaecologists, we are told, had abandoned the term by the early twentieth century.[10] Moreover, in Greece herbal emmenagogues were gradually abandoned in favour of medical methods and the use of curettage, as still recommended by physicians to their patients in some contemporary populations.[11] Although Van de Walle and others have discussed in depth the writings of Greek medical writers, they did so in relation to the ancient world.[12] I will argue that Greek women were eager to regulate their menses, because their irregularity was seen as pathology, but also because they thought it would enable them to become and/or remain fertile. This applied across Greek women in the nineteenth century and indeed up to the 1940s or even beyond in some rural areas.

'Bringing on the Menses': Greens, Herbs and Popular Knowledge of Emmenagogues

Greek women were well versed in the collection of wild greens and herbs, as these constituted a significant part of the Greek diet in the nineteenth and twentieth centuries. The required knowledge was acquired from an early age and it was, in most cases, an integral part of women's knowledge, embedded in their everyday activities, as was revealed for both the 1940s and the pre-World War II era by the oral histories collected on Mykonos, Syros and Hios.[13] Such knowledge varied depending on the local availability of greens, and was wider in rural areas, where opportunities for collecting wild greens were readily available.[14] Nevertheless, before World War II, townspeople were never that far away from the countryside, enabling those who wanted or needed such foods to find them.[15] Even among the affluent and educated, herbal and plant knowledge was considered important and desirable, presumably because plants and herbs were used in everyday life and in family/informal medicine. Thus in 1885 an Athenian schoolgirl created a plant-album that included specimens of plants and herbs with a short commentary.[16] Many of the herbs and plants mentioned in this chapter were included in her locally sourced collection. Even today many people continue to collect plants and practise this knowledge.[17]

Rue and Other Herbal Emmenagogues

A wide variety of plants could be used as emmenagogues or abortifacients. The best known and most widely available throughout Greece, in both wild and cultivated forms, was rue (apeganos, *Ruta graveolens*).[18] Its attributes were very well and widely known,[19] from ancient times up until the 1960s. Hippocrates referred to the plant in this context,[20] and there is also strong evidence that rue was available and in use in Byzantine times and thereafter.[21] In a tenth-century manuscript we learn how the plant is propagated and that 'this plant is by nature hostile to pregnant women'.[22] In the 1880s Tryfon Kontos, a physician, reported that pregnant women were not allowed to walk into a garden where the plant was present, let alone step on it, for fear of it causing miscarriage.[23] A recent discussion of the plant's appearances in Hippocratic treatises identifies its use as an abortive, as helping conception and as an emmenagogue.[24] Of those three uses, twenty-first-century Greeks, the paper argues, appear to be aware of only the first.

Whether twenty-first-century Greeks are aware or not of the emmenagogic properties of rue, those of the mid-twentieth century were well aware. Popular medicine, according to empirical practitioners interviewed in the 1970s, emphasised the strong and 'magical' powers of this plant[25] and advised that it should be planted in gardens in order to keep away unwanted demons and fairies (xotika). Considering the strong belief of the rural population in such creatures, and its fear of them, it would be expected that most rural gardens would have such a plant,[26] and therefore it would have been widely and readily available to all.[27] Indeed, Emm. Anases, an agriculturalist by training, gave details in his 1961 publication *The Medicinal Herbs of Greece* on how to cultivate and care for the plant in the garden, indicating that its cultivation in Greek gardens was common.[28] A century earlier a popular medical journal that addressed the educated non-physician discussed rue's wide availability in Greece and emphasised its importance as an 'excellent emmenagogue'. The author added that 'women use it as such everywhere with some success in many cases'.[29] Nevertheless, the author warned that its use often resulted in women bleeding and 'if it happened the woman to be pregnant, unknowingly to her, then the bad result [kakon, referring to the loss of the pregnancy] is terrible and unavoidable'. Therefore, the author proceeds to advise every 'wise' woman that they should not use rue and that they should consult a physician, since the retention of menstruation 'is not such a simple or innocent' affair.[30] Virtually the same advice was repeated in the 1890s in a pharmacology textbook, explaining that a weak rue infusion was used as an emmenagogue but a strong infusion was used as an abortifacient, in many cases killing the mother too.[31] The author of the book had first-hand knowledge, having examined women who, in their attempt to induce abortion, were poisoned by the herb.[32]

Although rue was the one plant identified consistently in all consulted sources, whether authored by qualified physicians or unqualified practitioners, a plethora of other plants and their products were mentioned in the various sources, some of them readily and widely available, some only locally available: savin (vrathy, *Juniperus sabina*), absinthe (apsinthi,

Artemisia absinthium), mugwort (artemisia, *Artemisia vulgaris*), *Aloe vera*, ergot (erysivodes olyra, *Claviceps*), saffron crocus (*Crocus sativus*); and, at later dates, apiol (extracted oleoresin of parsley), parsley (*Petroselinum sativum*), fennel (*Foeniculum vulgare*) and oleander (*Nerium oleander*). In addition, the sources mention drinks prepared with the leaves of the walnut (*Juglans*) tree, the root of the kermes oak (pournari, *Quercus coccifera*), spearmint (*Mentha spicata* or *Mentha viridis*) or, even more simply, onion leaves.[33] Among these, parsley and fennel have always been extensively used in Greek cookery, while oleander is a very common decorative plant, and therefore all three were widely and readily accessible without any effort.

Knowledge and Use of Emmenagogues, Abortifacients and Ecbolics/Expellants

Nineteenth- and twentieth-century iatrosophic books, as well as earlier ones, invariably refer to emmenagogic preparations. As many of the nineteenth- and twentieth-century iatrosophic manuscripts had been reproduced from earlier manuscripts, somewhat adapted over time, the information they contain is relevant to periods prior to the nineteenth century too. Almost without exception, such books included recipes to bring on the 'menses'. So the thirteenth-century *iatrosophion*, of which many variations and editions appeared subsequently, provides three possible therapies for the retention of the menses: blood-letting from the ankles; a wine drink with the 'Holy [medication]' and castoreum; and warm baths.[34] A later version of the same manuscript provides similar recipes for the same condition, including absinthe boiled in wine, the juice of pulverized rue, blood-letting from the ankles and warm baths,[35] as well as some additional methods, four of which involved herbs and the drinking of the produced infusion. A fifth method involved the creation of a pessary from myrrh and nettles, which was to be inserted into the vagina or placed just outside it.[36] In a third section within the same book are a further nine recipes to bring on the menses, including drinks made with the seeds of dill or fennel root, along with the leaves and seeds of the plant.[37] All the methods mentioned in the later edition are different from those of the earlier one except for blood-letting. Later iatrosophic books also consistently mention recipes for bringing on the menses. Thus, four such recipes are mentioned in a sixteenth-century iatrosophic book, three of which involved herbs brewed into drinks and one that was made from crabs in wine.[38] Another iatrosophic book, the *Geoponikon*, refers in passing to chickpeas, beans and fennel as aiding in bringing on the menses, whereas, it asserts, lentils retain the menses. Chickpeas have been identified as emmenagogues in the twentieth century too.[39] *Geoponikon* also provides a recipe that includes chickpeas, saffron and 'lots of oil' while also recommends fumigation of the patient.[40] A nineteenth-century iatrosophic book, written in Cyprus, provides the same recipes as the *Geoponikon*, though offering more specific dosage guidelines and clearer instructions.[41] Emmenagogues were available not only from such healing books but also from individuals, both laypersons and empirics.[42] Such knowledge is mentioned in a variety of publications compiled from oral reports collected around the mid-twentieth century.[43] Thus Mpimpe-Papaspuropoulou reports popular recipes for herbal infusions addressing menstrual delays and dysmenorrhoea from six different locations in Peloponnesos.[44]

Thus, healing recipes to 'bring on the menses' appeared regularly in the iatrosophic books and their reproductions, possibly with an increasing presence in the seventeenth and eighteenth centuries, at least in comparison to earlier times. As many of these iatrosophic books were reproduced, either copied or reprinted, and used in nineteenth- and twentieth-century Greece, we can expect that such knowledge would have been available to the owners and readers of those books (mostly empiric practitioners) and to all the people they advised.[45] That such knowledge was widespread among the population, or at least specific groups among the population, is reflected in both folklore studies and popular publications on herbs.

Euaggelia Fragkake, for example, collected popular medical cures of the pre-1960s period from her native Crete. Her informant, the daughter of an empirical/untrained midwife, emphasised the importance of the type and flow of menses for an unmarried girl and how it was the responsibility of the mother to make sure the flow was adequate and of good quality. If not, then specific herbal drinks were given to the daughter, fumigation with herbs was undertaken, poultices were applied and a drink with rust was administered. Since there was no possibility that an unmarried daughter could be pregnant, the issue here was exclusively to ensure the girl's regular menstruation, something that was considered inextricably linked to her future ability to procreate.[46]

Scientists too, such as the agriculturalist Anases, emphasised that his writings were based on first-hand knowledge that he collected 'from peasants or witnessed with my own eyes'.[47] His book, like the iatrosophic books, is organised by 'complaint/illness', followed by all the curing herbs. Under emmenagogues, Anases mentions ten different herbs in his first volume, one of which is absinthe (*Artemisia absinthium*).[48] Interestingly, rue is not included in this list, but when he discusses the plant later on in the book he makes it clear that it is indeed an emmenagogic plant and he proceeds to caution the reader about its use, as it can be poisonous.[49] It appears, therefore, that the plant's poisonous properties prevented the author from listing rue under emmenagogues, despite the fact that he acknowledges that it has such properties. In his second volume no fewer than seventeen herbs are listed as emmenagogues, whereas there is only one herb under abortifacients, *Aristolochia longa* (ampelokladoriza), which is also listed as an emmenagogue.[50] Another herb, *Aloe vera*, is mentioned only under emmenagogues, but in the detailed presentation of the plant its abortifacient properties are also mentioned.[51]

Folklore information from Thrace, in northern Greece, collected in the interwar period, mentions as emmenagogues boiled fennel in wine; the drink made from the boiled bark of a black mulberry tree, onion peels and hazelnut shells; and the first water with which sheared wool has been washed.[52] Pontic Greeks, a people who resided in Thrace after 1923 but originated from the Pontus region of the Ottoman Empire, employed fumigation with the hellebore (ellevoros, *Helleborus*).[53] Even in a 1952 popular women's magazine, we read in an article entitled 'Herbal Drinks' that chamomile, absinthe and *Origanum dictamnus* (erontas) were emmenagogic.[54] In the twentieth-century Santorini, women would gather rue or Italian arum (*Arum italicum*) and prepare an infusion that was taken on three consecutive days in the morning to induce their period.[55] And around 1970 a mother—who was also a trained nurse—would regularly prepare a cinnamon drink for her young daughters to take around their expected day of menstruation so that it would be painless.[56] Such folkloric, local knowledge and information continued to be reproduced in popular books praising the medicinal uses of traditional herbs and plants.

Thus, iatrosophic books, old and new, invariably provided a number of remedies in order to 'bring on the menses'. Similarly, books compiled in the twentieth century from the popular and/or folkloric knowledge and practice of the population also refer to plants with emmenagogic attributes. Significantly, the iatrosophic books also invariably refer to what needs to be done when a woman carries a dead foetus that needs to be expelled.[57] This always constitutes a separate section of the book and recommends recipes different from the emmenagogues.[58] In popular medicine, emmenagogues were thus differentiated from abortifacients/ecbolics used to expel a dead foetus, with distinct recipes provided 'to bring on the menses' or for 'expelling/aborting a child'.[59] The latter purpose referred primarily to expelling a dead foetus, and was articulated as such, rather than with the word 'abortion'.[60] Thus Theodoros Afentoules, a professor of pharmacology at Athens University, refers in his 1890–1891 pharmacology textbook to aloe as an emmenagogue but to ergot as a substance to be used to facilitate (natural) abortions and labours,[61] and cautions that aloe should not be used in pregnancy. Throughout 1938 the medical journal *Klinike* published a practical guide of poisonous substances and their effects and guidance on what the physician should do. Among the various substances, the usual abortifacients were mentioned, such as rue, ergotine, cantharides (Spanish fly) and quinine, with the clear indication that they provoke abortion.[62] Authors who published after 1950 provided, besides recipes for emmenagogues, lists of abortifacients. For example, Anases lists abortifacients separately from emmenagogues. Among the two lists of herbs there was only one overlap.[63] Only in the cases of *Aloe vera* (in his first volume) and *Aristolochia longa* (in his second volume) does he state that the herb is 'emmenagogic or it causes abortion too in pregnant women'.[64] Similarly, A. Arvanites distinguishes between emmenagogic and abortifacient herbs, although he indicates that *Arnica montane* and *Artemisia absinthium* can serve both purposes.[65] Furthermore, as noted above, most of the iatrosophic books also provide—in a separate section—recipes that would facilitate a woman's labour.[66] Only one case was traced in an iatrosophic book where the author refers to the desire to perform an abortion (as distinct from inducing menstruation or facilitating the birth of a dead foetus) and instructs the woman in what to do if she 'has conceived with the visitor'.[67] Yet, in another sixteenth-century one, there are instructions for the 'woman who wants to expel/miscarry (aporixei) the child'.[68] She is instructed to drink boiled wine with absinthe, after which she 'drops/aborts (rihnei) the child dead'. Considering that in the wider literature such a drink was expected not to bring death to the foetus but rather to initiate or facilitate its expulsion, I would argue that this specific recipe too refers to the expulsion of an already dead foetus.[69] The fact that all the existing iatrosophic manuscripts refer to emmenagogues or the expelling of a [dead] foetus indicates that the societal expectation was for a baby to be welcomed, except as indicated in the one case mentioned above, when a transgression had occurred. In the late nineteenth century, as mentioned above, Afentoules discussed the use of rue in a weak drink as an emmenagogic but in a strong drink as an *ektrotikon* (abortifacient).[70]

Writing along similar lines half a century later, Panteles Mpertsekas, in a study of induced abortion, emphasised that while savin is only emmenagogic rue is both emmenagogic and abortifacient.[71] Even in a 1952 popular women's magazine and in reference to emmenagogues, we read that *erontas*, a native herb of Crete, is emmenagogic but Hippocrates considered it an abortifacient and expellant of the placenta.[72] Thus in the written sources, a distinction was made between emmenagogues and abortifacients in the twentieth century; and emmenagogues and expellants/ecbolics in the nineteenth century.

Emmenagogues were therefore considered to be just that—not potions that would cause abortion—although, in all probability, and depending on how the emmenagogic mixture was prepared, some unplanned miscarriages would have occurred as a consequence of their use. The apparently high level of demand for them, as well as their failure rate, may be indicated by the sheer number of recipes and herbs seen in the sources. Most non-physician's lists of emmenagogues were significantly more populated than those either of preparations inducing the expelling of a dead foetus or facilitating labour, or of abortifacients. And it was emmenagogues that were invariably present in all books—old and new—and, more often than not, in more than one section of the book, presumably indicating their significant demand even in the 1960s. Thus, women, empirics and physicians were all familiar with emmenagogues; they used them, advised women to use them and generally did not link them to abortion. All that, mostly but not exclusively, when fertility was not within the 'calculus of conscious choice'.[73]

The wide variety of emmenagogic recipes and herbs provided in the books ensured that at least some of the proposed materials and herbs would be locally available. Thus, emmenagogues in the Greek world were part of popular medicinal knowledge and many women were aware of these potions or could be readily informed, if the need arose.[74] This knowledge was available widely from the eighteenth century onwards, and scant evidence suggests that it was also available in earlier centuries, although further work is required to ascertain this.

Why did Women Need to Use Emmenagogues?

Evidence for women's reasons for using emmenagogues, although circumstantial, comes from the numerous publications dealing with popular and herbal medicine in the twentieth century. Gymnasios Lauriotes, for example, an empiric who practised in the interwar period, offered a recipe for 'irregular menses' in his repeatedly published collection of popular medicine recipes,[75] as did Nikolaos Theodorakis, another empiric practising in Crete in the first half of the twentieth century.[76] Excess menstruation was also seen as a malady, with cures being recommended for both.[77] In the 1950s the *Household Guide*, along with food recipes and instructions on how to set up a household, offered nine herbs and corresponding recipes under the heading 'emmenagogues', with clear instructions on how to prepare an equal number of emmenagogic drinks.[78] As that guide addressed middle-class, educated readers, the inclusion of the preparation of emmenagogic drinks suggests that these were recipes intended to improve women's 'well-being', rather than anything else. In Fragkake's 1960s account of local Cretan traditional/popular medical practices we read that if a girl does not have 'sufficient blood' then her mother needs to give her a preparation that includes rue and absinthe. Moreover, a girl suffering from period pains, we are told, would be unable to bear children.[79] And if a girl gets cold, Fragkake states, she may be unable to have a child.[80] When young women wanted to attend church, because they had to be 'clean' (that is, not menstruating, which was regarding as polluting) they could take a drink made of black pepper pods in wine to suspend their menstruation.[81] But, the advice cautioned, 'if they do that a couple of times they will lose their [menstrual] order and they will never have a child'.[82] In yet another account of popular medicine we read that women's sterility was a result of an 'obstruction of the womb' that must be removed before the woman could become pregnant, and this could be achieved with emmenagogues.[83] Thus the twentieth-century evidence suggests a popular link between sterility, obstruction of the womb, irregularity of the menses and a desire to make the menses regular with the help of emmenagogues.

While the existing iatrosophic books consistently discuss how to overcome suspension of the menses, they do not discuss why such a suspension occurs. However, this is not specific to that ailment, but rather indicative of the nature of such books: they are compilations of cures of ailments, rather than discussions of why and how ailments developed. To identify contemporary understandings of the causes of the suspension of menstruation, we need to explore the writings of physicians, both those addressing other physicians and those addressing the public, as such writings reveal some of the thinking behind the actions recommended by the iatrosophic books.

Nineteenth-century evidence for the causes of amenorrhoea comes from De-Kigallas, a physician whose PhD was a *Study on menses and Chlorosis*. De-Kigallas argued that amenorrhoea led to chlorosis, an anaemia caused by iron deficiency.[84] Though De-Kigallas did not recommend any treatments, it is clear that he considered amenorrhoea to require attention.[85] Aside from the threat of chlorosis, irregular menstruation was by 1864 interpreted as an indication of an abnormal pathology that had to be medically treated.[86] Delayed menarche, too, was a matter of concern to physicians, Greeks and otherwise, as is illustrated in a *Lancet* article (translated into Greek) that focused on the efforts of physicians to induce menarche in an 18-year-old patient and to sustain regular menstruation thereafter.[87]

In the late nineteenth century the absence of menstruation did not necessarily indicate a pregnancy.[88] A midwifery textbook prepared by a physician in 1886 describes illnesses that mimic pregnancy, one of which is called *aimatometra*. In this, though the woman 'menstruates', the blood is not released because of some obstruction, either in the vagina or in the womb, so that the menstrual blood accumulates within the womb, enlarging it and mimicking pregnancy.[89] The textbook recommends that when the obstruction is vaginal, and thus easy to 'cure', the midwife should perform the necessary procedure, while other obstructions should be handled by physicians.[90] A contemporary treatise discussed obstructions and their relationship to women's sterility, explicitly linking *aimatometra* with sterility.[91] Moreover, healthy women, it was believed in the late nineteenth century, should be consistent in their menses; that is, while it was acknowledged that variation in the length of the cycle or the extent of their duration existed among women, each woman should be consistent in her own pattern throughout her life, except when there was a problem.[92] That this was a widely held belief and not one confined to physicians is evident in the many iatrosophic books that also offered advice on how to deal with excessive menstrual bleeding.[93] Timoleon Kardaras, who had advised that women should be consistent in their menstruation, also recommended that a few days prior to the expected date of their next menses, and if experiencing abdominal pains, breast discomfort or neurological disorders such as headaches and hysterical paroxysm, the affected woman should have a daily warm bath and use poultices and infusions of artemisia and absinthe.[94] Both these plants were well-known emmenagogues, and though neither was named as such in this source later on absinthe was named as a stimulant in cases of suppressed menstruation.[95] A medical publication of 1874 on women's ailments distinguishes among the different types of amenorrhoea and offers very different therapies for each case. This is probably the most detailed such account: the author, A. Vitsaris, recommended for trivial cases mild cathartics, foot-baths and externally used leeches, while for more serious cases sitz baths, leeches situated on the neck of the womb and douches with 'emmenagogues, aloe, savin, ergot, etc' were suggested.[96] The discussion of 'retention' of menstruation and the possible reasons behind it was even more complex, with no less than eight different explanations provided, ranging from a blocked vagina and an unperforated hymen to a stenosis. 'Retention', according to the author, meant that blood was produced by the body but not released, unlike the cases of amenorrhoea he had discussed earlier. The ultimate recommended therapy was surgery.[97] For dysmenorrhoea, the recommended therapies were somewhat less invasive, including douches and sitz baths but also dilation with 'rubber catheters or metallic ones or dilating articles'. Vitsaris adds that in cases where the patient suffers from metritis or parametritis leeches should be used instead,[98] and notes that the therapy should continue until a complete cure is achieved: 'that is, when the return of menstruation becomes regular'.[99] His recommendations for these include blood-letting and the use of leeches. It is interesting to note that Vitsaris frequently references non-Greek authors on many of the above ailments.

In the nineteenth century, Pyrros, an *iatrophilosophos*[100] who represented a fusion between popular and 'scientific' medicine,[101] attributed amenorrhoea and delay of menstruation to 'great fear, confusion, sorrow, major illnesses, obstructions of the liver and spleen, illness of the soul and also conception'.[102] Similarly, a 1900 textbook prepared for the training of midwives indicates that menstruation might be 'suspended due to various diseases of the reproductive organs'.[103] Thus, amenorrhoea was seen mostly as an indication of a disorder, except in the case of conception. To put the menses in order, advises Pyrros, the woman needs to drink 'emmenagogic medicines', '*anodynum*', 'maiden hair/Adiantum Capillus-veneris and chamomile' continuously.[104] The potions recommended for amenorrhoea included, among others, aloe, crocus, savin and *Aristolochia*, all familiar emmenagogues in popular, herbal medicine.[105]

Thus, emmenagogues were used by women suffering amenorrhoea and irregular menstruation to put themselves 'in good order' and, in doing so, prevent or overcome sterility, therefore enhancing their childbearing chances. This is very much in line with findings for eighteenth- and early nineteenth-century America, eighteenth-century England and contemporary populations in places such as Guyana.[106] Such advice, for the less severe medical cases, was in line with popular practices, and was forthcoming from the qualified physicians of the nineteenth century and the unqualified ones of the twentieth.

Emmenagogues, Abortifacients and Physicians

In the late nineteenth century some physicians started to disassociate reduced menstruation from sterility, indicating that women could conceive even when they had reduced menses. Nevertheless, they still saw the situation as one indicating a lack of health and where 'affected' women needed 'to be subjected to the suitable medical therapy'.[107] Afentoules describes the use of emmenagogues in medicine succinctly: 'Emmenagogues, that is medicines that bring on the menses, are many, as many are the damages of the procreative organs specifically or of the whole body, responsible for the suspension of the menses.' To make his point he lists a number of associated disorders, including anaemia, chlorosis, diseases of the uterus and ovaries, and the 'wandering' of the menses—that is, their discharge from places in the body other than the vagina (vicarious menstruation)—and points out that 'this is why emmenagogues are ubiquitously present in pharmacology'.[108] Despite this superfluity, however, he chooses to focus on only two, 'the strongest ones', after recommending that before administering emmenagogues the physician should make sure that the patient is not pregnant—something that, apparently, young, inexperienced physicians did not always ensure.[109] The two emmenagogues he discusses are savin and apiol, although he discusses at length only the former, which seems to have been the one more widely used in Greece. The use of savin to induce abortion was the cause of death in a number of women, and he cautions against its use for this purpose, pointing out that midwifery has other, safer means to perform an abortion when one is necessary.[110]

One such 'medicine' was ergot (erysivodes olyra, *Claviceps*), which must have been widely used by midwives and physicians alike during deliveries for one of its major properties—its ability to facilitate spontaneous abortion.[111] In 1849 a midwifery textbook authored by the Athens University professor of obstetrics states that when there is a threatened (spontaneous) abortion with excessive bleeding the physician may eventually decide to perform the abortion in order to save the woman's life.[112] To achieve this he would use ergot, hoping for the expulsion of both the foetus and the placenta.[113] In 1864, two new ways of preparing and conserving ergot were discussed in the professional medical journal *Ippokrates*, indicating its use by physicians and their concern for improving its preservation and quality.[114] A 1887 textbook of midwifery strongly advises midwives 'not to give in even to persistent requests of some of the labouring women who want through such [medicine], as was indeed very common in earlier times, to eliminate the delivery pains', recommending that ergot should be given only after the birth of the child and in order to facilitate the expulsion of the placenta.[115] In 1929 an eminent gynaecologist gave the same recommendation: that immediately after the delivery the labouring woman should be given two or three tablets of ergotamine, which was 'found in the trade as tartrate ergotamine or gynergene'.[116] Ergot and its by-products were thus used as an oxytocic, hastening parts of the delivery process.

The range and sophistication of emmenagogues were to expand in the twentieth century. In the 1920s medical preparations for this purpose were frequently discussed and advertised in medical journals. So, a gynaecologist writing on dysmenorrhoea recommended the use of capsules of apioline, which, the author informed the reader, was 'extracted from parsley whose emmenagogic properties had been proven by Siredey, Bouchardat and Dyjardin-Beaumetz'.[117] In the same year in the weekly medical journal *Klinike* eight advertisements for two different products appeared between October 20 and December 15, 1928.[118] The first product, *Ovarialhormon Folliculin*, was recommended for dysmenorrhoea and amenorrhoea but also for 'sterility when hypoplasia of the uterus was responsible for it'. The advertisement mentioned that samples and a bibliography were also available from the sellers.[119] The second, *Menstruol*, was advertised as 'effective and harmless' and recommended exclusively for dysmenorrhoea, to be taken two to three days before the start of the period due-date. This medicine was available throughout Greece.[120] Also in 1928, in the journal *O Praktikos Iatros*, an array of therapeutic methods were proposed in order to combat amenorrhoea, ranging across 'emmenagogic medicines' such as iron, arsenic and potassium permanganate; hormonal preparations such as Folliculine; physiotherapy; natural baths; and surgery. The author cautioned the reader against the use of 'old medicines' such as crocus, aloe, ergotine and apiol, all of which would cause 'congestion of the reproductive system'.[121] A few years later the translated summary of a foreign article brought to Greek medical readers of *Ellenike Iatrike* the latest on 'Progress in therapies of menstrual irregularities'.

There we read that reduced menstrual flow, though not associated with a pathology, 'makes women feel fatigued' and thus hormonal therapy is recommended.[122] Similarly, for amenorrhoea, although only under certain conditions, hormone therapy was again recommended.[123] However, this article's suggestion that menstrual irregularities could be disassociated from pathologies did not seem to have been adopted by either the Greek physicians or their clientele even in the 1950s. In responding to a query posed in a women's magazine about the woman's period, her ability to conceive and whether she could get married, the physician responded that she should not be discouraged, despite her irregular and modest period, but nevertheless recommended a five-month hormonal treatment with progynon or dimenformon and prolyton or progesterone.[124]

Other products not only targeted amenorrhoea but also reduced menstrual flow and dysmenorrhoea. '*Crinex*', we read, 'restores completely the endocrinal functions from which the woman's whole life benefits greatly'.[125] Pharmaceutical emmenagogic medications continued to be available in the 1950s and were advertised in medical journals such as *Klinike*.[126] Two products in ampoules, Estro-Prol and Estrovite, were recommended for all types of amenorrhoea, polymenorrhoea and oligomenorrhoea, and also for 'spontaneous abortion'.[127] Estro-Prol's main ingredient was progesterone, while Estrovite's main ingredient was oestradiol, a form of oestrogen.[128] Another emmenagogue, Hemagol, was explicitly advertised as such at least during the period 1949–1961.[129] The advertisement for it read 'Hemagol, the new emmenagogue, for menstruation pains; for delays of menstruation'. In the same issue the manufacturing company provided the ingredients of the drug and its recommendations: 'Valerianate de menthol, apiol, absinthe, armoise, aloes, protoxalate de fer, phenacetine, folliculine; recommended for amenorrhoea, oligomenorrhoea, delays, disorders of the menopause, painful periods.'[130] It is telling, perhaps, that most of Hemagol's ingredients were identical with the herbal emmenagogues that were widely known and used in Greece as a whole prior to 1950 and indeed also into the second half of the twentieth century in rural areas.[131] These 'modern' medicines were used in exactly the same ways as their herbal counterparts, as the numerous replies of the gynaecologist to the female readers of the fortnightly popular magazine *E Gynaika* ('The Woman') indicate—with the main aim of 'correcting' menstruation: one such piece of advice read 'You need to take measures to correct your period with hormone therapy', while another reader attributed the fact that she could not gain weight to her irregular period, and was duly advised to use prolyton.[132] In many cases, and when a pregnancy had been ruled out, menstrual irregularity was linked to inefficiency of the ovaries and therefore potential sterility, something that could be cured with the use of emmenagogues: 'we recommend that you have injections with estro-prol. From what you have written, since you have not had direct contact, you cannot be pregnant. [The problem] is about the inefficiency of the ovaries and therefore you should not worry.'[133] In a subsequent response the physician recommended treatment with etsron or progynon.[134] Of course, Greek women were not exceptional in being given hormone preparations by their physicians in order to 'bring on' their period. This was happening in 1970s Britain, for example, though only among less well-informed women, who were 'usually of lower socio-economic' status.[135]

But medical emmenagogues were not used only for that purpose, as the two following examples suggest. In the first case, the gynaecologist's reply to Triestina F. suggests that four to six Hemagol tablets could be taken, as 'they may have some effect'. But the reply continued by strongly recommending that the young girl tells her mother 'all that had happened' and that she should see a physician as soon as possible, although 'of course not there' (where she lived).[136] In the second case, again a pregnancy is insinuated and emmenagogues are recommended as a first attempt to bring it to an end; if not successful, however, a physician's help should be sought: 'The day is the right one as you wrote to me. Also the measures you took are correct. But if, despite that, your fear becomes reality then we recommend you take, in two doses, 400,000 thylacine (prozynone or estrovite). If you still do not get a result, then seek immediately a specialist physician.'[137] Thus, while emmenagogues were recommended as such by physicians, by 1950 they were also recommended occasionally for early abortion purposes.[138] In the latter case, as the expectation was that they might prove ineffective, concrete suggestions to approach a physician for further action were also made.

The very high frequency and the casual manner with which such medicines were recommended through the pages of a magazine indicates that urban women were very familiar with the notion of emmenagogues, and at some point in the mid-twentieth century swapped the traditional recipes for 'modern' drugs.[139] Rural women continued to use traditional herbal preparations at this time.[140] Emmenagogues continued to be readily recommended by those physicians who did not necessarily equate the suspension of menstruation with pregnancy. Thus, in a popular pregnancy textbook published in 1954, the obstetrician/gynaecologist author tells the female reader that 'when you fall pregnant ... in many cases it is not pregnancy but just a delay of the menses'. He advises her that she should face the situation calmly and take large doses of 'hormones of the ovaries, especially oothylacine', which 'offers good results just as do very hot baths' taken twice a day.[141] 'If, after all these, the period does not get regular and signs of pregnancy become evident', he continues, the woman should visit her physician. If a pregnancy is confirmed, then she should think very hard before 'asking her physician for an abortion'. In the preceding paragraphs the author was at pains to emphasise that when women fall 'pregnant' they should not go to 'old ladies, that is, unqualified midwives' and follow their advice in taking folk medicines, even though his own advice differed little from that given by such women to some of our informants. The physician is clearly the preferred solution, according to the textbook. Yet again, for women who had undergone an abortion and were bleeding, the author recommends that they use 'ergotin'—a preparation that the pharmacist would make up. Ironically, this was one of the main 'folk-medicines' women would use to procure abortions,[142] and one of the very few medicines that midwives were allowed to provide to women, although—in theory—only during delivery.[143] It was also widely accessible, at least in the first half of the twentieth century, to physicians, who prescribed it for 'menstruation ailments'.[144]

So, physicians recommended modern emmenagogues just as unqualified practitioners recommended herbal ones before them and in parallel to them in rural areas. They were well aware that women used them extensively, and did not present any objections to their use; indeed, they recommended them when medical preparations in the form of pills became available, and women did use them as such.[145] Equally, ecbolics/abortifacients were used by midwives to facilitate the expulsion of the placenta in the nineteenth and twentieth centuries. These were also used and prescribed by physicians too, though mostly in their 'modern' form, especially in the twentieth century.

Thus the twentieth-century urban evidence, like that of the nineteenth century, indicates a link between sterility, inefficiency of the ovaries, irregularity of the menses and a desire to make the menses regular with the help of emmenagogues, all recommended by qualified physicians. The term 'emmenagogues' was employed by the educated in the middle of the nineteenth century and throughout the twentieth century, while the lay population referred to the 'regulation of the menses' or to 'bringing the menses on'.[146] It is references to abortifacients that become much more common in the twentieth century, on most occasions appearing along those to emmenagogues. So, in an encyclopaedia published in the 1920s we read under the entry 'abortifacients' the usual list of plants, with the clarification that these are really emmenagogues, that some are stronger than others and that their use is prohibited because they are dangerous,[147] and in a book published in the 1930s by a scientist on the popular, medicinal herbs of Greece there are two references to plants with 'emmenagogic' attributes.[148] In contrast, a publication of 1961 refers to three distinct plants that acted respectively as 'emmenagogic', 'abortifacient' and 'ecbolic'.[149]

When Should Someone Use Emmenagogues? The Difficulty of Knowing When a Woman Is Pregnant

Pyrros, writing in 1831, gives a detailed description of how to determine whether a woman is pregnant which is worth quoting at length:

> For the physician to find out if the woman is pregnant, he needs to fumble in the morning her pulse, and if the pulse beats continuously to 80 or 90 pulses … that is a sign that the woman is pregnant. But this is not sufficient evidence; the woman needs to have in the morning and before she eats, a restlessness and anxiety, to have little or a lot of vomiting, disgust towards some foods and appetite for others, now to like the sour foods and then the sweet, or even her menses to be delayed thirty or forty days; every day the laziness increases as well as the anxiety; her breasts enlarge, the nipples become pronounced and the abdomen becomes swollen because the womb swells … thus when the midwife inserts her finger underneath she traces the womb, whether it is closed or leaning upwards, whether she can reach it or not; if the woman experiences continual enuresis or constipation but mostly if the pregnant woman after a number of days, forty or fifty and beyond, feels an infant inside her abdomen and how she feels it, weakly or strongly, and as things progress she feels it more [stronger] and more often, with all these [signs] and the physician can still be fooled … And once the woman knows she is pregnant, without significant reasons she should not take medicines because the foetus is expelled, and then she dies too, as it has happened to many [women].[150]

Pyrros' description suggests that it was only the woman who could tell whether she was pregnant or not and in any case only with quickening.

Nineteenth-century midwifery textbooks, always authored by male obstetricians, continued to emphasise the difficulty of tracing a pregnancy with any certainty, even by the most experienced physician: 'During the early months, a definite diagnosis of a pregnancy is difficult because the phenomena, which are then presented, are vague and insignificant.'[151] One possibility was that the pregnancy was not real at all, despite the appearance of the observed signs of pregnancy; these were, instead, the result of various abnormalities and not of an 'enlivened ovum'.[152] Such pathological situations included, for example, hydrops/dropsy and the retention of menstruation.[153] Even in 1900 another such textbook advises midwives that the suspension of menstruation is one of the 'probable' signs of pregnancy, among many others, whereas the movement of the foetus in the fourth or later month of pregnancy is one of the 'certain' signs of pregnancy.[154] However, another textbook doubts even that, suggesting that the movements felt by a woman could not always be taken to indicate pregnancy, as some women, very eager to become mothers, mistook other muscular movements for those of a foetus.[155] Only the repeated tracing of movement by the midwife or the physician, the author advises, could be taken as a certain indication of pregnancy.[156] In this same work Pyrros goes on to caution women who feel themselves to be pregnant on what they should avoid doing and taking in order to avoid a miscarriage. He suggests the avoidance of purgatives and enemas, among others: women should stop 'taking medicines' when they realise they are pregnant—that is, at quickening.[157]

Delayed period, though one of the reported symptoms of pregnancy, it is only one of many and not much attention is paid to it in the literature as serious evidence of a potential pregnancy. Even in 1954 a gynaecologist, addressing the public, suggested that the stopping of the menses was merely one of the probable signs of pregnancy, the latter becoming certain when the limbs of the foetus could be felt/traced.[158] Pyrros' guide to diagnosing pregnancy was the first to express the difficulties involved: in a midwifery textbook from 1887 detection of pregnancy in the early months is described as 'difficult since the phenomena associated with it are vague and insignificant', and, even for the later months, the same author asserts, many physicians misdiagnosed pregnancy.[159] Similarly, a 1895 publication concluded that the only 'certain' sign of pregnancy is delivery of the baby.[160] It was not only Greek physicians who expressed so clearly these difficulties: a manual published in the USA in 1900 explains that if the physician is consulted in 'supposedly in the first or second month' of a possible pregnancy, the 'tactful physician will study her [the woman's] own wishes in the matter' and then, in a non-committal way, he 'should allow his opinion to lean in the direction of her desires'.[161]

It seems, therefore, that delay of menstruation was seen much more often as evidence of some disorder rather than as evidence of pregnancy, and the cure for the disorder was emmenagogues, which were not to be consumed once a pregnancy was established, mostly by quickening. Before quickening—that is, around the fourth month of pregnancy—the use of emmenagogues was permissible and even advisable in order for a woman to restore normal menstruation. Yet, even when a woman was diagnosed as pregnant in those early months before quickening, the outcome was not necessarily a foetus—rather, she might have been experiencing a molar pregnancy.

Mole or Molar Pregnancies

One argument put forward by those accused of induced abortion in the first half of the twentieth century was that the induced 'abortion' was not of a foetus but of a molar pregnancy (myle)[162] and therefore the act of expelling it constituted neither an abortion proper nor a criminal act.[163] Though this was the argument advanced in the first half of the twentieth century, discussions of molar pregnancies were taking place in the previous century too. Thus, the molar, or mole, Kontos explained in 1883, 'is called a fertilised ovum that [internally and naturally] degenerated or modified during its development' and which, by the time its expulsion was attempted, was not alive.[164] Nikolaos Kostes in 1849 and Alexandros Triantes in 1887 clarified that the degenerated egg was reabsorbed and that therefore there was no visible 'egg' in what was expelled at a later stage.[165] However, while most authors agreed that the death of the foetus was a prerequisite to a molar pregnancy, some referred to a molar pregnancy involving a live foetus.[166] In all cases, the mole resembled a fleshy watery mass.[167] If not interfered with, according to the contemporary understanding, the molar pregnancy would be expelled naturally sometime 'in the third or fourth month or sometimes later', accompanied by bleeding.[168] However, it could last 'as long as a year and maybe longer'.[169] Nineteenth- and twentieth-century Greek physicians were very familiar with molar pregnancies, which were invariably included in their obstetric textbooks.[170] Presentations of such pregnancies were repeatedly brought before the Athens Medical Society, including, for example, the discussion in 1842 presented by the Bavarian physician Rezer and the instance in 1883 of a 'myle' delivered after eight months of 'pregnancy'.[171] One of the responsibilities of forensic medicine in relation to pregnant women was to establish whether the pregnancy had been a molar one or not.[172] Similarly familiar with this phenomenon were British and USA physicians: references to molar or 'false pregnancies' can be found in the literature from both countries from before the nineteenth century and into the twentieth.[173]

As noted above, the usual outcome of a molar pregnancy, as stated by Kontos, was that it 'comes out during the 4th or 5th month and thus a woman would not have put herself through the use of violent procedures to achieve an abortion', if her intention was not to get rid of a foetus.[174] Kondos' view was that there was no actual need to intervene with a molar pregnancy and facilitate the expulsion of the mole, and he disagreed with the lay understanding of the mole and the importance for women of taking action to 'put things right' rather than waiting for things to take their natural course. In contrast, other physicians were advocates of a proactive approach. Thus, Vitsares explains that once a molar pregnancy is diagnosed the only recommended course of action is its extraction. While, he added, 'nature may sometimes do that', the physician needs to be vigilant and react immediately to any pathological indications by performing the extraction himself. This is achieved, he continued, 'with tamponade, dilation of the [cervical] neck with a prepared sponge, and in particular ergot [administered] internally, all of which cause contractions of the uterus and cause the automatic expulsion of the mole'.[175] Following the expulsion, the procedure should be the same with that following a delivery, which among other, included the use of ergot.[176] Yet another physician, writing 30 years later, suggested that, while waiting for the natural expulsion to happen, fairly warm douches should be performed. If abundant bleeding occurred, tamponade was recommended. Following the expulsion, further douching should take place and if necessary curettage and tamponade too.[177]

Women may have had good reason to attempt to bring to an early end a molar pregnancy, since the natural end of such a pregnancy was expected, according to Nikolaos Kostes, 'to be accompanied by strong pains and heavy bleeding, which often poses great danger, sometimes causing even the death [of the woman]'.[178] Other obstetricians gave much grimmer predictions for the mother's fate in cases of molar pregnancy, with Mihael Kaires citing a 13% chance of death occurring owing to complications during the delivery, while the natural expulsion of the molar pregnancy was seen as a rare phenomenon.[179] And though British physicians also seemed to have advocated the 'wait and see' approach, they too expressed their uneasiness about it: 'the health is more broken after molar pregnancy than by the results of simple abortion [done by the physician to end the molar pregnancy]'.[180] In contrast, an American case study shows a physician who immediately, upon his diagnosis of a 'vesicular mole', 'ordered ergot to be given with a view to expel it'.[181] Similarly, in 1891 a Greek professor of pharmacology, who indicated that ergot could be used in non-pregnant women to expel what is inside them, had used the substance on a woman he though was pregnant and was having a miscarriage in order to facilitate the spontaneous abortion; however, much to his surprise, what was expelled was a mole.[182] A 1908 obstetrics textbook, although emphasising that the diagnosis of a mole pregnancy was very difficult, stipulated that as soon as bleeding becomes significant 'the evacuation of the uterus is mandatory'.[183] By 1924 physicians were advised that in cases of '*hydatidiform* mole' they should proceed to 'immediate abortion and a complete evacuation of the uterus'.[184] The danger, the author warned, lay in the malignant degeneration of the mole and a consequent cancerous growth.

Not surprisingly, most women adhered to such recommendations and proceeded to evacuate what they perceived to be molar pregnancies. Since there was no foetus involved no criminal act was committed by performing such a procedure.[185] Two separate sources from the 1920s, one an academic legal journal, the other an encyclopaedia, argue that the expulsion of 'mole, according to *common understanding* (koine doxa), cannot be subject to the crime of abortion', presumably because there was no live foetus involved and in most cases there was no discernible foetus either.[186] Equally interesting is the public argument in a 1932 newspaper debate on abortion by a physician—a VD/dermatologist specialist—that, prior to quickening, all a woman carries is a mole (myle), which may or may not proceed to a pregnancy.[187]

Thus, all in all, it was extremely difficult, if not outright impossible, for the afflicted woman, her physician or her midwife to determine whether she was pregnant with a child or whether she carried a mole.[188] This could be determined with some confidence only by quickening—that is, around the fourth month of pregnancy. Before that, some physicians may had been inclined to 'wait and see', while women may have felt anxious to 'cleanse' themselves of a suspected mole, especially those eager to become pregnant with a child. Furthermore, while in English the term employs the word 'pregnancy', in Greek the reference is simply to a 'mole' (myle), thus somewhat disassociating it from a normal pregnancy. However, those eager to remove an early pregnancy were in a position to argue that they carried a mole and were taking steps to expel it early, in most cases resulting in the expulsion of substances similar to those of a mole. Thus mole pregnancies provided women with a feasible reason, legally and ethically, to take action against an unwanted pregnancy. However, in many more cases it would have been the fear of an actual molar pregnancy that would have led women to take action. Interestingly, references to molar pregnancies became significantly rarer from the 1930s, exactly the time when induced abortions became increasingly common, suggesting that the actions taken to remove molar pregnancies in earlier times were aiming in most cases to do just that: remove a perceived molar pregnancy.

Medical Discussions of Methods of Abortion: Emmenagogues, Abortifacients and Others

Some of the earliest explicit discussion of abortion in Greece comes from the PhD thesis of Tryfon Kontos, a physician who, being born in the Ottoman Empire, albeit of Greek origin, had perhaps fewer qualms than others in discussing abortion and its practice in the modern Greek state.[189] Kontos provides an exhaustive list of the means that were used to obtain an abortion, which he categorises as 'direct' and 'indirect' methods. The latter, which he considers ineffective, included blood-letting (with or without the use of leeches placed around the genitals or even on the cervix), warm baths, violent movements and 'drinks' or 'medicines reputed to have abortifacient properties'.[190] The last, according to Kontos, included purgatives and diuretics, although 'women did not like either of those' because they would become exhausted after their use.[191] Interestingly, Kontos declares that it is well known pharmacologically that all purgatives, especially the drastic ones, and diuretics could be used as abortifacients.[192]

Within the category of abortifacients, Kontos discussed those most preferred by women, giving clear descriptions of how these should be used, what the effects would be and when these should be recommended or not.[193] The five abortifacients, four of which were plants, are potassium iodide (***kali iodatum***) (also considered to be an emmenagogue, according to Kontos), savin, yew (*Taxus baccata*), rue and ergot (erysivodes olyra, *Claviceps*). Kontos' evidence that these substances were indeed used by women comes from the work of Afentoules, who examined three pregnant women who employed rue and died as a result.[194] Savin, Kontos explained, was also used by physicians, although only externally, because of its well-known abortive properties.[195] Kontos' evaluation of these methods was that they were not actual abortifacients, as they did not target the pregnancy but rather poisoned the mother. If all the above failed, we are told, women would resort to midwives who would use direct means—that is, a prepared sponge, laminaria, gobbler quill or the release of carbonic [sic] acid into the womb with the use of rubber catheters, which 'have replaced everything else because they are the most safe'.[196] The use of metallic or wooden sticks is also mentioned, but Kontos states that their use 'is the most dangerous of all'.[197]

Kondos because of his cosmopolitan background also discusses the methods used in Istanbul by Ottoman, Greek, Armenian and Jewish women, who all resorted to midwives from their own ethnic group. Each group employed some distinct methods in addition to those used commonly across all groups. The indirect methods utilised in Istanbul were, however, identical to those used in Greece and so Kontos' main discussion is of the direct methods.[198] It is difficult to assess to what degree Kontos' discussion and knowledge comes from sources from Istanbul, Greece or the West. While his knowledge of abortifacients seems first-hand—whether it originated in the Ottoman Empire, his native Lesvos or Athens—his knowledge of some of the direct methods clearly originated in Western writings, as revealed by his mistranslation of carbolic acid (properly translated as fainiko oxy), a solution utilised in performing abortions in the West, as anthrakiko oxy (carbonic acid). His cursory discussion of the direct methods, which is essentially confined to a paragraph outlining the use of the catheter, also points to his lack of knowledge of such methods. Considering he was the first to publish on this subject, this suggests that knowledge of the rubber catheter method was not widespread in Greece at this time, and that it was certainly not practised by Greek physicians in the nineteenth century. However, in 1914 the medical publication *Iatrike Proodos* described in detail how a single pregnant woman, a servant, employed this exact method, but using a gunpowder solution rather than an acid one. The young woman regularly undertook the whole operation on her own, on or around 'the days she was expecting her regular menstruation, in the absence of pregnancy'. When there were no results after the first attempt, she repeated the procedure. In all the instances—except for one—she was successful in 'expelling the egg'.[199] The second method discussed involved the heavily pregnant woman employing violent movements and applying external pressure to her abdomen in an attempt to injure the foetus.[200] While the author presents these two methods of abortion as 'new', it is interesting that the first is essentially the same as that mentioned by Kontos in the 1880s.

By the 1930s the methods discussed seem in the main similar to those described by Kontos in 1883, although by now curettage had become the 'scientific' method.[201] Leaving this method aside for the moment, we see in Kamboure's book of 1933 all the common abortifacients, such as ergotine, apiol, rue and artemisia, as well as purgatives. In addition, however, he included arsenic, quinine and cantharides, along with the indication that 'other medicines' were also employed.[202] The wide use of emmenagogues and abortifacients in the 1930s that we have already seen is further corroborated by two sets of medical evidence: admissions to one of the largest gynaecology clinics in Athens, part of the Aretaieion Hospital; and the results of forensic examinations of the bodies of women brought into the public morgue.[203] Though the study based on these datasets was written in 1944 by Panteles Mpertsekas, a highly trained Athenian gynaecologist who practised in the hospital where the women were admitted, and published in 1948, the data were collected in the years 1932–1936. None of those women whose bodies were sent to the public morgue by the police had sought hospitalisation after abortion and while alive. All the hospitalised cases, a total of 19, were women who had attempted abortion, and though they all had been successful, there were serious enough complications for them to seek hospitalisation. All but two of these women, with ages ranging from 26 to 40, were married. None of them had more than five live children, while a third of them reported that they had had an abortion before, with one patient admitting having had four. A very clear distinction emerges between the married and the unmarried women: the former attempted abortion when 4, 6 or 8 weeks pregnant; the latter as late as 12 and 24 weeks. Of the 19 women admitted there were two deaths: that of the unmarried woman in her third month of pregnancy and one of the married women in her second month of pregnancy. According to the study's author, the majority of the abortions were taking place in the early stages of the pregnancy and before the foetus was clearly formed.[204] Of the 18 women admitted to the hospital, all but one explained the methods they used. Of these, only seven mentioned the involvement of a midwife, with two-thirds referring to advice from other women along with medicines recommended by the pharmacist. Many of those women had inserted various objects into their vagina, including wax and matches.[205] Although it could be argued that women generally tried to avoid incriminating a third party when they did not mention a midwife, this cannot be the case, as the same women mentioned the involvement of a pharmacist.

Mpertsekas, in his discussion of abortion methods, devotes a separate section to 'medicinal and other drinks', these methods being included under what he terms 'empirical methods' (as opposed to scientific ones).[206] Among the abortifacients 'used and advertised' are the 'strong purgatives': ergot, apiol, cantharides, absinthe, savin, rue, arsenic and mercury, as well as lead and phosphorus. The last two, he clarified, were used mostly in England and Germany. He also mentions the 'empirical drinks made by infusion of ivy (*Hedera*), tobacco, various fruits, roots and leaves of bushes and plants',[207] singling out savin and rue as widely cultivated throughout Greece and as 'known and famed by the populace' as abortifacients. He differentiates between the two, however, explaining that although savin is known to be an emmenagogue science disputes its value as an abortifacient, while rue is accepted as both an emmenagogic and an abortifacient. Two points should be made here. First, Mpertsekas acknowledges the use of traditional, non-medical methods of abortion in Athens. His own patients in the mid-1930s clearly outlined the extensive use of such methods, especially in the first two months of pregnancy.[208] Unlike Kontos, writing 50 years before, he seems to accept the abortive properties of these traditional, herbal methods, although both agreed on the potentially lethal effects of some.[209] Second, Mpertsekas clearly distinguishes between emmenagogues and abortifacients and categorises them separately, as did the eighteenth- and nineteenth-century writers of the iatrosophic 'medical recipes' and the lay women who employed them, as he explains in the case studies he cites. That women were thinking along similar lines to Mpertsekas is evident in oral accounts from elderly Greek women, this one from Rhodes, referring to a time around or before 1965:

> When we were late, and we might be pregnant, but we didn't want it, after a few days we boiled onion skins or cinnamon, and we'd drink it on an empty stomach every morning for two or three days so that the blood would come. If you drink [the infusion of] onion skins, you'll see a period. But if there was a child [if pregnant], though, the blood wouldn't come [i.e. emmenagogues would not harm the pregnancy].[210]

Interestingly, Georges observed that among her informants those in their 70s and 80s referred to such drinks as emmenagogics, while the subsequent generation called them abortifacients, indicating a change over time in how they were used or perceived.[211] Since Georges conducted the interviews in the early 1990s, the older generation is made up of women born before 1920; the younger generation included women born after 1920. The above quote represents the bringing together of the ideas and vocabularies of two worlds—one in which emmenagogues were used to bring on the menses when they were delayed 'a few days' but before a foetus had formed, so that the action was not ethically problematic. Since the foetus was perceived to form much later, using emmenagogues soon after a missed period was not expected to interfere with a foetus; emmenagogues were not perceived as powerful enough to affect a foetus—hence the assertion that 'if there was a child' the emmenagogues would have been ineffective. Members of the post-1920 generation, in contrast, were clear that they were using abortifacients right from the start of a potential and unwanted pregnancy. These two perspectives raise the possibility of diverse understandings of when it was permissible to take action and when not.

In the late 1950s and early 1960s a trained midwife established in rural mainland Greece reported to Blum and Blum that local women resorted to induced abortion regularly. To achieve this, women 'sit in hot water, and use suppositories and local medicines'.[212] The midwife also reported a case of a local woman who inserted a wooden stick into her uterus, following her neighbour's advice, only to die in hospital.[213] The midwife reported that induced abortions—almost certainly curettages—by midwives and physicians were also taking place, but in Athens and not locally, if anything because of the need for secrecy.[214]

Conclusions

Much of this chapter has evolved from McLaren's, Riddle's and van de Walle's views on whether women employed herbal and other preparations as abortifacients or emmenagogues. Riddle argued that some remnants of the medieval knowledge of abortifacients survived to the twentieth century. In Greece, it was more than remnants that survived. Greece's tardiness in abandoning empirical and popular medicine—especially in rural areas—provided women with access to and knowledge of emmenagogues until the end of the studied period and, although the use of the term 'emmenagogues' was abandoned by mainstream gynaecologists in much of Europe and the USA by the early twentieth century, in Greece it continued to be used well into the twentieth century by both laypeople and physicians. Knowledge and use of emmenagogic preparations, for the wellbeing of women, to avoid or cure sterility and in many cases to enhance fertility and ensure that all was in order for the next pregnancy to occur, was widespread in the nineteenth and twentieth centuries—at least up to the early 1960s—and had certainly existed in earlier centuries too. It was also understood that some herbs and substances could be used to speed up part of the delivery. I would argue, therefore, that the knowledge of using herbal infusions as abortifacients was also widely available in the nineteenth and early twentieth centuries and in all probability earlier on. These do not seem to have been in use as such in the nineteenth century, though for those in 'need' an abortion could always be procured.

Physicians were accommodating and supportive of the need to use emmenagogues for women's health and to guard against sterility. Naturally, they delineated their expertise and modernity by using pharmaceutical preparations and, later on, hormonal ones. However, the aims were similar to those of earlier, herbal preparations. It has been argued here that Greek women in both the nineteenth and the early twentieth centuries were eager to regulate their menses not only because irregularity was seen as pathological but also because it would enable them to become and/or remain fertile. However, physicians' most recommended therapy for many women's pathologies in the early twentieth century was curettage, which we will examine next.

Notes

1. Angus McLaren (1981) '"Barrenness against Nature": Recourse to Abortion in Pre-Industrial England', *The Journal of Sex Research*, 17(3), pp. 224–37; John Riddle (1998) *Eve's Herbs: A History of Contraception and Abortion in the West* (London; Cambridge, MA: Harvard University Press), p. 26.
2. Riddle, *Eve's Herbs*, pp. 8, 257.
3. Riddle, *Eve's Herbs*, pp. 179–80.
4. Etienne van de Walle (1997) 'Flowers and Fruits: Two Thousand Years of Menstrual Regulation', *The Journal of Interdisciplinary History*, 28(2), 201.
5. Van de Walle, 'Flowers and Fruits', 202.
6. Joan Cadden (1993) *Meaning of Sex Differences in the Middle Ages* (Cambridge: Cambridge University Press), pp. 173–4. Also see Van de Walle, 'Flowers and Fruits', 185; and Sangeetha Madhavan and Alisse

Diarra (2001) 'The Blood that links: Menstrual Regulations among the Bamana of Mali' in Etienne van de Walle and Elisha P. Renne (eds), *Regulating Menstruation: Beliefs, practices, interpretations* (Chicago: The University of Chicago Press), pp. 176–8 for a similar view in a modern population.

7. Roy Porter (1989) *Health for sale. Quackery in England 1660–1850* (Manchester: Manchester University Press). His chapter on 'Quacks and sex' is peppered with such references (pp. 148–9, 161–2, 166–7).
8. Jennifer Evans (2011) '"Gentle Purges corrected with hot Spices, whether they work or not, do vehemently provoke Venery": Menstrual Provocation and Procreation in Early Modern England', *Social History of Medicine*, 25(1), 2.
9. See, for example, Susan E. Klepp, 'Colds, worms, and hysteria: menstrual regulation in eighteenth-century America'; Madhavan and Diarra, 'The Blood that links', both in Van de Walle and Renne (eds), *Regulating Menstruation*, pp. 39–63, 176–8.
10. Etienne van de Walle and Elisha P. Renne (2001) 'Introduction', p. xxiii citing Stefania Siedlecky (2001) 'Pharmacological properties of emmenagogues: A biomedical view' in Van de Walle and Renne (eds), *Regulating Menstruation*, pp. 93–112.
11. Elisha Renne (2001) '"Cleaning the Inside" and the regulation of Menstruation in Southwestern Nigeria'; Terence H. Hull and Valerie J. Hull (2001) 'Means, Motives and Menses: Use of Herbal Emmenagogues in Indonesia'; Heidi Bart Johnston (2001) 'Regulating Menstruation in Matlab, Bangladesh: Women's Practices and Perspectives', all in Van de Walle and Renne (eds), *Regulating Menstruation*, pp. 193, 206–7, 225, referring to Nigeria, Indonesia and Bangladesh respectively.
12. Etienne van de Walle (2001) 'Menstrual catharsis and the Greek physician' in Van de Walle and Renne (eds), *Regulating Menstruation*, pp. 3–21.
13. Violetta Hionidou (2011) 'What do starving people eat? The case of Greece through Oral History', *Continuity and Change*, 26(1), 113–34. See also A. Karanastases (1952) 'Oi Zeugades tes Ko, e Zoe kai oi Asholies ton', *Laografia*, 14, 245–6, referring to the island of Kos (cited in Maria Antoniou (2006) 'Paradosiake Diatrofe sten Ellada kai hrese Lahanikon kai Frouton apo tis Arhes tou 20ou Aiona' (postgraduate dissertation, Harokopeion University), p. 145, who also cites many similar cases from other areas of the country).
14. See, for example, Maria Verivaki, 'Identifying wild greens in the Cretan landscape', http://www.organicallycooked.com/2013/01/identifying-wild-greens-in-cretan.html (accessed 13 October 2018); Antonia-Leda Matalas and Louis E. Grivetti (2007) 'Non-food food during famine. The

Athens famine survivor project' in Jeremy MacClancy, Jeya Henry and Helen Macbeth (eds), *Consuming the Inedible: Neglected Dimensions of Food Choice* (New York: Berghahn).

15. This was certainly the case in Athens during the famine, but also in Hermoupolis, Hios town and Vrontados. See also George Horton (1902) *In Argolis* (London: Duckworth), pp. 65–6.
16. ELIA Athens, A.E. 44/01, 1885, Fytologion Kalliopes Trapantzale (pupil in the 4th year of secondary school).
17. For the contemporary use of such greens, and knowledge and scientific assessment of their nutritional value, see Logan Strenchok, Panayiotis G. Dimitrakopoulos, Thanasis Kizos and Taxiarchoula-Maria Pitta (2018) 'Local knowledge of selected wild plant species collected in Agiassos, on Lesvos, Greece', *Norsk Geografisk Tidsskrift—Norwegian Journal of Geography*, 72(5), 273–86; and Eleni V. Mikropoulou, Konstantina Vougogiannopoulou, Eleftherios Kalpoutzakis, Aimilia D. Sklirou, Zoi Skaperda, Joëlle Houriet, Jean-Luc Wolfender, Ioannis P. Trougakos, Dimitrios Kouretas, Maria Halabalaki and Sofia Mitakou (2018) 'Phytochemical Composition of the Decoctions of Greek Edible Greens (Chórta) and Evaluation of Antioxidant and Cytotoxic Properties', *Molecules*, 23(7), 1541.
18. Among many others are the following: Dem. Zaganiares (1935) *Ta Farmakeutika Futa tes Elladas* (Athens: Apatside), p. 57; Xen. G. Anagnostopoulou (1961) *Ta Votana. Laike Farmakologia kai Therapeutike Laografia* (Athens: n.p.), p. 25; E. Georges (2008) *Bodies of knowledge: The Medicalisation of Reproduction in Greece* (Nashville, TN: Vanderbilt University Press), pp. 107–11; Paulos Drandakes (1929) *Megale Ellenike Egkyklopaideia*, vol. 9 (Athens: Pyrsos); Dionysios Pyrros o Thettalos (1831) *Egkolpion ton Iatron Etoi Praktike Iatrike, Periehousa ten Ylen tes Iatrikes, ten Farmakopoiian, ten Ygieinen*, vol.2 (Naupleion: Konstantinou Tompras), p. 260.
19. Rue was one of the herbs included in the 1885 herbal album of an Athenian schoolgirl (ELIA Athens, A.E. 44/01, 1885, Fytologion Kalliopes Trapantzale).
20. M.M. Moyseides (1928) *E Ektrosis kata ten Elleniken arhaioteta. Melete Iatrodikastike, Klinike kai Farmakologike* (Athens: Ad. Gerardon), pp. 45, 40–1, mentioning artemisia (*Artemisia campestris* L.), savin (*Juniperus sabina*), absinthe (*Artemisia absinthium* L.), etc.
21. Vassos Kassianos (2008) *Geoponika*, translated by Epameinondas Malainos (Athens: Koultoura), originally printed in 1930. The original work is a compilation of older works focused mostly on agriculture that was prepared in the tenth with the encouragement of the Byzantine emperor Constantine VII Porphyrogenitus. This was translated into the vernacular

Greek (Demotike) and published in 1930. An old edition of the published book was used as iatrosophic by a traditional healer in twentieth-century Neneta, Hios: Sevaste Haviara-Karahaliou (1993) *E Laike iatrike tes Hiou* (Athens: GasciHellas), p. 384.

22. Kassianos, *Geoponika*, p. 222.
23. Tryfon K. Kontos (1883) *Peri Examvloseos e Amvloseos* (Athens: Enosis), pp. 11, 14. Similarly, Argenti and Rose report from early twentieth-century Hios that folkloric accounts urged that rue should be avoided by pregnant women because it is 'dangerous both to her and to her unborn child' (Philip P. Argenti and H.J. Rose (1949) *The Folk-lore of Chios* (Cambridge: Cambridge University Press), vol. 1, p. 415).
24. However, the conclusion concerning Greece is based on a small study. The populations that still consider it an emmenagogue are Algeria, Libya and Turkey: A. Pollio, A. De Natale, E. Appetiti, G. Aliotta and A. Touwaide (2008) 'Continuity and change in the Mediterranean medical tradition: *Ruta* spp. (rutaceae) in Hippocratic medicine and present practices', *Journal of Ethnopharmacology*, 116, p. 478.
25. Aglaia Mpimpe-Papaspyropoulou (1985) *Paradosiake Iatrike sten Peloponneso* (Athens: Ethniko kai Kapodistriako Panepistemio Athenon), p. 63. The sources that this book was based on are oral histories collected from empirics or persons related to empirics and thus it depicts the actual practices of the population. Such practitioners would have been of advanced age, since young persons can rarely be considered empirical practitioners. Moreover, considering that practising as an empiric was illegal at the time, the experience of these practitioners would be referring to earlier years, certainly before 1960.
26. See, for example, C. Stewart (1991) *Demons and the Devil: Moral Imagination in Modern Greek Culture* (Princeton, NJ: Princeton University Press); Richard Blum and Eva Blum (1970) *The Dangerous Hour: The Lore of Crisis and Mystery in Rural Greece* (London: Chatto & Windus), pp. 127–9, 173–5, 192–5; and the many relevant references in both these books.
27. The plant regularly appears in botanical searches on Greek territory: Th. De Hellreich (1898) *E Chloris tes Aiginas* (Athens: K. Maisner and N. Kargadoure), p. 23; Th. De Hellreich (1899) *E Chloris tes Theras* (Athens: K. Maisner and N. Kargadoure), p. 10; Michael Defner (1922) *E Chloris tes Tsakonias* (Athens: Staurou Hristou), p. 11.
28. Emm. S. Anases (1959) *Ta farmakeutika Votana tes Ellados*, vol. 1 (Athens: n.p.), pp. 239–40.
29. Anonymous (November 1860) 'Proheiros Farmakapotheke', *O Iatros tou Laou*, 1(21), 349.
30. Anonymous, 'Proheiros', 349.

31. Theodoros Afentoules (1891) *Farmakologia: Etoi peri Fyseos kai Dynameos kai Hreseos Farmakon*, vol. 1 (Athens: Paliggenesia), p. 635.
32. Kontos, *Peri examvloseos*, pp. 11, 14 referring to Prof Afentoules in the 1880s. The knowledge of the ecbolic properties of wild-rue infusion was available from the tenth century (Kassianos, *Geoponika*, pp. 221–2).
33. Pyrros, *Egkolpion*, vol. 1, p. 21; Afentoules, *Farmakologia*, vol. 1, pp. 113, 635; Drandakes, *Megale Ellenike*; Zaganiares, *Ta Farmakeutika*, pp. 4, 14–15; Anagnostopoulou, *Ta Votana*, pp. 322–3; A. Arvanites (ed.) (2006) *Laike Paradosiake Iatrike* (Ahaia: n.p.), pp. 68–87; Mihael Malamas (1982) 'E Laike votanotherapeutike sto Zagori' (unpublished PhD: Ioannina University), pp. 38–9; Georges, *Bodies of knowledge*, pp. 109–11. Other authors identify some of the above as abortifacients. See, for example, Arvanites, who names secale cornitum and crocus sativus as exclusively abortifacients (*Laike*, pp. 68, 87). Again, all the above are mentioned in the ancient Greek texts as abortifacients and emmenagogues (Moyseides, *E Ektrosis*, p. 33).
34. Barbara Zipser (2009) *John the Physicians's Therapeutics. A Medical Handbook in Vernacular Greek* (Leiden: Brill), p. 98 (edition N).
35. Zipser, *John*, p. 208 (edition ω).
36. Zipser, *John*, p. 288.
37. Zipser, *John*, p. 284.
38. Lamprine Manou (2008) *Giatrosofia 16ou aiona* (Thessalonike: Adelfoi Kyriakide), p. 24 where manuscript 181 of the Iveron Monastery is used.
39. G.K. Hatzopoulos (1977–78) 'Laike Iatrike sto horio Antreaton Amisou Pontou', *Arheion Pontou*, 34, 226, 244. While Hatzopoulos refers to a Pontic village situated in today's Turkey, this population was moved into Greece in 1923 and one can only assume that they continued following the same beliefs and practices.
40. Agapios Monahos o Kres (2002) *Geoponikon. Giatrosofia kai Palies syntages* (Athens: Koultoura), pp. 70–2, 76, 147, reprint from the 1850 publication. Original publication 1643.
41. K. Filaretos (ed.) (1924) *Iatrosofikon, syntahthen ypo tou skeuofylakos tes en Kypro Ieras Mones Mahaira Metrofanous 1790–1867* (Nicosia: D.H. Kyriakidou), p. 112.
42. A twentieth-century Cretan empiric recommended as an emmenagogic douching with seawater or a warm drink made with wine, absinthe and saffron: Patricia Ann Clark (2011) *A Cretan Healer's Handbook in the Byzantine Tradition: Text, Translation, and Commentary* (Farnham: Ashgate), pp. 56, 100. Recipes for bringing on the menses are repeatedly cited in the printed version of the healing book that was used by the empiric Georgios Tourikes in the village of Augonuma, which was transcribed on 5 October 1874 (Haviara-Karahaliou, *E Laike*, pp. 150–249).

This book was self-described as a compilation of 'medical notes of old and new scientists and is used by the empiric doctor Georgios Tourikes' (Haviara-Karahaliou, *E Laike*, p. 150). Since the 'illness' (as described in the book) of retained menstruation is often referred to in the book, the cures mentioned there would have also been recommended to the empiric's patients.

43. Haviara-Karahaliou, *E Laike*, pp. 448, 463, 467; also pp. 47–8, citing oral accounts from four different villages on Hios. Mpimpe-Papaspuropoulou collected her material in the 1970s (*Paradosiake Iatrike*).
44. Mpimpe-Papaspuropoulou, *Paradosiake Iatrike*, pp. 322–3. The author does not name these as emmenagogues, although her description suggests exactly that.
45. For example, we are told that some of the seventeenth-century iatrosophic books do not differ substantially from Pyrros' 1818 publication (Malamas, 'E Laike', p. 10). Moreover, a copy of Pyrros' book was utilised as an iatrosophic book by a traditional healer in Neneta, Hios, and another in the town of Hios. Both healers practised in the twentieth century (Haviara-Karahaliou, *E Laike*, pp. 384).
46. Euaggelia K. Fragkake (1978) *E Demodes Iatrike tes Kretes* (Athens: n.p.), p. 33.
47. Anases, *Ta farmakeutika*, vol. 1, p. 9. Just like the iatrosophic books, Anases discusses plants and their use in addressing medical problems. Unlike them, the book is well organised, in a 'scientific' manner, facilitating the search of cures for specific ailments but also presenting the herbs individually.
48. Anases, *Ta Farmakeutika*, vol. 1, pp. 31, 84.
49. Anases, *Ta Farmakeutika*, vol. 1, pp. 239–40.
50. Emm. S. Anases (1962) *Ta Farmakeutika Votana tes Ellados*, vol. 2 (Athens: n.p.), pp. 24–5.
51. Anases, *Ta Farmakeutika*, vol. 2, pp. 38–9.
52. Hrysoula Hatzetake-Kapsomenou (2001) 'Gynaikeies hreseis votanon: sto metahmio therapeutikes kai mageias' in *Farmakeutika kai Aromatika futa, Kypros, Paralimni, 21–25 Martiou 1997* (Athens: Politistiko Idruma omilou Peiraios), p. 171 citing E. Stamoule-Sarante (1938) 'Pos giatreuan sten Thrake', *Thrakika* 9, 197.
53. Hatzetake-Kapsomenou, 'Gynaikeies hreseis votanon', p. 171 citing Hatzopoulos, 'Laike Iatrike', 226, 244. Arvanites also cites this as an emmenagogic (*Laike*, p. 71).
54. Anonymous (23 March 1952) 'Ta Vrastika', *Gynaika*, 3(57), pp. 36–7. On origanum dictamnus, for example, see Nikos Krigas, Diamanto Lazari, Eleni Maloupa and Maria Stikoudi (2015) 'Introducing Dittany of Crete (*Origanum dictamnus* L.) to gastronomy: A new culinary con-

cept for a traditionally used medicinal plant', *International Journal of Gastronomy and Food Science*, 2(2), 112.

55. Kyriake Hrysou-Karatza (2006) *Trofe kai Diatrofe stis Kyklades (19os–20os ai.)* (unpublished PhD: Athens University), p. 448.
56. The family resided in Athens, where the mother had been born and raised (personal communication, March 2019).
57. Filaretos, *Iatrosofikon*, p. 111 (absinthe, leek leaves, leek seeds); Agapios Monahos o Kres, *Geoponikon*, pp. 145–6 (bay leaves, poultices made with leek leaves, leek seeds); Zipser, *John*, version ω, pp. 288–9, suggesting thirteen different recipes, all varying from the recommended emmenagogues.
58. Only occasionally there is a further section that refers to both bringing on the menses and 'to expel[ling] a child from the womb' (Zipser, *John*, version ω, p. 321).
59. On the 'medical recipe books' see Christos Papadopoulos (2009) 'Post-Byzantine Medical Manuscripts: New Insights into the Greek Medical Tradition, its Intellectual and Practical Interconnections, and our Understanding of Greek Culture', *Journal of Modern Greek Studies*, 27(1), 107–30. Also Hionidou, 'Popular medicine'.
60. Zafeires Vaou (1982) *Mageies, Getemata, Laike Therapeutike tes Melou (18os–19os aionas)* (Athens: n.p.), pp. 81, 82; Kontomihes Pantazes (1988) *E Laike Iatrike sten Leukada* (Athens: Gregore), pp. 85, 123, 206. The one reference to aborting a child comes from Vaou, *Mageies*, p. 81. A similar distinction seems to have been made in the writings of the ancient Greek authors: Moyseides, *E Ektrosis*, p. 36. Moyseides cites Hippocrates, Aetios and Galenos.
61. Afentoules, *Farmakologia*, vol. 2, pp. 60–1, 361–4.
62. Anonymous (1 March 1938) 'Dia ten Praxin. Deleteriaseis', 'Kantharides', *Klinike*, 14(5), 112; Anonymous (15 February 1938) 'Ergotine', *Klinike*, 14(4), 8–67; Anonymous (1 February 1938) 'Vrathy', *Klinike*, 14(3), 65; Anonymous (1 March 1938) 'Kinine', *Klinike*, 14(5), 113.
63. Anases, *Ta Farmakeutika*, vol. 2. Under emmenagogues nine different herbs are mentioned, one of which is absinthe (*Artemisia absinthium*) (vol. 1, pp. 31, 84). Of *Aristolochia longa* it mentions that it was used by the ancient physicians as an emmenagogue and abortifacient (vol. 2, pp. 51–2). Similarly, Arvanites distinguishes between emmenagogic and abortifacient herbs, although for some—*Arnica montane* and *Artemisia absinthium*—he indicates that they perform both functions: Arvanites, *Laike*, pp. 86–7.
64. Anases, *Ta Farmakeutika*, vol. 2, p. 39.
65. Arvanites, *Laike*, pp. 86–7.

66. Filaretos, *Iatrosofikon*, p. 110 (insert into the vagina a root of cyclamen or lily); Clark, *A Cretan*, p. 48 (to facilitate the delivery 'even if the baby is dead'), 104, 132 (a magic spell is employed rather than herbs (geteia)).
67. Kypros Hrysanthes (1951) 'Ena Kypriako giatrosofi', *Kypriakes Spoudes* 15, η. As the author mentions, this is not a purely Cypriot text; rather, he argues, it was transcribed by a Cypriot (στ).
68. Manou, *Giatrosofia*, p. 55.
69. The same drinks that were used to expel a dead baby or to facilitate a delivery were used by empiric midwives in order to expel the afterbirth. So, for example, Oikonomopoulos and Oikonomopoulou refer to wine-based drinks made with, among other ingredients, wild fennel (*Foeniculum vulgare*, marathon), dittany of Crete herb (*Origanum dictamnus*, diktamo), mandrake or oregano: Hristos Th. Oikonomopoulos and Alexandra H. Oikonomopoulou (2006) 'O toketos, oi dystokies, ta "eutokia" kai e ananepse tou apnoikou neogennettou ste demode iatrike kata ta metavyzantina hronia tou neou Ellenismou (1453–1953)', *Themata Maieutikes-Gynaikologias*, 20(2), 151.
70. Afentoules, *Farmakologia*, vol. 1, p. 635: 'Rue is used as emmenagogic (weak drink) by the populace; but also as abortifacient [ektrotikon] (strong drink) though occasionally kills the mother too.'
71. Panteles D. Mpertsekas (1948) *Oi Kindynoi kai ai Epiplokai tes Amvloseos kai ta Iatrodikastika Provlemata autes* (Athens: Euth. Hristodoulou), p. 15.
72. Anonymous (23 March 1952) 'Ta Vrastika', *Gynaika*, 3(57), pp. 36–73. Fragkake also refers to *erontas* (*E Demodes*, p. 32).
73. Ansley J. Coale, 'The demographic transition', in *International Population Conference, London 1969* (Liege: IUSSP), Vol. 1, pp. 53–72.
74. It should be made clear that such knowledge would be shared by those somehow involved with 'caring', such as empirics, midwives, wise women, giatrises (female 'doctor') and so on. Married women would also discuss and exchange information. Single women would not have had access to such information, as becomes clear in the oral interviews conducted on Mykonos. Moreover, when I interviewed women there, they would not divulge any information related to childbearing and sex to me until I assured them that I was already aware of all these issues.
75. P. Gravigger (1970) *Iatrosofia* (Athens: Vivliotheke Sfiggos), vol. 1: 'For irregular menses' there is a recipe by Gumnasios (no. 82), p. 474; G.I. Koukas (ed.) (1975) *Gymnasios Lauriotes. O Kalogeros kai oi syntages tou* (Athens: Leon), 'About the menses', p. 32.
76. Clark, *A Cretan*, chapter 4. See also a folklore recipe for irregular menstruation on early twentieth-century Hios, although this one outlined how to prepare and consume 'slag from a smithy' (Argenti and Rose, *The Folk-lore of Chios*, vol. 1, p. 409). Yet another one instructed the con-

sumption of freshwater crabs in wine (Argenti and Rose, *The Folk-lore of Chios*, vol. 1, p. 414).

77. Clark, *A Cretan*, p. 66.
78. Emm. S. Anases (1961) *Odegos tes Noikokyras: Aparaiteto Voethema gia tis Agrotisses, agrotoneanides klp* (Athens: Spyros Spyrou), p. 122.
79. Fragkake, *E Demodes*, p. 33.
80. The same belief is strongly expressed in Timoleon Kardaras (1894) *Praktike Iatrike ton Oikogeneion*, 2nd edn (Athens: Georgiou D. Fexe), p. 191. Kardaras was a physician and this is stated in his volume on practical family medicine. This is a popular belief that remains strong in Greece.
81. On the polluting powers of menstruation see Blum and Blum, though the references to it among anthropological works on Greece are abundant (Richard Blum and Eva Blum (1965) *Health and Healing in Rural Greece* (Stanford, CA: Stanford University Press), pp. 33–4, 50, 138. On similar contemporary practices among Muslims in Indonesia during the Ramadhan and pilgrimages to Mecca see Terence H. Hull and Valerie J. Hull (2001) 'Means, motives, and menses: Use of herbal emmenagogues in Indonesia' in Van de Walle and Renne (eds), *Regulating Menstruation*, p. 213.
82. Fragkake, *E Demodes*, p. 34; Haviara-Karahaliou, *E Laike*, p. 448, describing an incident that occurred in 1927 on Hios.
83. 'Female sterility: the womb has closed up, it needs to be opened up': Kostas D. Moutzoures (2003) 'Laike iatrike sto Akroteri Hanion', *Laike Iatrike, Diethnes Epistemoniko Synedrio Rethymno 8–10 Dekemvriou 2000, Praktika* (Rethymno: ILEP), p. 288. Moreover, in Hatzetake-Kapsomenou's review of the use of herbs for 'female' reasons she refers to one plant as emmenagogic, only to add later on that the same plant was used by women who had difficulty conceiving (Hatzetake-Kapsomenou, 'Gynaikeies hreseis votanon', p. 171).
84. Iosef De-Kigallas (1838) *Diatrive peri emmenon kai Hlorioseos* (Hermoupolis: Georgios Polumeres), p. 8 and 16. At the time De-Kigallas was writing, the causes of chlorosis were not known. Only late in the nineteenth century was it linked to iron-deficiency anemia: John K. Crellin (2012) 'Revisiting Eve's Herbs: Reflections on therapeutic uncertainties' in Anne Van Arsdall and Timothy Graham (eds), *Herbs and Healers From the Ancient Mediterranean Through the Medieval West: Essays in Honor of John M. Riddle* (Farnham: Ashgate), pp. 311–12. Chlorosis was frequently mentioned in seventeenth-century literature (Van de Walle and Renne, 'Introduction', p. xxiii).
85. De-Kigallas, *Diatrive*, p. 16. When De-Kigallas' work was presented to the Athens Medical Society (Iatrike Etaireia Athenon) a heated debate took place as to whether a link did exist between menarche/menstruation

and chlorosis, with many of the participants disagreeing with De-Kigallas: Tryfon K. Andrianakos, *E Maieutike kai Gynaikologia kata ten diadromen tou viou tes Iatrikes Etaireias Athenon 1835–1908* (Athens: S.K. Vlastou, 1929), pp. 33–5.

86. Anonymous (1864) 'Fysiologia kai Nosologia. Peri emmenon ypo fysiologiken kai nosologiken apopsin', *Ippokrates*, 2(11), 273–9.
87. K. Thomas Chambers (1862) 'Peri aimaterou idrotos, anaplerountos ten emmenon katharsin', *Ippokrates*, 1(8), 199–200, anonymous translator. The article was focused on non-vicarious menstruation, a topic that attracted the attention of physicians at the time.
88. Alexandros E. Triantes (1887) *Egheiridion Maieutikes pros hresin ton Maion kai ton Mathetrion tou Maieuteriou* (Athens: Vlastou), pp. 127, 316.
89. Triantes, *Egheiridion*, pp. 139–40. A similar description is in Antonios I. Kindynes (1889) *E Steirosis para te Gynaiki kai Therapeia Autes* (Athens: Vlastos Varvaregos), pp. 53–5.
90. Triantes, *Egheiridion*, pp. 139–40.
91. Kindynes, *E Steirosis*, pp. 53–5, 124–6. Endometritis was considered a prime cause of sterility (Dem. Antonopoulos, *E Steirosis para te Gynaiki* (Athens: Koronaiou-Denaxa, 1926), pp. 42–3).
92. Kardaras, *Praktike Iatrike*, p. 190. See also Anonymous (1864) 'Fysiologia kai Nosologia. Peri emmenon ypo fysiologiken kai nosologiken apopsin', *Ippokrates*, 2(10), 225–30.
93. See, for example, Manou, *Giatrosofia*, p. 24.
94. As the term used in Greek is artemisia, this can be referring to any of this diverse genus of plants though in all probability it refers to *Artemisia vulgaris* i.e. mugwort. Absinthe is usually referred to as apsinthi and so artemisia is almost certainly not referring to *Artemisia absinthium*.
95. Kardaras, *Praktike Iatrike*, pp. 88, 192. He also indicates that these are self-help remedies and that the patient should see the doctor in order to overcome the cause of the mentioned symptoms.
96. A. Vitsares (1874) *Nosoi ton Gynaikon*, vol. 1 (Athens: Ermou), pp. 75–9.
97. Vitsares, *Nosoi*, pp. 80–98.
98. Vitsares, *Nosoi*, pp. 104–9.
99. Vitsares, *Nosoi*, pp. 198–9.
100. An *iatrophilosophos* was a physician who also studied the arts. S.G.S. (1926–34) 'Iatrophilosophos', in *Megale Ellenike Egkyklopaideia*, ed. Paulos Dandrakes, vol. 12 (Athens: Pyrsos), p. 829.
101. Pyrros was a bishop and a physician, trained in Padua, who returned to his homeland at the outbreak of the Greek Revolution in the 1820s. He remained in Greece and, in the 1830s, along with other qualified physicians in the newly created Greek state, set up the Athens Medical Society. Thus, while he represents the educated, qualified physicians, his priesthood suggests that he also had a very good knowledge of the medicine

practised by his contemporary empirics. He used both magic and herbs in his practical medicine book, unlike other physicians of his time: Dionysios Pyrros o Thettalos (1840) *Egkolpion ton Iatron: Etoi Praktike Iatrike*, 1st edn 1831, vol. 1 (Athens: Aggelos Aggelides). In addition, in his writings he both referred to and praised various empirics: Pan. Kretikos (1961) 'O Mandragoras', *Laografia*, 19, 402–5.

102. Pyrros, *Egkolpion*, vol. 1, p. 20. As elsewhere, the sixteenth-century iatrosophic book indicates that the menstrual blood was released when women were not pregnant but, when pregnant, it was retained and used by them in order 'to feed the children in their wombs' (Manou, *Giatrosofia*, p. 22). Also, for similar ideas in eighteenth-century France, see Cathy Clive (2002) 'The Hidden Truths of the Belly: The Uncertainties of Pregnancy in Early Modern Europe', *Social History of Medicine*, 15(2), 209–27.
103. D.K. Konsolas, *Egheiridion Maieutikes pros hresin ton Maion kai Mathetrion tou Maieuteriou*, 3rd edn (Athens: S.K. Vlastou, 1900), p. 41.
104. Pyrros, *Egkolpion*, vol. 1, p. 196. Pyrros recommends no fewer than twenty-one therapies for amenorrhoea. Elsewhere polytrihi is mentioned: a simple made of it is used by the people (laos) for women who had just given birth, for its positive effect on the uterus: Anonymous (15 July 1860) 'Proheiros Farmakapotheke', *O Iatros tou Laou*, 1(14), 224.
105. Pyrros, *Egkolpion*, vol. 1, pp. 20–1.
106. Klepp, 'Colds, worms, and hysteria', pp. 22–38; Janet Farrell Brodie, 'Menstrual Interventions in the Nineteenth-century United States' in Van de Walle and Renne (eds), *Regulating Menstruation*, pp. 39–63; Van de Walle and Renne, 'Introduction', p. xiii; Evans, '"Gentle Purges"'.
107. Kardaras, *Praktike Iatrike*, p. 192.
108. Afentoules, *Farmakologia*, vol. 2, pp. 91–2.
109. Afentoules, *Farmakologia*, vol. 2, p. 92.
110. Afentoules, *Farmakologia*, vol. 2, p. 93–4.
111. Afentoules, *Farmakologia*, vol. 2, pp. 361–4.
112. Nikolaos Kostes was appointed in 1837 as Professor of Obstetrics, Botanology, Pharmaceutical Chemistry and Pharmacology (Tryfon Andrianakos [1937] 'Exelixis kai proodoi tes maieutikes kai gynaikologias en te neotera Ellada', *Ellenike Iatrike*, 11, 14). He studied medicine in Heidelberg.
113. Nikolaos Kostes (1849) *Egheiridion Maieutikes* (Athens: S.K. Vlastos), pp. 331–4.
114. X. Landerer (1864) 'Peri tou Tropou tes Skeuaseos tou Vammatos tes Erysivodous Zeias', *Ippokrates*, 2(8), 197–8; X. Landerer (1864) 'Peri Neas tinos Methodou pros Diateresin tes Erysivodous Zeias', *Ippokrates*, 2(8), 198. X. Landerer, probably a Bavarian, was the Royal pharmacist.

115. Triantes, *Egheiridion*, pp. 367–8.
116. G.K. Lameras (August 1929) 'Therapeia tes epiloheiou endometritidos', *Praktikos Iatros*, 7(8), 27.
117. D. Theodoridou (1928) 'E therapeia tes Dysmoinorroias', *Praktikos Iatros*, 6(4), 184–5.
118. (1928) *Klinike, Evdomadiaia Epistemonike kai Epaggelmatike Epitheorese*, 4(16–24), published weekly.
119. Anonymous (20 October 1928) 'Advertisement of *Ovarialhormon Folliculin*', *Klinike, Evdomadiaia Epistemonike kai Epaggelmatike Epitheorese*, 4(16), 519.
120. Anonymous (20 October 1928) 'Advertisement of *Menstruol*', *Klinike, Evdomadiaia Epistemonike kai Epaggelmatike Epitheorese*, 4(16), 519.
121. Nikolaos Vasileiades (August 1928) 'Peri Amenorroias', *O Praktikos Iatros*, 6(8), 354.
122. Anonymous (1930) 'Maieutike Gynaikologia: Siebke. Ai proodoi tes therapeias ton anomalion tes emmenou roes. (Fort d. Ther. No 14, 1930)', *Ellenike Iatrike*, 4(11), 1223–4.
123. Anonymous, 'Maieutike Gynaikologia: Siebke', 1223–4.
124. Anonymous (13 December 1950), 'O Gynaikologos Apanta: Hrysanthemo, Mika N.', *E Gynaika*, 1(23), p. 19.
125. Anonymous (February 1939) 'Efeveia epivradyntheisa', *Hera*, 1(2), 31.
126. There were five advertisements of two products in *Klinike*, 22(17–24) (September–December 1951).
127. Anonymous (15 September 1951) 'Estro-Prol', *Klinike*, 22(17); Anonymous (1–15 October 1951) 'Estrovite', *Klinike*, 22(19–20).
128. The Estro-Prol advertisement read: 'Estro-Prol. Mixed preparation progesterone 10mg Estradiol 15,000 dm. For primary amenorrhoea. For functional amenorrhoea and spontaneous abortion. Polymenorrhea, oligomenorrhea. For functional haemorrhage of the uterus. For the most persistent cases of secondary amenorrhoea. 1c.c intramuscularly for 5 days or according to the physician's instructions. Note: We are informing the honourable physicians that a substantial amount of the above preparation has been received.' Anonymous (15 September 1951) 'Estro-Prol', *Klinike*, 22(17).
129. Anonymous (April 1949) '*Hemagol.* To Ariston Emmenagogon Skeuasma', *To saloni tou Giatrou*, 15(1); 15(2) (May 1949); 15(3) (June 1949); 16(13–14) (April–May 1950); 16(32–33) (August–September 1952); 24(81) (March 1961).
130. Anonymous (April 1949) '*Hemagol.* To Ariston Emmenagogon Skeuasma', *To saloni tou Giatrou*, 15(1), 13.
131. See, for example, Fragkake, *E Demodes*, pp. 32–3.

132. Anonymous (21 September 1950) 'O Gynaikologos Apanta: reply to Katerina K.', *E Gynaika*, 1(17), p. 52; Anonymous (9 May 1951) 'O Gynaikologos Apanta: reply to Athenaia K.A.', *E Gynaika*, 2(34), p. 40. For reasons of 'normalising the period' emmenagogues are recommended also in the cases: Anonymous (7 March 1951), 'O Gynaikologos Apanta: Mia dystyhismene E.K', *E Gynaika*, 2(29), p. 30; Anonymous (7 March 1951) 'O Gynaikologos Apanta: E Dystehismene', *E Gynaika*, 2(29), p. 30. The reply to MSG recommends estro-prol or prosyclo and, once the period returns, progynon etc. (Anonymous (19 April 1951) 'O Gynaikologos Apanta: MSG', *E Gynaika*, 2(32), p. 52).
133. Anonymous (6 September 1950), 'O Gynaikologos Apanta: Veatrike', *E Gynaika*, 1(16), p. 49.
134. Anonymous (13 December 1950) 'O Gynaikologos Apanta: Veatrike A.K.', *E Gynaika*, 1(23), p. 19.
135. Elphis Christopher, *Sexuality and Birth Control in Social and Community Work* (London: Maurice Temple Smith, 1980), pp. 252–3. GPs were subsequently advised not to prescribe such tablets because of the possibility of foetal abnormalities.
136. Anonymous (9 May 1951) 'O Gynaikologos Apanta: Triestina F.', *E Gynaika*, 2(34), p. 40.
137. Anonymous (29 November 1950) 'O Gynaikologos Apanta: Mia Kastoriane', *E Gynaika*, 1(22), p. 61.
138. The use of pills by women who wanted to abort was also mentioned in an interview with an elderly physician, although she called these abortifacients (ektrotika farmaka) (No. 3D, Athens 2010). The physician graduated in the late 1960s and referred to that and later times. See also Ioannes Danezes (1969) 'E tehnete ektrosis os diethnes kai Ellenikon provlema', *Iatrike*, 15(3), 195; Antonia Polychronopoulou (1967) 'E en Elladi Syhnotes ton Apoxeseon tes Metras' (unpublished PhD thesis: Athens University), p. 11. Danezes argued that the use of abortifacients and emmenagogues in the 1960s was very rare.
139. For such a shift taking place in Bangladesh, where both traditional and modern methods are available in parallel, see Heidi Bart Johnston (2001) 'Regulating menstruation in Matlab, Bangladesh: Women's practices and perspectives' in Van de Walle and Renne (eds), *Regulating Menstruation*, pp. 220–40.
140. See Georges, *Bodies of Knowledge*, pp. 103–7; Mpimpe-Papaspuropoulou, *Paradosiake Iatrike*; Haviara-Karahaliou, *E Laike*. Herbal emmenagogues were on sale in France until the early 1960s (Van de Walle, 'Flowers and Fruits', 197).

141. Konstantinos Metropoulos (1954) *Ygieine tes Egkyou. Pleres Parousiase tes Viologias tes Syllepses* (Athens: Papademetriou), pp. 142–3. Diamantopoulos also cites the case of an unmarried young woman who, having fallen pregnant, took a number of 'pills in the hope that I would be saved'. She haemorrhaged and, after resorting to a doctor, had an abortion (D. Diamantopoulos, *Iatrike Egkyklopaideia tes Gynaikas* (Athens: Gerolympou, 1957), p. 36)
142. Metropoulos, *Ygieine*, pp. 134, 137, 144, 148. Similar advice provided in K. Louros (1926–34) 'Ektrosis', in *Megale Ellenike Egkyklopaideia*, ed. Paulos Dandrakes, vol. 9, 2nd edn (Athens: Pyrsos), p. 850.
143. Tryfon Andrianakos (1937) 'Exelixis kai Proodoi tes Maieutikes kai Gynaikologias en te Neotera Ellada', *Ellenike Iatrike*, 11, 49.
144. Anonymous, 'Maieutike Gynaikologia: Siebke', 1223. In 1943 it was one of the items confiscated by the goverment (Mykonos Library, Mykonos Archive DAM/B/30, 5 May 1943, Egkyklioi Ypourgeiou Oikonomikon pros Teloneiakes Arhes 1940, 1942–44, Arithmos Protokolou E 4878, Arithmos Egkykliou 53, Ypourgeio Oikonomikon pros tas Teloneiakas Arhas tou Kratous).
145. No. 11 Athens. The informant referred to 'pills that you take when the period is late; you take a couple of pills for the period to come' (No. 11, interview in Athens; informant lived most of her life in mainland Greece in one of the Epirus towns, born in 1938, married in 1959).
146. Pyrros utilised both terms (Pyrros, *Egkolpion*). Colloquial use: Mpimpe-Papaspuropoulou, *Paradosiake Iatrike*, p. 323. The author used oral history in her investigation of popular medicines prescribed by untrained empirical practitioners. The recommendation was to use boiled rye and to drink the potion; No. 11 Athens.
147. Drandakes, *Megale Ellenike*.
148. Zaganiares refers to *Artemisia absinthium*, *Petroselinum sativum* and *Ruta graveolens* (Zaganiares, *Ta Farmakeutika*, pp. 14–15, 49, 57). As the author says, 'its fruit constitutes in the popular therapeutics a known emmenagogue' (p. 49).
149. These were rue, oleander and fennel respectively (Xen. G. Anagnostopoulos (1961) *Ta Votana. Laike Farmakologia kai Therapeutike* (Athens: n.p.)).
150. Pyrros, *Egkolpion*, vol. 1, p. 195.
151. Triantes, *Egheiridion*, p. 125.
152. Kostes, *Egheiridion*, p. 68.
153. Kostes, *Egheiridion*, p. 68.
154. Konsolas, *Egheiridion*, pp. 55–7.
155. Triantes, *Egheiridion*, pp. 130–1. Similar doubts over women's judgement of quickening were expressed by Kostes, *Egheiridion*, p. 101.

156. Triantes, *Egheiridion*, pp. 130–1.
157. Pyrros, *Egkolpion*, vol. 1, p. 196. Earlier works also caution pregnant women to avoid some, otherwise regular, treatments such as enemas (Manou, *Giatrosofia*, p. 54).
158. Metropoulos, *Ygieine*, p. 51. Identical with M. Moyseides (1927) *Ygieine tes Egkyou, Epitokou, Lehoidos, kai tes Galouhouses* (Alexandreia: Kasigone), p. 7.
159. Triantes, *Egheiridion*, p. 125.
160. Vasileios Parlapanes (2014) 'E Iatrodikastike sten Ellada Mesa apo Demosieumata tou 19ou kai ton Arhon tou 20ou Aiona' (unpublished P h D thesis: Aristoteleio University Thessaloniki), p. 117, citing D.A. Kallivokas (1895) *Iatrodikastike (kata A. Lutaud): Kata ten Elleniken Nomothesian*, 3rd edn (Athens: N. Tzaka).
161. Joseph Brown Cooke (1900) *A manual of obstetrical technique as applied to private practice; with a chapter on abortion, premature labor, and curettage* (Philadelphia and London: J.P. Lippincott), p. 18. Similar difficulties existed in late Imperial China (Yi-Li Wu (2010) *Reproducing Women: Medicine, Metaphor, and Childbirth in late Imperial China* (Berkeley: University of California Press), pp. 123–7). For early modern Europe, when much was in doubt to the very end of a pregnancy, see Clive, 'Hidden Truths', pp. 209–27.
162. The colloquial name of such a pregnancy was *arpahtra* (the snatcher) (Tryfon K. Andrianakos (1907) *Ai aimorragiai en te Maieutike kai Gynaikologia* (Athens: A. Sakellarios), p. 51).
163. L. Mantas (1945–60) 'Amvlosis', in *Evdomadiaia Egkyklopaidike Epitheorese O Elios*, vol. 2 (Athens: Elios), p. 480. This would refer to the first half of the twentieth century.
164. Kontos, *Peri Examvloseos*, p. 7. Similar definition is provided by W. Tyler Smith, according to whom moles 'are the result of impregnation … consisting of different forms of degeneration of the membranes of the ovum' (W. Tyler Smith (5 April 1856) 'Molar pregnancy—Blighted Ova', *The Lancet*, 67(1701), 361).
165. Triantes, *Egheiridion*, p. 306. Kostes, *Egheiridion*, p. 68.
166. Mihael G. Kaires (1909) *Praktikos Odegos tou Iatrou kai tes Maias. E Maia anaplerousa ton Iatron* (Athens: Raftane-Papageorgiou), p. 471.
167. M. Venizelos (1881) *Maieutike* (Athens: n.p.), pp. 276–8. Tyler, a British physician, adds that only occasionally a 'small embryo of two or three weeks' growth' would be discernible in a molar pregnancy (Smith, 'Molar pregnancy', 361).
168. Konsolas, *Egheiridion*, pp. 64–5.

169. Triantes, *Egheiridion*, p. 306; Vitsares, *Nosoi*, p. 417. Again, these remarks are in agreement with those by Smith, 'Molar pregnancy', 361–2.
170. For example, a case was reported in 1837 in the Greek medical journal *Asklepios*, translated from a British journal (Anonymous (1 July 1837) 'Myle ragoeides (mola vesicularis) me syneparhousan kyesin. Ek tes efemeridas tou Kasperou', *Asklepios*, IB, 416). See also earlier references and Venizelos, *Maieutike*, p. 8; Konsolas, *Egheiridion*, pp. 64–5; Konstantinos Louros (1916) *Maieutike* (Athens, P.A. Sakkelariou), p. 420.
171. Cases of 5 December 1842, 11 November 1857, 2 August 1858, 13 February 1882 and 22 January 1883, all cited in Tryfon K. Andrianakos (1929) *E Maieutike kai Gynaikologia kata ten diadromen tou viou tes Iatrikes Etaireias Athenon 1835–1908* (Athens: S.K. Vlastou), p. 51.
172. Parlapanes, *E Iatrodikastike*, p. 118 citing A.D. Kallivokas (1895) *Iatrodikastike (kata A. Lutaud): Kata ten Elleniken Nomothesian*, 3rd edn (Athens: N. Tzaka); A. Lacassagne (1897) *Ypodeigmata Iatrodikastikon Ektheseon kai Autopsion: Parartema 'Iatrikes Proodou'*, translated Ioannes A. Foustanos (Syros: Renieres-Printezes).
173. See, for example, M. Andral (5 January 1833) 'Mental Alienation', *The Lancet*, 19(488), 462; E. Tilt (1851) *On the diseases of menstruation and ovarian inflammation* (New York: Samuel S. and William Wood), p. 237; Edward Calthrop (3 April 1869) 'On the diagnosis of accidental haemorrhage from placenta praevia', *The Lancet*, 93(2379), 458–9. Patricia Crawford (1981) 'Attitudes to menstruation in seventeenth-century England', *Past and Present*, 91, 64, especially fn 103, referring to seminal works such as *Aristotle's Master-piece*, discussing molar pregnancies.
174. Kontos, *Peri Examvloseos*, p. 7. Kostes argued that this happened between the third and fifth month (p. 101).
175. Vitsares, *Nosoi*, p. 417. Vitsares' book is a compilation of translated French, German and English gynaecology texts (p. γ).
176. Vitsares, *Nosoi*, p. 418.
177. Kaires, *Praktikos Odegos*, p. 472.
178. Kostes, *Egheiridion*, pp. 105–6.
179. Kaires, *Praktikos Odegos*, p. 471.
180. Smith, 'Molar pregnancy', 363.
181. Clement Godson (1878/1879) 'Remarks on two cases of Vesicular Mole', *Obstetrics Journal of Great Britain and Ireland*, 6, p. 703.
182. Afentoules, *Farmakologia*, vol. 2, pp. 361–4.
183. Anna Katsigra (1908) *E Maieutike en te praxei* (Athens: Auge Athenon), pp. 164–5.
184. V.A. Fotakes (January 1924) 'Ypo poias peristaseis dikaiologeitai e iatrike amvlosis?' *Iatrike Proodos*, 39(1), 8. The difficulty of detecting molar pregnancy remains to date. The two main methods are a blood test and

an ultrasound scan (https://www.ouh.nhs.uk/patient-guide/leaflets/files/5266Pmolarpregnancy.pdf, p. 3, accessed 6 July 2019). Hydatidiform mole refers to a mass of grapelike vesicles.

185. See chapter 6 on Law in Greece.
186. Haralapos Tzortzopoulos (1926) *Sholia eis ton Ishyonta Ellenikon Poinikon Nomon, Teuhos 1, Egklemata kata tes zoes kai tou somatos* (Athens: Athena), p. 185. Also Mantas, 'Amvlosis', p. 480.
187. I. Pontikopoulou (10 January 1932) 'Einai Egklema e Ektrosis?' *Makedonia*, 22(6969), p. 3.
188. Triantes, *Egheiridion*, p. 307; Katsigra, *E Maieutike*, pp. 163–4.
189. Kontos, *Peri examvloseos*. On the extensive use of abortion in the Ottoman Empire see Alan Duben and Cem Behar (1991) *Istanbul Households: Marriage, Family and Fertility, 1880–1940* (Cambridge: Cambridge University Press), pp. 81–3, 188; and Tuba Demirci and Selçuk Akşin Somel (2008) 'Women's bodies, demography, and public health: abortion policy and perspectives in the Ottoman Empire of the nineteenth century', *Journal of the History of Sexuality*, 17(3), 417–18. Induced abortion is also explicitly mentioned in a medical publication of 1894, although the author does not elaborate beyond the statement that 'this crime is not rare' in Greece (Kardaras, *Praktike Iatrike*, 47).
190. Kontos, *Peri Examvloseos*, pp. 10–15.
191. Kontos, *Peri Examvloseos*, pp. 10, 11.
192. Kontos, *Peri Examvloseos*, p. 11. Kontos does not indicate which those purgatives are. In 1944 Mpertsekas lists what he considers to be purgatives: aloe, ergot, apiol, absinthe, savin, rue and so on (Mpertsekas, *Oi Kindynoi*, p. 15).
193. Kontos, *Peri Examvloseos*, pp. 12–15.
194. Kontos, *Peri Examvloseos*, p. 14.
195. Kontos, *Peri Examvloseos*, pp. 12–13. Kontos cites Dioskourides here as the source of knowledge.
196. Kontos, *Peri Examvloseos*, p. 20. The insertion of a sponge was reported as the reason for the death of a woman, owing to perforation of the uterus. The doctors who performed the autopsy reported to the Athens Medical Society meeting of 15 December 1884 that this was done 'for criminal reasons' (Tryfon K. Andrianakos (1929) *E Maieutike kai Gynaikologia kata ten diadromen tou viou tes Iatrikes Etaireias Athenon 1835–1908* (Athens: S.K. Vlastou), p. 30).The use of goose quill is also mentioned by Malcolm Potts, Peter Diggory and John Peel ((1977) *Abortion* (Cambridge: Cambridge University Press), p. 258). Treated (waxed) sponges and laminaria were used as cervical dilators by physicians (Afentoules, *Farmakologia*, vol. 3, pp. 272–4). Historically we are aware of the use of dried seaweed in Japan, dried asparagus in China and slippery elm in London (Potts et al., *Abortion*, pp. 261–2).

197. Kontos, *Peri Examvloseos*, pp. 15, 16.
198. Kontos, *Peri Examvloseos*, p. 20.
199. Konstantinos Merkourios (1914) 'Dyo Neai Methodoi Egklematikes Ektroseos', *Iatrike Proodos*, 19, 1.
200. Merkourios, 'Dyo neai', 2.
201. Hristodoulos Ant. Kampoures, *Therapeutikai kai Koinonikai Endeikseis tes Tehnetes Ektroseos* (Athens: Georgiou Vasileiou, 1933), pp. 8–9; Konstantinos N. Louros (15 May 1896) 'Peri apoxeseos tes metras kai ton pros tauten endeikseon', *Galenos*, 26, 8–9.
202. Kampoures, *Therapeutikai*, p. 8.
203. B Obstetrics and gynaecology clinic, University (Aretaioion Hospital) (Mpertsekas, *Oi kindynoi*, p. 39).
204. Mpertsekas, *Oi Kindynoi*, p. 11.
205. The information available for the dead women was too scarce to enable their inclusion in the discussion.
206. Mpertsekas, *Oi kindynoi*, p. 14.
207. Mpertsekas, *Oi kindynoi*, p. 14.
208. See also such a case for Rhodes, revealed through oral history, referring to the pre-World War II period (Georges, *Bodies of knowledge*, p. 111).
209. Mpertsekas, *Oi kindynoi*, pp. 14–15.
210. Georges, *Bodies of knowledge*, p. 109. I changed the author's translation at the very start of the quote from 'When we were delayed, *kathisterimeni*' to 'When we were late'. Women in Rhodes were also aware of rue and were employing it as both an emmenagogue and an abortifacient (Georges, *Bodies of knowledge*, pp. 110–11).
211. Georges, *Bodies of knowledge*, p. 109.
212. Blum and Blum, *Health and Healing*, p. 76.
213. Blum and Blum, *Health and Healing*, p. 154.
214. Blum and Blum, *Health and Healing*, p. 76.

CHAPTER 5

The Physician's Method: Curettage

In the previous chapter we saw how physicians supported women's desire to regulate their menstruation by providing them with modern emmenagogues. And, while there is no evidence that they were ever involved in the provision of abortifacients, they played a pivotal role in the provision of curettage.

The earliest reference to curettage (apoxesis) comes in a meeting of the Athens Medical Society on May 28, 1888, where the physician Alexandrogiannos presented the beneficial effects of curettage on a woman who suffered from haemorrhagic endometritis.[1] The subsequent discussion focused on whether dilation was necessary or not. Another late-nineteenth-century author, Antonios Kindynes, in his 1889 book discussing sterility, recommended dilation for those patients suffering from vaginal stenosis, a condition that, it was believed, led to dysmenorrhoea and sterility but could also cause metritis and parametritis.[2] Candles, metallic pessaries and laminaria were among the methods Kindynes suggested.[3] The use of laminaria and candles in order to treat stenosis and aplasia of the uterus, both seen as causes of sterility, continued well into the twentieth century.[4] On December 14, 1891, Alexandrogiannos again discussed the beneficial effects of the use of curettage, in this case for puerperal infection, in front of the Athens Medical Society.[5] K. Louros, who observed it being 'frequently' practised in Berlin and Munich, and where he had performed it

V. Hionidou, *Abortion and Contraception in Modern Greece, 1830–1967*, Medicine and Biomedical Sciences in Modern History,
https://doi.org/10.1007/978-3-030-41490-0_5

himself, also discussed curettage in 1896.[6] Many Greek gynaecologists were trained in Germany and thus they would have been familiar with the methods practised there.

Louros recommended curettage for patients suffering from endometritis, but only after the more benign therapeutic methods had been applied: namely, douching, tampons and scarification.[7] He also recommended curettage for cases of metritis and menorrhagia.[8] He was clearly at the forefront of his profession in Greece, as J.W. Ballantyne, in his short history of curettage written at the end of the nineteenth century, identified 1878 as the watershed year when the method started to become known among physicians worldwide.[9] Already in 1899, in a book entitled *On the Curettage of the Uterus in Obstetrics and Gynaecology*, we are informed that 'curettage is not unknown in Greece'; indeed, it was 'a daily incident today in Greece both in midwifery and gynaecology'[10] and had been performed by Professor Theodoros Aretaios, who had died as early as 1893.[11] Starting with the statement that it would not be an exaggeration to suggest that for most of the illnesses of the uterus the physician should 'have the curette in hand', Th. Saktoures explained in detail how and when to perform curettage.[12] He recommended curettage for metritis and sterility, specifying in detail their possible causes, among them endometritis, salpingitis and atresia.[13] For midwifery, like some of his colleagues, he argued that curettage was recommended during the early months of a 'pathological pregnancy when we are certain that the pregnancy threatens the life of the mother and that the only way to save the mother is to expel the egg from the uterus'.[14] Illnesses that endangered the mother's life included, according to Saktoures, pernicious vomiting, jaundice, nephritis, corruption of the nervous system and heart conditions. He stressed that the decision to perform an induced abortion had to be taken 'in conference with a colleague, except for emergencies'.[15]

Both Louros and Saktoures emphasised that there were no dangers in performing curettage, especially when the rules of the procedure were followed. Saktoures was explicit in indicating that it did not cause sterility, as some suggested, while Louros detailed the responsibility of the physician to detect an early pregnancy, if there was one, and avoid using the method in such cases: 'There is no doubt that curettage can result in abortion .... But this is a proof of the lightness with which in many occasions physicians approach gynaecological surgery.' And Louros added, 'The physicians should be responsible and knowledgeable so that they can recognise pregnancy in its early stages; they should examine thoroughly the patients to find out if she is pregnant or not.'[16]

Such enthusiastic support for the potential of this method in resolving sterility and many other gynaecological problems continued into the following decades. For example, in 1904 D. Theodorides, a practising physician in Athens, published a short paper on curettage in a French medical journal,[17] while in 1930 Vasos Verges published a very detailed textbook on curettage, although he chose to focus only on gynaecological issues. His introduction presents curettage as a panacea to women's problems: 'Curettage is a simple and very useful operation, removing many and diverse illnesses of the uterus (bleeding, growths, changes in the walls due to an infection, etc.) and restoring health to its natural state.'[18]

While some hailed curettage as a ground-breaking method, others saw it only as the continuation of earlier practices, such as using hands to clean the uterus, a very common practice according to Nikolaos Petsales.[19] Introduced by Doleris in the 1880s, dilation, curettage and douching were perfected by Pozzi and Pinard, producing 'today's accepted' and widely practised therapy for sterility.[20] Dilation and curettage (D&C) was, as intimated above, the method suggested to overcome the most common gynaecological ailments in turn-of-the-century Greece. But while eminent authors—Saktoures, Verges, Petsales and Louros among them—offered their support to this method, to what degree was it adopted in the practice of gynaecology and obstetrics?

The published summary reports of inpatients of the Athens University Surgery clinic in 1892–1893 list, under urinary and reproductive organs of women, 21 inpatients, 12 of whom were suffering from 'acute and chronic inflammation of the uterus' and two with abortion-related issues.[21] Among the twelve women mentioned above, six were diagnosed with endometritis. All were treated with dilation, curettage and douching 'successfully, none of them returned showing further complications'.[22] Three other women suffering from post-partum metritis and uterus abscesses were treated with douching. For the two abortion cases—both noted in the report as 'natural abortions', that is miscarriages—no curettage was employed. Interestingly, the three women suffering from acute metritis were treated with leeches 'applied locally'.[23] The 1904 report cites 166 women who were treated in the hospital for illnesses of the reproductive system. In thirteen cases curettage was performed, although in all cases this was done after a long list of other, somewhat less invasive treatments.

Thus, five women were treated by curettage for chronic metritis (out of fifteen suffering from the condition); 5 (out of 20) for catarrhal metritis; and three (out of fourteen) for haemorrhagic metritis.[24] In two cases of natural abortion, curettage was performed.[25] The private clinic of Papaioannou during its operation and until the end of 1908 treated 79 (out of 91) cases of chronic inflammation of the uterus, two cases of polypus and a case of natural abortion successfully with D&C.[26] The sources suggest that curettage was increasingly known and practised only in hospitals and private clinics from at least 1892 onwards. It was utilised almost exclusively for women's ailments and only rarely for post-abortion or post-partum operations prior to 1909.

The patients' book of the private obstetrics and gynaecology clinic of Soterios Sofianopoulos in Patras gives us a picture of how and when curettage was employed in the period April 1909 to November 1928.[27] An advertisement placed in the local press in 1910 informs the reader that the director of the clinic was educated in Paris and that the clinic treated female ailments and particularly sterility. The advert also indicated that facilities existed to care for pregnant women, who would reside in private rooms in the clinic.[28] Indeed, deliveries took place there, although these involved less than 5% of all patients treated in the clinic. The most common diagnoses among the patients were abortion/*ektrosis* (this did not refer to induced abortion), metritis and endometritis, all of which were treated with curettage in the clinic.[29] In only three cases do the notes mention that an abortion had been initiated—in one case by the woman (patient no. 88, 14 weeks pregnant) and in another by a midwife (patient number 1033); in the third case the patient was diagnosed with haemorrhagic metritis and her notes indicate that this could have been a result of induced abortion, as her husband had long been absent (patient no. 145). It is interesting to note that many of the deliveries were of illegitimate children, all of who were taken to the local asylum within 24 hours of their birth. For almost all of those deliveries the notes were written in French, which we can assume was done in an effort to protect the single mother and to conceal, to a degree, the embarrassing situation. No such effort was made for the cases recorded as abortions, which were all recorded in Greek.

The treatments women received in the Sofianopoulos clinic reflected the practical application of Saktoures' textbook, in which metritis and endometritis (51% of all admissions when deliveries are ignored) and incomplete abortions (9% of all admissions when deliveries are ignored) were invariably treated with curettage; polypus was treated only occasionally with curettage; and post-partum infections (17%) were treated through cleansing the uterus with the fingers, followed by douching. In the cases of abortion the month of pregnancy was noted as well as the reason for entering the clinic (e.g., 'retention of the egg' or 'retention of the placenta' is the most common diagnosis). Some of the incomplete abortions mentioned may well have been induced ones. A significant percentage of the 'metritis' cases are accompanied by comments indicating the woman's sterility or comments that suggest that sterility—in many cases secondary—was the problem.[30] The single most common treatment performed in the Sofianopoulos clinic was thus curettage (52.5% of cases), irrespective of the cause.

A similar situation can be seen in the hospital records of Hios. Though this was a general hospital, gynaecological problems were also treated there. Our sample of records covers the years 1938–1943 and is a systematic sample of one in every ten patients entering the hospital.[31] Again, the records demonstrate that curettage was routinely used as a therapeutic method. It was employed in every single case of endometritis, and was invariably used where a miscarriage (apovole) or abortion (ektrosis) (whether induced or spontaneous was not clarified) was mentioned, usually indicating an 'incomplete' abortion (hence the necessity of curettage).[32] Among the 483 records concerning women aged 15–50 who entered the hospital in that period for any reason, 42 curettages were performed.

It seems, therefore, that Greek physicians were very familiar with curettage and were able to manage the after-effects of natural and induced abortions that took place outside the hospital.[33] They also used D&C readily and extensively for the most common gynaecological problems, such as metritis and endometritis. In the 1930s, curettage (or the use of fingers/hands for those who preferred the old ways—for example, in 1908 Katsigra insisted that curettage should be used only if the prior use of hands had not resolved the problem[34]) was utilised widely by physicians, especially in hospitals and clinics.[35]

The figures cited above demonstrate that only a proportion of the curettages performed were for the purposes of induced abortion. The close association between metritis/endometritis and sterility and the adoption of curettage as a cure for those conditions, and therefore sterility, was well known and widely accepted; even the eminent gynaecologist and committed anti-abortionist N.K. Louros recommended curettage in his 1948 textbook for cases of menorrhagia, aiming to ultimately cure the patient and enable her to conceive.[36] However, in 1940 and in the 1950s concerns were raised about the intensive use of curettage as a cure for sterility. V. Maroule, in his presentation to the Obstetrics and Gynaecological Association of Athens in 1940, suggested to his fellow gynaecologists that they should be more restrained in 'performing curettage which should be performed only in those cases where there is immediate danger to the life of the woman due to heavy bleeding and in no other case, let alone in cases of sterility and with the aim to cure [sterility]',[37] while in a 1950 issue of the popular women's magazine *E Gynaika* the gynaecologist advised the reader who wrote expressing her concerns about potential sterility that 'we do not recommend curettage, worse things can happen [as a result]'.[38] Interestingly, the reader had not even tried to become pregnant at that point; however, she was aware that curettage could help 'cure' sterility. A 1955 publication focusing on curettage stressed that 'in the past, curettage as a cure of sterility had many supporters'—but no more, the author added.[39] Nevertheless, the same author recommended the method as a treatment for metritis, employing both candles and laminaria for dilation.[40] By 1957 curettage was no longer recommended in a lay medical encyclopaedia as a treatment for metritis.[41] It is probably safe to say that sometime in the 1960s curettage stopped being used for such reasons; already by 1957 one gynaecologist was recommending vaginal suppositories.[42] However, since earlier in the twentieth century private clinics had emphasised in their advertisements their services to those who suffered from sterility, it would be safe to say that it was widely known as a 'cure' for sterility and a significant proportion of patients who were treated with curettage were seeking ways to overcome sterility and become fertile.

Curettage was thus an obstetric method that from an early point in time was readily adopted by Greek physicians of the highest standing. Detailed textbooks were published around 1900 and thereafter, and the method was recommended as a possible cure for sterility throughout the first half of the twentieth century; as a possible therapy for many women's ailments during the same period; and as a necessary operation for incomplete natural abortions (a practice that still continues). Almost certainly, this meant that it was also performed for incomplete induced abortions, although it is the above reasons that are presented as the causes for the treatment provided to female patients in the hospitals for which we have sources. That performing curettage on a woman who, unbeknown to all, was pregnant would result in abortion was also well known and stressed in all publications, so that such incidences would be avoided as far as possible. Indeed, Sofianopoulos discussed three such cases, naming these cases 'Grossesse méconnue'. It is possible, too, that some women may have sought to have an induced abortion carried out under a camouflaged diagnosis such as endometritis or metritis. This is what Valaoras argued for the 1950s and 1960s, as explained below, but there is no direct supporting evidence in the sources. Yet again, in many cases induced abortions were prescribed by physicians themselves for therapeutic reasons. Excessive vomiting was one such reason;[43] for example, in the 'Correspondence' column of the medical journal *Ellenike Iatrike* a question concerned a pregnancy of three months with excessive vomiting for which 'antiemetics, orexine, teint. [sic] noix vomiques, cocaine' had been prescribed by the attending physician without any result. Another physician suggested that the pregnant woman proceed with an 'interruption' of the pregnancy, leading the attending physician to seek advice from the journal.[44] The reply suggested an array of further substances that should be tried (ovoglandol, ringer, insulin) and that, if all those failed—but also if other symptoms were to appear, such as palpitations, change of the patient's colour and so on—then an interruption should take place.[45] Sofianopoulos did perform one such induced abortion after a diagnosis of 'excessive vomiting', although interestingly the notes referred to the 'emptying of the uterus' rather than to curettage. Earlier on, in 1900, Saktoures and, before him, Venizelos clearly articulated the reasons for carrying out therapeutic-induced abortions, which were performed in order to save the mother's life when it was threatened by the pregnancy.

As noted above, Valaoras, writing in 1969, stated that induced abortions (referring exclusively to curettages) were performed under the diagnosis of menorrhagia or menstrual disorders, effectively arguing that physicians misreported the illegal abortions they were performing.[46] It may well have been the case that virtually all reported curettages in the 1960s were cases of unwanted pregnancies and induced abortions but this was certainly not the case earlier in the century, when many women sought to be cured of sterility with the method that later on would become synonymous with the termination of pregnancy. However, even in the 1960s women employed curettage in order to 'cleanse' their uterus, enhance their fertility or stop menorrhagia.[47]

Greek gynaecologists in the twentieth century were very well versed in the provision of curettage and had the necessary training to perform it if required.[48] It was, as physicians writing prior to 1940 stated, a method used almost exclusively by trained medical professionals (indeed, its adoption by some midwives seems to have had grave consequences[49]). And, though he emphasised the 'scientificity' of curettage, in 1954 Konstantinos Metropoulos admitted that, even when performed by the most able physician, there were still potential dangers. Therefore, the exclusivity of the method to trained physicians was in sharp contrast, he argued, to the non-qualified practitioners and their methods.[50] So, after World War II physicians offered their clients 'scientific' methods, whether emmenagogues or abortion, in contrast to the 'traditional' methods of the midwives and of the women themselves, performed by female practitioners (abortionists) and midwives who were only interested, according to physicians, in their own enrichment.[51]

Who, When and How?

Despite its illegality from the moment of the Greek legal system's creation, abortion was neither prosecuted nor publicly discussed, as—some argued—such a discussion would further spread knowledge of it. A newspaper article from 1901 argued that, while fertility control occurred frequently in Athens, 'abortion occurs rarely, because it is more dangerous'.[52] Twenty years previously, however, the first physician to explicitly discuss induced abortion, Tryfon Kontos, had attempted to explain why it was so common in the early 1880s by quoting Tradieu, who had claimed that induced abortion in 'the east' was morally acceptable to that populace.[53] Kontos argued, rather exceptionally, that 'there are already physicians, midwives and others engaging in it' and that, therefore, they already possessed the necessary knowledge to perform abortions.[54] Timoleon Kardaras, in his 1894 *Family Medicine*, similarly suggested that criminal abortion was 'not rare',[55] although, unlike Kontos, he did not discuss methods of induced abortion. However, Kontos went further still in arguing that abortion was widely practised in the late nineteenth century. In discussing induced abortion in the 1890s, criminal forensic experts focused extensively on non-appliance methods, such as abortifacients, herbal and chemical preparations (cantharides, rue, arsenic and so on), leeches and violent blows to the abdomen,[56] although textbook methods, such as the use of catheters and needles, but also simply the insertion of the midwife's finger, were also mentioned. At the same time, 'most forensics', we are told, reported the use of abortifacient drinks and substances, but as they did not believe that these could actually cause an induced abortion—since science does 'not know whether any of those substances are effective'[57]—they were not categorised as such and presumably prosecution was not sought for those. Essentially, the use of popular methods of abortion was ignored by the medical elite as inefficient, unscientific and unmodern.[58] The confusion and lack of familiarity with the various methods that existed at this time, however, even among medical professionals, is exemplified by a 1914 article in a medical journal that presented two 'new' methods of induced abortion, the first involving the use of rubber catheter and a solution (the same method as presented 30 years earlier by Kontos as one that was widely used)[59] and the second involving the use of violence by the mother towards the foetus.[60] This indicates that the use of appliance abortion methods was very limited at the start of the twentieth century, and that methods such as curettage were not then used to procure abortions. In the mid-1920s an archimandrite discussing induced abortion referred to women who 'in many cases murder themselves too through the intake of drugs or other artificial means', clearly indicating the use of both sets of methods, old and new.[61]

Certainly, therefore, induced abortion occurred, but most such procedures were carried out on women carrying an illegitimate child. So, for example, in 1848 there is a reference in the minutes of the Medical Society to an induced abortion that a midwife performed on a single girl; the comment appeared more concerned with the 'uneducated midwife' than with the inappropriateness of the action, with the author, a physician, marvelling that 'empiricism has reached its ultimate degree'.[62] Further references to abortions of unmarried women are available, such as the one from Kos in 1867 and examples from early 1910s Athens.[63] In the early twentieth century the press referred to the fruits of illegitimate relationships in matter-of-fact language, whether the discovery of the bodies of twin foetuses in the sixth or seventh month of development, along with the 'pharmaceutical preparations that were used' to procure their abortion, or the physician who performed abortions on his servants who he had impregnated himself.[64] The memoirs of a gynaecologist practising in 1940s Athens also illustrate that such transgressions happened at all levels of society. He cites the case of a 18-year-old from a well-off family who visited him with her mother; on being found to be three months pregnant, the mother immediately proposed an induced abortion.[65] Similarly, a physician informant replied to my question about abortions on the island of Hios, where he had practised from the 1950s onwards, by outlining the 'necessity' of abortion in order to cover up serious transgressions:

> I can say to you, without feeling ashamed, yes. There was illegal love. There was illegal relationship. And with the sailors, when the sailor was away etc. There was the illegal relationship and there had been occurrences, occurrences, occurrences. And of course, abortion always existed. Abortions, so that something bad would not happen and [to avert the] breaking up of the family.[66]

Similar comments were made in the 1930s press and are numerically expressed in the illegitimacy rates of Greece, which have never been higher than 1.5% of all births from the mid-1920s onwards (Table 5.1).[67] In the absence of national figures, the illegitimacy rates of Mykonos provide a guide as to what the levels may have been prior to that. In the period from 1854 to 1928 the illegitimacy rate for Mykonos was consistently below 2.5%, while after 1928 the rate was below 1.5—that is, in line with the national figure.[68] This decline in the illegitimacy rates from the 1930s is most certainly associated with the wider availability of induced abortion, not necessarily on Mykonos but in Athens.

Table 5.1 Illegitimacy rates in Greece, 1926–1969

Year	*Illegitimate births per 1000 live births*	*Illegitimate births per 1000 married women aged 15–44 years*
1926–1928	12.3	–
1936–1938	13.2	–
1956	14.5	1.2
1957	15.1	1.2
1958	13.5	1.1
1959	13.0	1.1
1960	12.3	1.0
1961	12.2	1.0
1962	11.5	0.9
1963	11.9	0.9
1964	10.9	0.8
1965	10.5	0.8
1966	9.9	0.8
1967	9.8	0.8
1968	10.8	0.9
1969	11.2	0.9

Source: Charalampos Zianicas (1976) *Evolution Démographique de la Grèce Contemporaine. Etude de la Nuptialité* (unpublished PhD thesis: University de Dijon), p. 111

References from the mid-1920s onwards and without interruption until the 1980s refer to the epidemic of abortions taking place. In the 1930s, medics and others referred to the 'heap' of abortions among all social classes in urban places.[69] Glaringly clear in the existing sources is the widespread incidence of abortions in urban centres. The first editorial in *Macedonia* in 1930 referred to the high number of induced abortions taking place in Thessaloniki—where the newspaper was based—while one of the authors, a gynaecologist based in Athens, remarked that if the secrets of physicians' professional archives were ever to be revealed they would unfold an 'innumerable multitude of cases demonstrating that abortion had become a great social necessity'.[70] The authors, and the overwhelming majority of physicians, argued that when they had to refuse an abortion because it was illegal the pregnant women would seek one from midwives or possibly even their own neighbour, often with grave consequences.[71]

Although the wide availability and practice of abortion in urban areas was thus not disputed by anyone from 1925 onwards,[72] its availability and frequency in rural areas were much less clear. Some professed that none happened in rural areas;[73] others, referring to exactly the same time period, argued that among those practising birth control in villages situated near a town abortion was also used, provided it could be afforded.[74] In 1930 A. Doxiadis suggested that the members of the 'lower class' were not using abortion often, but that this was not due to their lack of interest in it but rather to the difficulties associated with its performance.[75] Furthermore, the author argued that, while well-off women received abortions from gynaecologists in their private clinics—the whole process being termed 'a small surgery'—the poor were 'paying with their own lives' for any such attempt, and their acts were called 'crimes'.[76] It can only be assumed that physicians such as Doxiadis, like the forensic experts of earlier decades, did not classify the use of abortifacients as 'abortion'.

Finding a physician or midwife to perform it in urban areas in exchange for a relatively small payment (which would nevertheless have been substantial for rural dwellers) appears, thus, not to have been an issue. The oral interviews also articulate the availability—through either physicians or midwives—and practice of abortion on Hios from the 1920s onwards, and in the town of Hermoupolis, on the island of Syros, during the early 1940s, where abortions were performed by midwives in the hospital, although for nearby Mykonos the only evidence of women obtaining abortions was in the cases of those who were living in or travelled to Athens from the 1930s onwards.

Q. Did you know women who did something? …
A. Yes, yes, I did not use those.
Q. Others? Where were they going? Here on Mykonos? Or …
A. They would go to Athens, they had abortion, they did curettage … around 1940. Around that time. Many were going … You asked me if I went. I did go and had curettage. I went once. Around 1960 [it was actually in the late 1930s] it was … because my husband did not want. He did not want me to go and he was saying 'so many years we have not had a child. Let's have one now'. But I would not have been able to carry on with my job! … Anyway, I tell him I have a pain, I will go to the physician. So he [my husband] let me go and I left. And I went and I found a friend and I told her and straight away …
Q. Was it still early?
A. There had been 20 days [delay of the period]. And I said [to the physician] 'Am I pregnant after all? And he said you are. He cleansed me [me katharise].[77] That is my sin. You are the first one I said it to …
Q. Was it a physician? Was it not a midwife?
A. No.
Q. Did you have any problems or were you all right?
A. No, nothing bothered me. I sat for half an hour, an hour on the bed in the hospital, then I got up and went home.[78]

Writing 15 years after Doxiadis, Panteles Mpertsekas argued that, among Athenians, the poor employed abortion in order to control their childbearing, whereas the affluent employed contraception.[79] Thus, he signals the increased uptake of induced abortions by the lower socio-economic groups as a method of controlling their fertility within the period 1930–1944. However, for quite some time old and new methods co-existed, as uptake of new ideas and preferences varied across the population. Alexandros Tsakires comments on the case of a servant girl, probably one who originated from rural Greece but resided at the time in an urban centre:

> She will seek help from a midwife 'an angel maker'. An abortion will be doubly dangerous since it will take place in secrecy, without skill and not in time, that is, when the foetus has advanced development, usually after the second month. This happens because precious time was wasted in order to experiment unsuccessfully with abortifacients, the drinks and prozynon injections.[80]

Abortions among single women were a relative commonplace in Greek society. What was new, at least to some, in the 1920s were abortions among married women. Referring to induced abortion in 1924, an archimandrite condemned the 'hedonistic spirit ... that teaches and convinces women to avoid the family burdens of childbearing'.[81] Among the nineteen women who were admitted to the gynaecology hospital in the years 1932–1936 following an attempted abortion seventeen were married, and some of those had had previous abortion experiences.[82] That married women were the ones having induced abortions after World War II as well is clear from all sources, including contemporary physicians: 'It was also because it would happen by chance to have too many children and maybe one delivery after the other, then a termination of the pregnancy would take place.'[83] Even in the late 1970s, among sampled single Athenian university students, including those who originated from rural areas, only 10% admitted to have had experienced an induced abortion.[84] The percentage among married women in the early 1960s was 45.1.[85]

By 1950 it was not unusual for women to have had repeated experiences of abortion, indicating that it was not a one-off 'accident'.[86] The gynaecologist advising women through a women's magazine column 'The gynaecologist replies' had no doubts about that when he replied to one correspondent: 'The neurosis of the stomach, the psychological shock etc. are due to repeated abortions.'[87] At the same time, Metropoulos clearly differentiates between villages, where traditional methods of inducing abortion were used (such as warm baths, 'traditional' medicines, inserting objects and/or hands into the uterus), and urban places, where curettages and physicians performing them seemed to have been the norm, although midwives did continue to practise there too.[88] Others corroborated Metropoulos' assessment. For example, in the mainland villages that Blum and Blum studied in late 1950s and early 1960s women used such traditional methods extensively but abortions by physicians and midwives were also sought, although these would take place in Athens, to which pregnant women would travel.[89] The ethical code of the Greek countryside did not permit curettages to take place in rural areas, since this would become quickly public knowledge. Both the trained and non-trained midwives practising in the villages would consult young pregnant village women in Athens, where they would invite those villagers in need of discretion, mostly to perform abortions in secret.[90]

In the rich study on induced abortion conducted by V.G. Valaoras, Antonia Polychronopoulou and Dimitri Trichopoulos in the early 1960s, the authors chose to focus on curettage as the abortion method.[91] However, Polychronopoulou, the only female physician of the team, outlined in her own thesis the existence of 'traditional' abortion methods and noted that she chose to ignore them because of their ineffectiveness: 'pharmaceutical or chemical means act mostly as emmenagogues; only exceptionally or in toxic doses can these achieve the interruption of an existing pregnancy.'[92] Moreover, she added that 'induced abortions achieved through mechanical or chemical means are part of the popular tradition and are performed by numerous and irresponsible people'.[93] In contrast, curettage—performed, according to Polychronopoulou, exclusively by physicians and trained midwives—impacted on medical ethics, according to the author, and thus, she felt, 'was of far greater importance'.[94] Thus it was the interests of those physicians who conducted the survey that led to its focusing exclusively on curettage, rather than examining what was happening in Greece, what the women themselves thought they were trying to achieve and how they went about it. This is also demonstrated by the exclusive use of a non-Greek bibliography employed in the co-authored article. Thus, Polychronopoulou's and the survey's estimates of induced abortion are certainly underestimates of total induced abortions, especially so prior to the 1950s and for rural areas. An important part of rural women's reasoning in continuing to use traditional methods, even in the early 1960s, was the impossibility of accessing locally a physician willing to undertake curettage, the difficulty involved in finding a midwife who was able to perform a surgical procedure in a village, and the consequent need to travel to the nearby urban centre for an induced abortion, with the considerable travel and professional expenses involved.[95] Even in the early 1980s one of the reasons put forward for the legalisation of abortion was the 'inconvenience of going to a doctor in the main town (40 miles away) and incurring travel costs as well as the cost of the operation', something that certainly continued to happen at the time, but also after the liberalisation of abortion.[96] Interestingly, a lack of information about where to find a physician willing and able to perform abortions has never been put forward as a problem, despite the fact that advertising related to abortion was illegal from 1950.[97] However, it was never illegal for physicians to advertise their gynaecological practice and this was very widespread throughout the study period.

The work of Valaoras et al. reveals that in the urban populations of Athens and Thessaloniki more women admitted having abortions, and more abortions, than in the rural areas. The estimated number of abortions in the urban centres equalled that of live births.[98] When looking at the women who admitted having had a curettage, 31.6 of rural women did so while 39.7 of urban women did (the preponderance of urban women was consistent across all age groups).[99] The corresponding percentages for women aged 45 and over were 36.8 and 40.3%, respectively. Valaoras et al. further differentiated between Athens, Thessaloniki and the smaller urban centres. The corresponding percentages of women admitting to abortion were 44% and 39%, respectively. Thus, more than a third of all women, urban and rural, of that age group had had at least one curettage, which presumably had taken place sometime in the proceeding 20 years—that is, roughly from 1940 onwards.[100] Valaoras, in his assessment of the reasons for the fertility decline in Greece, identified abortions as one of the two main reasons. Using the same survey as the other authors in the 1960s and offering the figure of 100,000 abortions per year, he asserted that abortions were performed 'in almost every village, town or city of Greece', and that, although their incidence was higher in urban areas, they were 'also extensively performed in rural areas'.[101] Such a conclusion contradicts those of all contemporary observers. When rural women had curettages, these were performed in urban centres. Travelling to urban centres for health reasons was a common occurrence in the 1960s despite the expense as most families had some connections in nearby cities owing to the extensive in-migration that had taken place in towns and cities from at least the 1950s. Those women who did not have access to curettage in urban centres, it can only be assumed, continued to use the traditional, familiar methods in most cases, with the occasional help from untrained midwives who still practised in such places. The subsequent disappearance of empiric midwives must have also resulted gradually in the disappearance of the use of traditional methods thereafter.

In 1969 Ioannes Danezes quantified induced abortions by curettage to a 'few tens of thousands' and concurred with Valaoras' estimated figure of 100,000 for the total number of abortions by curettage annually.[102] Konstantinos Roukas, writing a decade later, explained that Valaoras et al., using the actual numbers provided by their informants, had estimated that 54,000 curettages for the purposes of abortion were performed annually among married women.[103] However, he added, the use of unreliable contraceptive methods by the women in their sample, such as condoms and withdrawal, could not explain the rapid decline in fertility and thus Valaoras, and also N. Louros, revised the figure upwards to 100,000 to make up for the perceived discrepancy.[104] Valaoras himself, writing two decades later, during the legalisation of abortion, questioned the 'imaginary' abortion figures that were circulating at the time, which ranged from 200,000 to 400,000 abortions annually.[105] Using the data he and his colleagues had compiled in the 1960s, Valaoras revised the total figure of induced abortions for the 1960s down to 75,000, which included abortions of unmarried women and (estimated) non-disclosed abortions too.

The methods used were the curettage by the physicians, increasing their presence in the market from the 1930s onwards but significantly in the post-World War II era. From 1960 onwards, other methods would have only exceptionally been used. Midwives also used appliance methods until they were made to stop practising. However, women in the 1930s and beyond, and in all probability before that, were using abortifacients. These they would either pick up from their environment or purchase from the pharmacist. Most of these were herbal and some would have been used in earlier times as emmenagogues since some emmenagogues were also abortifacients. It is the regular and legitimate use of emmenagogues throughout the nineteenth century that had made women familiar with such preparations. Once the women desired and decided to curtail their childbearing, it was easy for them to adopt and use abortifacients. They were well versed in the use of their 'sisters', the emmenagogues, and the switch from one to the other was easy to make.

The use of abortifacients was not risk-free, as already noted. But they were available to all, rural and urban women, and did not necessitate much exposure to the curious social gaze. Midwives, in addition to delivering children, would also at times offer advice on what to do at the early stages of a possible pregnancy or would even perform an abortion in urban areas. Physicians also participated, but only in urban areas, offering more experience and prestige, mostly to the well-off. Physicians, and increasingly the newly qualified gynaecologists, were available to offer their services in post-World War II Greece and also moved to provincial towns, offering 'scientific' abortion to the town residents but also to the population of the town's hinterland. Thus, in the 1960s abortion became 'easily' and safely accessible to virtually all, offered by the trustworthy hands of a gynaecologist. The latter seemed only too happy to offer their services, in the hope, presumably, that their clients would return to them when they needed medical assistance in the birth of their child as well. Since abortion was illegal for the majority of cases, this source of income was untaxed and over and above the salary they received from their hospital employment, if they were so employed. Those practising privately would usually set up their own private surgeries and even clinics in order to attract and retain clients who would return for future abortions or help with other gynaecological matters. Curettages were thus performed in the gynaecologists' private practices[106] or in private clinics,[107] as well as in hospitals.[108]

Conclusions

The existing evidence suggests that, prior to 1910, abortion was overwhelmingly undertaken for pregnancies out of wedlock. The desperate attempts to conceal such an ethical transgression were acceptable and understandable to virtually all. Curettage had been available and practised as a therapeutic method since the end of the nineteenth century and continued to be used throughout the first half of the twentieth century as a treatment for female ailments and ultimately sterility, allowing physicians to gain expertise in its practice. From the mid-1920s, things changed. Curettage was also employed to provide abortion to affluent urbanites and gradually to those few poor urbanites and rural inhabitants who could afford and were able to make the trip to the urban centre. Those rural women and poor urbanites who did not desire a potential pregnancy continued to employ abortifacients and traditional emmenagogues if they were determined or desperate enough. Many who were aware of the available methods chose not to use them, fearing the health and/or ethical implications. In the 1950s, with rapid urbanisation and improved infrastructure, many more could travel into towns and cities and pay for the 'efficient' curettage that took place there. The increasing numbers of gynaecologists and the safety of the method, performed mostly by gynaecologists, must have become known to interested parties, despite the apparent—and not always evident—illegality of the method and the prohibition on advertising. Rural women continued to employ traditional methods of abortifacients after World War II, though increasing numbers also travelled in order to have a curettage, the modern medical method of abortion. Twenty-five years after the full legalisation of induced abortion in 1986 women continued to seek discretion in private clinics rather than have a free procedure in public hospitals, indicating not only the continued need for discretion but also the power and importance of social networks in seeking the 'best' physician.[109]

Notes

1. Endometritis was considered a prime cause of sterility (Dem. Antonopoulos (1926) *E Steirosis para te Gynaiki* (Athens: Koronaiou, Denaxa and Co), pp. 42–3).
2. Antonios I. Kindynes (1889) *E Steirosis para te Gynaiki kai Therapeia Autes* (Athens: Vlastos Varvaregos), pp. 96–102.
3. Kindynes, *E Steirosis*, pp. 102–6. See also Th. A. Saktoures (1899) *Peri apoxeseos tes metras en te maieutike kai gynaikologia* (Athens: Sp. Kousoulinou), pp. 12–13. Their use is mentioned extensively in most if not all relevant books until, at least, the mid-twentieth century.
4. Antonopoulos, *E Steirosis*, pp. 33–9.
5. Tryfon K. Andrianakos (1929) *E Maieutike kai Gynaikologia kata ten Diadromen tou viou tes Iatrikes Etaireias Athenon 1835–1908* (Athens: S.K. Vlastou), p. 28.
6. Konstantinos N. Louros (15 May 1896) 'Peri Apoxeseos tes Metras kai ton pros Tauten Endeikseon', *Galenos*, 26, 8.
7. Louros, 'Peri apoxeseos', 9–10. In the same context it is mentioned in the meeting of the Athens Medical Society (Iatrike Etaireia Athenon) of 28 May 1888 (Andrianakos, *E Maieutike*, p. 28).
8. Louros, 'Peri apoxeseos', 10.
9. J.W. Ballantyne (1896) *Curettage of the Uterus: History, Indications and Technique* (Edinburgh: Oliver and Boyd), p. 5.
10. Saktoures, *Peri apoxeseos*, Introduction and p. 8.
11. Indeed, the report on the inpatients of the hospital where Aretaios practised indicate the performance of curettage in the years 1892–3 (D.S.P. Mpalanou (1895) *Peri ton en aute kata to akademaikon etos 1892–1893 Noseleuthenton Arroston. Statistike Ekthesis* (Athens: Georgiou Fexe)).
12. Saktoures, *Peri apoxeseos*, pp. 29–33, prologue.
13. Saktoures, *Peri apoxeseos*, pp. 75, 83.
14. Saktoures, *Peri apoxeseos*, pp. 71–2.
15. Saktoures, *Peri apoxeseos*, p. 72. A very similar statement—although curettage is not mentioned as the recommended method—is made in Mihael G. Kaires (1909) *Praktikos Odegos tou Iatrou kai tes Maias. E Maia Anaplerousa ton Iatron* (Athens: Raftane-Papageorgiou), pp. 725–6.
16. Louros, 'Peri apoxeseos', 9; Saktoures, *Peri apoxeseos*, p. 83.
17. D. Theodorides (1904) 'Nouvelle curette special pour les curettages «post-abortum» où «post partum»', *Progrès Medical*, 20, 1–5.
18. Vasos Verges (1930) *Heirourgika. E Apoxesis tes metras* (Rhodes: n.p.), p. 1.

19. Nikolaos Alex. Petsales (1902) *Peri tes ton Ymenon Episheseos. Symvole eis ten Aitiologian Auton* (Athens: Estia), pp. 60–1. Petsales adds that there is no reason for him to elaborate on the hands method because it is well known. Anna Katsigra (1908) *E Maieutike en te Praksei* (Athens: Auge Athenon).
20. Antonopoulos, *E Steirosis*, pp. 11, 39.
21. Mpalanou, *Peri ton en aute*.
22. Mpalanou, *Peri ton en aute*, pp. 73–4.
23. Mpalanou, *Peri ton en aute*, pp. 74–6.
24. D.S.P. Mpalanou (1904) *Heirourgike kai Gynaikologike Klinike Theodorou kai Elenes Aretaiou. Peri ton en aute noseleuthenton arroston apo 1es Maiou 1899–31 Augoustou 1903* (Athens: Estia), pp. 44–9.
25. Mpalanou, *Heirourgike*, pp. 60–1.
26. Theodoros Papaioannou (1909) *Arheia Heirourgikes kai Gynaikologikes Klinikes Theodorou Papaioannou* (Athens: P.D. Sakellarios), pp. 339–41.
27. ELIA Archive Athens, A.E. 6/06, April 1909 to November 1928, *Maieutike kai Gynaikologike Klinike Soteriou Sofianopoulou, Patras.*
28. Anonymous (1910) 'Maieutike kai gynaikologike klinike en Patrais Soteriou Sofianopoulou', *Odegos ton Patron*, 1(1) (http://daniilida.lis.upatras.gr/index.php/svetsou/article/view/2861/2636, accessed 29 September 2018). The same advert appeared in 1912, in *Panahaikon Emerologion*, 1(1), 110 (http://daniilida.lis.upatras.gr/index.php/panax_hmer/article/view/3089/2864 accessed 29 September 2018). A very similar advertisement appeared in the same issue of the 1910 *Odegos ton Patron* journal advertising a clinic operating in Athens, under the direction of a female physician, again stressing the therapy of 'sterility (CHILDLESSNESS)' (capitals in the original).
29. Pyrros describes metritis as an 'inflammation of the utero'. He attributes this to the incomplete emptying/clearing of the utero, conceptions, 'french passions' and 'midwives' pessaries'. Pyrros explains that metritis could lead to swelling and ultimately death (Dionysios Pyrros o Thettalos (1840) *Egkolpion ton Iatron Etoi Praktike Iatrike, Periehousa ten Ylen tes Iatrikes, ten Farmakopoiian, ten Ygieinen*, vol. 1, 1st edn 1831 (Athens: Aggelou Aggelidou), p. 142). Gravigger describes metritis in similar terms and one of the methods of treatment he suggests is curettage (P. Gravigger (1970) *Iatrosofia*, vol. 1 (Athens: Vivliotheke Sfiggos), pp. 489–90). Metritis and endometritis were also seen as indirect causes of sterility, cured either with bloodletting performed with leeches or with cauterisation (Kindynes, *E Steirosis*, pp. 138–40).
30. See, for example, case 139 of 1909 and 389 of 1915. In the second case the notes state: "Married for 10 years. Had one delivery only, six years

ago. 'After the therapy she became pregnant'". The presentation of the original was retained. Identical was case 370 of 1914.

31. For more on the hospital and its records see Violetta Hionidou (2009) '"It was a bridge from life to death": Hospitals during the Food Crisis, Greece 1941–1944', *Social History of Medicine*, 22(2), 361–85.
32. Metropoulos, writing in 1954, recommends curettage for an incomplete spontaneous abortion (Konstantinos Metropoulos (1954) *Ygieine tes Egkyou. Enas Polytimos Odegos gia ten Ygieine Diaviose tes Egkyou* (Athens: Papademetriou), p. 134).
33. Panteles D. Mpertsekas (1948) *Oi Kindynoi kai ai Epiplokai tes Amvloseos kai ta Iatrodikastika Provlemata Autes* (Athens: Euth. Hristodoulou); ELIA Archive Athens, A.E. 6/06, April 1909 to November 1928, *Maieutike kai Gynaikologike Klinike Soteriou Sofianopoulou, Patras*; General State Archives of Hios (hereafter GSAH), ABE 1256 78, *Metroo Asthenon kyrios Nosokomeiou 1937–1938*; GSAH ABE 1256 79, *Metroo Asthenon kyrios Nosokomeiou 1.1.1939–8.10.1941*; Skylitseio Nosokomeio of Hios, Hios, *Metroo Asthenon kyrios Nosokomeiou, 1941–1943.*
34. Katsigra, *E Maieutike*, p. 228.
35. K. Louros (1926–34) 'Ektrosis', *Megale Ellenike Egkyklopaideia*, ed. Paulos Dandrakes, vol. 9 (Athens: Pyrsos), p. 850. On the use of hands rather than the curette see Katsigra, *E Maieutike*, p. 228; G.K. Lameras (August 1929) 'Therapeia tes Epiloheiou Endometritidos', *Praktikos Iatros*, 7(8), 26–7; and Petsales, *Peri tes ton Ymenon*, pp. 60–1.
36. N.K. Louros (1948) *Gynaikologia* (Athens: Ellenike Ekdotike Etaireia), p. 270.
37. V. Maroule (15 September 1951) 'E Gonimotes tes Gynaikos eis ta Steira Zeuge', *Klinike*, 22(4), 84. See also M. Moyseides (1 September 1947) 'Meno-Metrorragiai en te praxei', *Klinike*, 18(21), 654, 656. A similar argument was put forward by Alexandros Tsakires (1954) *Megale Sexologia. Anikanotes, Steirosis kai e Syghrone Therapeia ton*, 3rd edn, first published 1947 (Athens: n.p.), p. 604.
38. Anonymous (20 November 1950) 'O Gynaikologos Apanta: reply to *Polyvasanismene*', *E Gynaika*, 1(20), p. 31.
39. D. Diamantopoulos (1955) *E Apoxesis tes Metras* (Athens: n.p.), p. 31.
40. Diamantopoulos, *E Apoxesis*, pp. 32–6.
41. D. Diamantopoulos (1957) *Iatrike Egkyklopaideia tes Gynaikas* (Athens: Gerolympou), pp. 195–8.
42. Diamantopoulos, *Iatrike*, pp. 196–8.
43. Hristodoulos Ant. Kampoures (1933) *Therapeutikai kai Koinonikai Endeikseis tes Tehnetes Ektroseos* (Athens: Georgiou Vasileiou), pp. 8, 22.

44. A.E. (April 1930) 'Allelografia tou Praktikou Iatrou, 3h erotesis', *Ellenike Iatrike*, 4(4), 435.
45. Kerameus (April 1930) 'Allelografia tou Praktikou Iatrou, Eis to 3on erotema', *Ellenike Iatrike*, 4(4), 546.
46. Vasilios Valaoras, A. Polychronopoulou and D. Trichopoulos (1969) 'Greece: Postwar abortion experience', *Studies in Family Planning*, 1(46), 14.
47. Marlene Sue Arnold (1985) 'Childbirth among Rural Greek Women in Crete: Use of Popular, Folk and Cosmopolitan Medical Systems' (unpublished PhD thesis: University of Pennsylvania), p. 250.
48. No. 6D. The informant studied at the Athens medical school 1959–65.
49. Mpertsekas, *Oi Kindynoi*, p. 15, 17. Kontos had reported in the 1880s that midwives were using the catheter methods, though he seems to be unique in supporting this (Tryfon K. Kontos (1883) *Peri Examvloseos e Amvloseos* (Athens: Enosis), p. 45).
50. Metropoulos, *Ygieine*, p. 142.
51. Mpertsekas, *Oi Kindynoi*, p. 19, 87; Metropoulos, *Ygieine*, pp. 134, 138, 142.
52. N.Sp. (11 December 1901) 'E Apotropaios Praxis', *Empros*, 6(1841), p. 1.
53. Kontos, *Peri Examvloseos*, p. 8.
54. Kontos, *Peri Examvloseos*, p. 9.
55. Timoleon Kardaras (1894) *Praktike Iatrike ton Oikogeneion*, 2nd edn (Athens: Georgiou D. Fexe), p. 47.
56. Vasileios Parlapanes (2014) 'E Iatrodikastike sten Ellada mesa apo demosieumata tou 19ou kai ton arhon tou 20ou aiona' (unpublished PhD thesis: Aristoteleio University Thessaloniki), pp. 122–3, citing A.D. Kallivokas (1895) *Iatrodikastike (kata A. Lutaud): Kata ten Elleniken Nomothesian*, 3rd edition (Athens: N. Tzaka).
57. Parlapanes, 'E Iatrodikastike', p. 124, citing Kallivokas, *Iatrodikastike*. For a modern assessment of their effectiveness see https://www.ncbi.nlm.nih.gov/pubmed/12807304 (last accessed 22 October 2018); and for the contemporary equivalent see C. Ciganda and A. Laborde (2003) 'Herbal Infusions Used for Induced Abortion', *Journal of Toxicology. Clinical Toxicology*, 41(3), 235–9.
58. Some of those 'popular' methods involved substances that had been used by physicians of previous generations. These had been adopted by the populace, who continued to use them for some time after they had ceased to be used by the physicians.
59. Konstantinos Merkourios (1914) 'Dyo Neai Methodoi Egklematikes Ektroseos', *Iatrike Proodos*, 19, 1.

60. Merkourios, 'Dyo Neai Methodoi', 1.
61. Athanasios Vettos Danielides Archimandrite (1924) *E Zoe ton Neon* (Athens: Paraskeuas Leones), p. 171.
62. Andrianakos, *E Maieutike*, quoting Epites, on the meeting of the Athens Medical Society that took place on 5 July 1848 (p. 31).
63. Panagiotes Savorianakes (2000) 'Oikogeneia kai Gamelies Praktikes sto Notioanatoliko Aigaio. E Kos sto 18o kai 19o Aiona', *Mnemon*, 22, 43, referring to a pregnancy that was the outcome of rape and where the alleged rapist had suggested that the midwife 'gives the girl medicines in order for her to lose the baby'; Athena Gaitanou-Gianniou, a socialist feminist who cohabited with her socialist partner, had an abortion before having a daughter in 1914 (Iris Aude-Kalkane (1997) *Mia antartissa tes Poles sten taragmene Athena. Athena Gaitanou-Gianniou 1880–1952* (Athens: ELIA), p. 44).
64. Anonymous (15 January 1929) 'Ptomata Emvryon entos tou Ilissou', *Skrip*, 32(9228), p. 2; Anonymous (3 January 1930) 'Oi ftohoi agrotes klevontai fanera apo tous tsormpatzedes kai to kratos', *Rizospastes*, 13(6389), p. 3.
65. N.K. Louros and K.N. Alivizatos (1979) *Dyo Giatroi Thymountai* (Athens: Filippote), p. 71.
66. No. 7D.
67. Mpertsekas, *Oi Kindynoi*, p. 67.
68. Violetta Hionidou (1993) 'The Demography of a Greek Island, Mykonos 1859–1959: A Family Reconstitution Study' (unpublished PhD thesis: University of Liverpool), Figure 7.8.
69. Kampoures, *Therapeutikai*, p. 32.
70. Hr. Papatheofilou (6 January 1932) 'Einai Egklema e Ektrosis; E Apopsis tou Hr. Papatheofilou', *Makedonia*, 23(6965), p. 1 (the author was a gynaecologist); Kampoures, *Therapeutikai*, pp. 30–1; M. Moyseides (1925) *E Gyne. Ygieine tou Gamou kai tes Eggamou Gynaikos* (Alexandreia: A. Kasigone), p. 68.
71. Georgios K. Zouraris (24 December 1931) 'Einai Egklema e Ektrosis e Apeleutherotikon Kinema?' *Makedonia*, 22(6955), p. 5; Hr. Papatheofilou (6 January 1932) 'Einai Egklema e Ektrosis; E Apopsis tou Hr. Papatheofilou', *Makedonia*, 23(6965), p. 1; Mpertsekas, *Oi Kindynoi*, p. 79.
72. See, for example, M. Moyseides (1927) *Ygieine tes Egkyou, Epitokou, Lehoidos, kai tes Galouhouses* (Alexandreia: Kasigone), p. 66, who comments that induced abortion 'is widely performed and with light consciousness'. Moyseides maintained that it was done by midwives or women themselves.

73. Kampoures, *Therapeutikai*, p. 31 According to the author, women in the countryside remain ethical/honourable (timies) because they are still under the supervision of society and their parents. A more liberal abortion law would have no effect in rural Greece, he asserts.
74. Euaggelos An. Averof (1939) *Symvole eis ten Ereunan tou Plythesmiakou Provlematos tes Ellados* (Athens: n.p.), p. 72. The author investigates couples married after 1922 and areas that experienced high fertility. Within the studied populations, the subgroups that were employing birth control also sought abortions, 'provided the couple could afford' it.
75. Apostolos Doxiadis (12 September 1930) 'E thesis tes Gynaikos. Seira semeiomaton tou k. Ap. Doxiadi', *Eleutheron Vema*, pp. 1–2.
76. Doxiadis, 'E thesis tes Gynaikos', pp. 1–2.
77. See Van de Walle's discussion of the principle of periodic catharsis within the Hippocratic tradition (Etienne van de Walle (2001) 'Menstrual Catharsis and the Greek Physician' in Etienne van de Walle and Elisha P. Renne (eds) *Regulating Menstruation: Beliefs, Practices, Interpretations* (Chicago: The University of Chicago Press), pp. 3–21).
78. No. 20 Mykonos.
79. Mpertsekas, *Oi Kindynoi*, p. 73.
80. Tsakires, *Megale Sexologia*, p. 538.
81. Danielides, *E Zoe*, p. 171.
82. Second Obstetrics and Gynaecology Clinic, University (Aretaieion Hospital) (Mpertsekas, *Oi Kindynoi*, p. 39.).
83. No. 7D. Also No. 3D and No. 6D. For later dates see H. Lovel and C. Bakoula (1985) 'Lack of family planning leading to induced abortion in rural Greece', *International Planned Parenthood Federation Medical Bulletin*, 19(3), 1.
84. Figure calculated by author from the data provided in Konstantinos I. Roukas (1979) *Genetesiai Sheseis kai Prokletai Ektroseis eis Spoudastikon Plethysmo ton Athenon* (Athens: n.p.), pp. 41, 45. As this was self-reported abortion, it is very possible that this is a minimum rather than the real percentage.
85. The figure includes miscarriages, stillbirths and abortions. V.G. Valaoras, Antonia Polychronopoulou and Dimitri Trichopoulos (1965) 'Control of Family Size in Greece (The Results of a Field Survey)', *Population Studies*, 18(3), 273.
86. No. 24 Mykonos; No. 5 Syros; No. 7D; No. 12 Athens; Mpertsekas, *Oi Kindynoi*, p. 39. Richard Blum and Eva Blum (1965) *Health and Healing in Rural Greece* (Stanford, ca: Stanford University press), p. 76, relying on information from the local midwife, who estimated that some women may have aborted as many as thirty times, though using 'traditional methods'.

87. Anonymous (21 September 1950) 'O Gynaikologos Apanta: Reply to *Dystyhismene Syzygo*', *E Gynaika*, 1(17), p. 52.
88. Metropoulos, *Ygieine*, p. 141.
89. Blum and Blum, *Health and Healing*, p. 76.
90. The untrained midwife in this instance performed a caesarean on a five-month-pregnant local unmarried girl in her Athens clinic (Blum and Blum, *Health and Healing*, p. 150).
91. Antonia Polychronopoulou (1967) 'E en Elladi Syhnotes ton Apoxeseon tes Metras' (unpublished PhD thesis: Athens University), p. 25; Valaoras et al., 'Control', 265–78.
92. Emphasis in the original.
93. Polychronopoulou, 'E en Elladi', pp. 25–6.
94. Polychronopoulou, 'E en Elladi', p. 27.
95. Blum and Blum cite prices ranging from $10 to $175, reaching $230 for a professor of obstetrics (Blum and Blum, *Health and Healing*, p. 76).
96. Lovel and Bakoula, 'Lack of family planning', 1. Personal observation on Mykonos in the late 1980s, from where women would invariably travel to Athens.
97. George Siampos (1975) 'Law and Fertility in Greece' in Maurice Kirk, Massimo Livi Bacci and Egon Szabady (eds) *Law and fertility in Europe: A study of legislation directly or indirectly affecting fertility in Europe*, vol. 2 (Belgium: Ordina Editions), p. 344. However, abortion was never advertised before 1950 either.
98. Polychronopoulou, 'E en Elladi', p. 48
99. Polychronopoulou, 'E en Elladi', p. 45, table 12.
100. Polychronopoulou, 'E en Elladi', p. 45, table 12; Valaoras et al., 'Greece: Postwar', 13. This study took place in 1966–7 and therefore women older than 45 would have been in their prime reproductive years around 1945 and later.
101. Vas. G. Valaoras (1971) 'Changing Patterns of Fertility Differentials (The Case of Greece)' in *International Population Conference, London 1969* (Liege: IUSSP), p. 2080.
102. Ioannes M. Danezes (1969) 'E Tehnete Ektrosis os Diethnes kai Ellenikon Provlema', *Iatrike*, 15(3), 201.
103. Roukas, *Genetesiai*, p. 36.
104. Roukas, *Genetesiai*, p. 36.
105. Vasilios G. Valaoras (1987) 'The Present and the future of the Population of Greece', *Praktika tes Akademias Athenon*, 62, 310.
106. No. 3D; this is also confirmed by informant No. 12 Athens, who had two such abortions in Athens in the late 1960s under general anaesthetic; No. 6D; No. 11 Athens.

107. No. 3D; No. 6D; No. 11 Athens; Arnold, 'Childbirth', pp. 117–19.
108. Informant No. 6D argued that abortions could not have occurred in hospital 'since these were controlled'. However, other informants suggested that they did happen there too. No. 23 Mykonos, referring to the 1930s.
109. Elizabeth Ioannidi-Kapolou (2004) 'Use of Contraception and Abortion in Greece: A Review', *Reproductive Health Matters*, 12(24), Supplement: Abortion Law, Policy and Practice in Transition, 180.

CHAPTER 6

Abortion: Law and (Dis)order, Physicians and Midwives

The earlier chapters examined the availability, timing and geographical spread of the various methods of induced abortion throughout the existence of the Greek state, referring where appropriate to the lack of prosecution for what was, for the chronological span investigated here, an illegal act. This chapter will examine the letter and practice of induced abortion law in Greece.

The Greek state was created in the early 1830s and its penal system was designed by the Bavarian Georg Ludwig von Maurer, who arrived in Greece with the country's first king, Otto, and was instructed to create the legislative system of the new state. Although for many aspects of the law Maurer went to some trouble to become informed of the 'customs' of the people and to shape the law accordingly, in the case of abortion the new Greek law followed the Bavarian example almost word for word, even being written initially in German and only subsequently being translated into Greek. The new penal code came into force in 1835.[1] Three main articles of the penal code, 303, 304 and 305, addressed abortion, covering the performance of abortion by the pregnant woman or by a third party. These short articles read as follows:[2]

> Article 303. If the mother who gave birth to a premature or dead infant (vrefos) used prior to that, knowingly, alone or with someone else, internal or external means, [means that] can cause a premature delivery or the death

V. Hionidou, *Abortion and Contraception in Modern Greece, 1830–1967*, Medicine and Biomedical Sciences in Modern History,
https://doi.org/10.1007/978-3-030-41490-0_6

of the foetus (*emvryo*) in the mother's abdomen, she is punished with imprisonment (eirkte).

Article 304. The same penalty is imposed on the midwives or pharmacists or others in the medical service who cause abortion with the consent of the pregnant woman or by recommending or by providing the means for performing such a felony.

The sentences were a maximum of ten years both for the mother who committed the act herself or caused it to be committed and, if performed by a third party, for that individual as well.[3] This law remained unchanged and in force for 90 years, although amendments were made in the first half of the twentieth century.

The 1835 law refers to an infant (vrefos), a foetus (*emvryo*) and a delivery. It is worth exploring what the lawmaker and his contemporaries meant when using these terms. Nikolaos Kostes, the first professor of obstetrics of Athens University, writing in 1849, explains that some use the term *emvryo* (foetus) after the 'conceived has been developed', whereas when the body parts of the *embryo* cannot be discerned 'this is called by some' *kyema* ('that which is conceived') or *gone* (elsewhere, Nikolaos Kostes calls semen 'gone').[4] Nikolaos Kostes places the time at which the body parts become discernible at around the sixth week of pregnancy.[5] Elsewhere he refers to 'the egg', denoting the early stages of the fertilised ovum, and explains that prior to the third week the 'egg shows no signs of the *embryo*', while by the start of the second month the head is discernible.[6] The legislation, in the article considering infanticide, uses the term 'new-born child' (neognon teknon) to refer to the newly born baby, indicating that '*neognon*' is the term applicable to the period of time immediately after birth.[7] Thus, *vrefos* seems to be referring to the foetus in the late stages of pregnancy.[8]

It was not only Nikolaos Kostes who perceived the early pregnancy as *not* constituting a foetus.[9] The lay population and also, at times, physicians referred to the *embryo* in the first three months as 'the egg', implicitly disassociating the early stage of the foetus from what the law referred to: that is, a visually discernible foetus. Women in the early 1930s explicitly made the point that what was expelled after their abortion was an 'egg', and thus that any action they may have taken could not be punishable by law.[10] This did not escape the attention of observers. The author of a short newspaper article dating to 1901, discussing a working-class woman's attempted abortion, noted that, 'according to her minimally developed intellect, the foetus (*emvryo*) is not a ***human***, it does not have the rights of a human', while in an earlier sentence he referred to 'the conceived in her belly'.[11] His view was that the penal justice (poinike dikaiosyne) system had been too slow to realise that the foetus is human.

Therefore, if what the woman carried in those early months of pregnancy was not considered an actual foetus, while the law referred specifically to a foetus, it followed that any action taken in those early months to end a pregnancy was not punishable by law. Considering the extreme ambiguity in determining pregnancy, especially before quickening, there was no legal reason to prevent women from considering the reasons for the suspension of their menstruation and, if they believed that there was reason for action, taking emmenagogues to 'put themselves right'. If the treatment taken was successful, the lack of a discernible foetus when bleeding would have meant to them that they had simply succeeded in bringing their menses on.

Furthermore, women would have understood the possibility of a molar pregnancy (discussed in Chap. 4), and would have wished to expel what they carried in such a case. As the condition could not result in the birth of an infant, women who were keen to have a child would have taken measures to expel the mole rather than wait for months for that to happen naturally. Molar pregnancies were impossible to detect at the time; even today their detection requires blood tests and ultrasound scans. Frequent references to them by physicians in their writings, however, indicate their preoccupation, and that of women, with such 'pregnancies'. The existence of the term and condition, the difficulty in tracing such a 'pregnancy', the observable outcomes in terms of what was expelled and the wording of the law—expecting a formed foetus and a delivery—meant that a woman who took action in order to resolve such a condition could not be punished. This common understanding (koine doxa) that the expulsion of a 'myle'[12] was not a crime and was not associated with abortion was articulated in the authoritative interpretation of the law in 1877 and by numerous authors in the 1920s.[13] Efforts to terminate such a 'pregnancy' would have occurred both when women wanted to be rid of a 'myle' in order to proceed with a more promising pregnancy but also when women did not want a pregnancy at all. This 'liberal' interpretation of molar pregnancy did not escape the attention of the lawmakers and those interpreting the law, however. By 1892 Konstantinos Kostes, a law professor, had added a footnote to his interpretation of the law to the effect that women were not permitted to argue that they had performed an abortion believing that they carried a molar pregnancy. However, he added that, if after the abortion it was proved that the pregnancy was molar, then such an act was not punishable[14]—suggesting the common use of the molar pregnancy as an excuse or reason for abortion. However, the complexity of Konstantinos Kostes' argument also suggests that an implementation of his understanding of the law was impossible in practical terms.

Simply put, abortion in the early months of pregnancy could not be and was not punished simply because at the time it would have been impossible to prove that in every case a pregnancy existed that would have led to anything resembling 'giving birth' or that taking action had caused 'a premature delivery', as the law indicated.[15] However, in his 1877 interpretation of the law, Konstantinos Kostes explicitly stated that the abortion law covered the period from the moment conception took place to the time of the delivery, while consistently referring to the '*embryo*'.[16] While Kostes' interpretation attempted to bring Greek law into line with European legislation more widely, the actual practice of the law continued to follow the strict letter of the law even at the turn of the twentieth century. So, in a Supreme Court case of 1905 the judge emphasised that article 303 of the penal code considers as a 'necessary element of the offence of abortion' that 'the mother gave birth to a dead or premature foetus'. Without such evidence, the Supreme Court judge, N. Momferatos, determined that the law could not be applied and that further consultations had to take place on the specific case.[17] However, in 1927 another court case clarified that, despite the letter of the law, it was not necessary for the court to have knowledge that the foetus was alive before the attempted abortion. The judge clarified that the law applied 'even when the conception is recent and the foetus had not started giving signs of life yet'.[18] So, only after 1927 was an induced abortion in the first three months of pregnancy actually punishable.

To complicate matters further, article 106 of the penal code indicated that 'a person who undertook an illegal act in order to urgently protect their own or someone else's life' should not be punished. As early as 1872 this law was explicitly linked by forensic judges to the action of induced abortion when it was performed in order to save the mother's life.[19] Discussing his interpretation of article 106 in 1871, Konstantinos Kostes acknowledged the necessity for physicians to perform an induced abortion when the mother's life was in danger. He unambiguously articulated the mother's right to request action (referring to the cutting or perforation of the foetus head while in utero, or a caesarean delivery) that would ensure her survival.[20] If the mother was not in a position to make a choice it was to be left exclusively to the physician.[21] The physician's obligation, Konstantinos Kostes stated, was 'to save the birthing woman'. Only when 'every possibility' of achieving this had vanished should he then try to save the baby, if possible.[22] Ioannes Pyrlas clarified in 1872 that an induced abortion was also justified in cases of extensive haemorrhage and serious illness of the mother.[23] At the same time eminent obstetricians explicitly defined 'artificial abortion' in their midwifery manuals (inducing the birth of a non-viable foetus perceived to be prior to 28 weeks of pregnancy) and noted that its purpose was the 'preservation of the mother's life'.[24] M. Venizelos explained that 'if there are such circumstances which the continuation of the pregnancy will certainly lead to the death of the mother, then [artificial abortion] is recommended'.[25] That the right to abortion had de facto expanded to include issues related to the health of the mother is observed in the revised edition of Konstantinos Kostes' interpretation of the Penal Code. This by 1892 explains that abortion is not punishable not only when it aims to protect the life of the mother but also when it aims to 'prevent damage to her health'.[26]

This interpretation was actually embedded in the new Draft Penal Code of 1924, when for the first time the 'medical justification (endeikse)' for induced abortion was introduced to the penal system, allowing induced abortion when the mother's life or health was in significant danger: 'Unpunished remains the abortion performed by a physician with the purpose of avoiding an otherwise unavoidable endangerment of her life or significant and constant impairment of the health of the pregnant woman.'[27] While the sentences remained the same as before, extenuating circumstances could be taken into account that reduced the sentence both for the mother and for the person performing the abortion to a minimum of six months' imprisonment (article 282).[28] The primacy of the mother over the foetus was reiterated and emphasised in medical publications dealing with the law, articulating that under certain medical conditions 'the physician was obliged to sacrifice the foetus in order to save the mother'.[29]

The 1930s and to a lesser extent the 1940s proved a time of active engagement of the law with induced abortion, but only at the level of legislation. Further draft laws were introduced in 1934 that proposed the change of abortion from a felony (kakourgema) to a misdemeanour (plemellema) and in 1939 that incorporated the 'moral justification (endeikse)', thus making abortion unpunishable when pregnancy was the result of rape, abuse of a person unable to resist, seduction of a minor younger than 15 years or incest; and in 1947 draft law laid out that a self-induced abortion was punishable with a maximum of three years' imprisonment, while an abortion performed by someone else with the woman's consent attracted a sentence of a minimum of six months, with the repeated performance of abortion deserving of the highest sentence of ten years.[30] Interestingly, medical authors who were dealing with the question of abortion, such as Panteles Mpertsekas, were not fully aware of all the draft laws and their various amendments that had been prepared.[31] However, whether officially enforced or not, in effect these draft laws were followed and used for guidance in the application of the law. So, for example, the 'medical justification' included 'malignant vomiting'—that is, excessive vomiting on the part of the pregnant woman—which was considered as endangering her long-term health. In 1929 an eminent gynaecologist published an article entitled 'Indications for interruption of pregnancy due to malignant vomiting' in which he argued that, following an extensive, detailed and repeated assessment of the pregnant patient, in some circumstances the physician 'not only … has the right to intervene but he has the obligation to do so'.[32] In 1930 we read in the question-and-answer section of the medical journal *Ellenike Iatrike* about a patient who suffered from 'fairly frequent vomiting'. Though her physician had prescribed an array of medicines in order to overcome the vomiting, this nevertheless continued. Another physician advised the patient to terminate the pregnancy. The corresponding physician asked his 'expert' colleagues in the medical journal for the best course of action[33] and received a reply suggesting a series of alternative medications and concluding that only if those did not work and further symptoms were evident an abortion should take place.[34]

Thus, despite the draft legislation not having been passed into law, it was essentially in effect: that is, medical and legal practices were in fact guided by these draft laws. In 1950 the new penal code, which was identical to the draft law of 1947, was finally voted into law, coming into force in 1951.[35] Both medical and moral reasons were accepted as reasons for the removal of the 'injustice' from the act of abortion as articulated in the earlier draft laws, thus allowing physicians to perform abortion for a good number of reasons (the 'medical' and the 'moral' clauses being incorporated as paragraphs 4 and 5 of article 304 of the penal code).[36] Prior to 1950, article 106, on the defence of human life, provided the opportunity to permit abortion for 'therapeutic reasons' when undertaken by a physician.[37] After 1950, induced abortion was permitted when the pregnant woman suffered from tuberculosis, syphilis, heart conditions, diabetes, psychopathic disorders, schizophrenia, haemophilia or 'malignant vomiting', provided that two physicians would certify the condition(s).[38] The 1950 penal law prosecuted self-induced abortion with a maximum sentence of three years; performing abortion with the woman's consent was punished with a minimum imprisonment of six months; and the repeated provision of abortion carried a maximum of ten years' imprisonment.[39] The next change took place in 1978, with an amendment to the penal code that widened significantly the 'medical' clause, essentially permitting abortion up to the 12th week when there is 'danger to the psychological health of the pregnant woman' because of the pregnancy. This required certification by a psychiatrist employed in a public hospital.[40] Moreover, the 'eugenic' clause was introduced, permitting abortion for eugenic reasons such as thalassemia up to 20 weeks; however, it should be noted that haemophilia had been a legal justification for induced abortion since 1947.[41] Here, the new methods of detecting foetal abnormalities, especially in relation to thalassaemia, necessitated the expansion of the law. The 1986 law permitted 'termination of pregnancy' by demand until the twelfth week, provided that this took place within a medical establishment and was performed by a qualified obstetrician/gynaecologist.

But to what degree were transgressions of these laws punished? Lexouriotes indicates that the first two cases of abortion prosecuted were brought to justice in 1871.[42] Kontos in 1883, Kardaras in 1894 and others in the 1910s stated that the abortion law was not enforced and that cases came to court very rarely.[43] In the 1930s Tryfon Andrianakos lamented that, despite 'the heavy sentences prescribed for midwives and physicians ... these are extremely rarely implemented'.[44] At the same time Kampoures expressed the same sentiment, arguing that 'justice does not know [about the abortions] and therefore does nothing about it'.[45] The very few cases that reached the courts up to 1930 exclusively concerned illegitimate pregnancies, mostly where the abortion had been or was intended to be performed against the will of the pregnant woman.[46] Mpertsekas, writing in 1945 and referring to the 1934 draft law, indicates that the draft law had not come into force and that the physician was still accountable; nevertheless, he added that 'the criminal courts do not deal usually or they do not enforce the prosecution of the physician'.[47] Thus, despite this being a draft law, the courts and the judges were careful not to prosecute or punish physicians because of the prospect of the law soon changing. In 1954 Metropoulos argues that 'the law needs to be changed because it does not make sense since no one follows it', presumably referring to the lack of prosecution.[48] Things did not change in the 1960s: in 1967 the law professor G. Magkakes stressed that very few cases ever reached the courts—approximately ten per year in Athens and Thessaloniki—the main areas in which abortion took place—invariably cases involving the death of the woman.[49] According to Valaoras et al. in the period 1956–1965 there were fewer than three deaths per year due to abortion (induced and spontaneous) because 'all the abortions reported in the sample were performed by licensed physicians', whereas in the period 1933–1938 a total of sixty-five deaths was attributable to the same cause.[50] Considering that the number of abortions per year for the 1960s had been estimated at around 100,000, this is a minuscule percentage and one that could possibly be explained as the result of medical negligence and/or the patients' health circumstances. The prosecution of those involved in abortion did not change in the following decades, either. Konstantinos Roukas, for example, referred to 20–30 abortion cases per year brought to court in the 1970s.[51] Of those, only a few were convicted: eight in 1974, two in 1976, nine in 1979 and three in 1981.[52] This continued to be the case in the 1980s, and most Greek women, myself among them, were as a consequence, not even aware of the illegality of abortion, although its availability was common knowledge and its practice widespread. Somewhat ironically, one of the driving forces in the amendment of the abortion law in 1986 was the need 'to preserve the integrity of the legal system, which was threatened by the increasing incidence of illegally performed abortions that were not prosecuted'.[53] This could well be true, but it would be interesting to investigate why it was not until 1986 that it became imperative to preserve the integrity of a system that essentially had *never* prosecuted abortion throughout the existence of the modern Greek state, no matter the letter of the law. As the jurist E. Symeonidou-Kastanidou remarked, when it comes to abortions the legal commodity [*nomiko agatho*] has never been protected in reality, irrespective of the existing legal frame of the time.[54] Rather, she emphasised, the legislation relating to abortion seems to have had only *symbolic* significance. It should be pointed out that this situation was not specific to Greece—France's experience seems to have been similar.[55]

It could be argued that Greece's first abortion law assumed that early-term abortion was not possible, given the non-existence of a discernible foetus, and thus it was meaningless for the state to try to police it. A discernible pregnancy could be one that a mother may have wanted to abort and the provision covered that possibility. Until the end of the nineteenth century, cases of early-term induced abortions thus remained an alien concept and attracted little attention, except for footnote references in academic interpretations of the law. This represented the understanding, ethics and practices of the populace, who had no desire to control their pregnancies or saw no major issue with an early 'expulsion' of the 'egg' during the first couple of months of pregnancy and before a discernible foetus was formed. The majority of the population understood that there were no major ethical problems with action taken in those early months—and so they did, when they needed to. Physicians—but also those who interpreted the law, at least many of them, especially those not educated in the West—shared to a large degree the understanding of the population and acted upon their requests. The precedent of the mother's life and health over that of the foetus was never contested and in interpreting the law this was explicitly declared in the late nineteenth and early twentieth centuries.[56] The letter of the law was followed during the first 90 years of its existence, with only a few abortions of discernible foetuses taking place and these being brought to justice during that time.

The Drive to Liberalise Abortion

Other than in the 1980s, feminist or women's groups were not involved in advocating a liberalisation of abortion law in Greece. Very few women discussed abortion, let alone demanded its liberalisation. Who, then, were behind the drive to liberalise induced abortion? It appears that one answer is men and, among them, as the citations in this study suggest, physicians, overwhelmingly gynaecologists. This is perhaps not surprising, as it was often, in the early days, and exclusively in the later ones, gynaecologists who performed abortions. In 1930 Tryfon Andrianakos, an eminent gynaecologist of his time, was invited to present his ideas in a conference that would shape Greece's hygiene policy.[57] He chose to discuss abortion and the issues surrounding it: that is, the medical speciality of obstetrics and gynaecology; the university education of physicians with an emphasis on gynaecology; and, most significantly, midwives. Andrianakos forcefully argued against the liberalisation of abortion, although he did support its liberalisation for therapeutic reasons, thus endorsing the 1924 'medical' clause—but only if it were to be performed by specialised obstetricians/

gynaecologists and not by *any* physician. He condemned the performance of abortion by midwives, who, he maintained, were performing it in secrecy, thus putting women's lives in further danger.[58] Andrianakos essentially argued for the ring-fencing of his medical speciality, obstetrics and gynaecology, as he felt that there were no clear boundaries defining who was a gynaecologist and who not: 'currently ... everyone can add a sign on his door [claiming to be a gynaecologist] without any knowledge'.[59] He went on to attack the state and its frequent interference in the 1920s with the university education of physicians, arguing that in the preceding decade it had 'offered' medical degrees to many Asia Minor refugees whose low quality of medical education presented a threat to public health. He urged the improvement of university education in general, and specifically in obstetrics and gynaecology, for which new clinics were necessary for the students' training.[60] Most of all, however, Andrianakos took issue with midwives, simply calling them a 'social stigma'.[61] One of the major problems with them, he said, was their lack of education, which led him to recommend the purging of the profession in an attempt to 'clean' it, something already prescribed by the law.[62] This would mean the removal of those midwives who lacked education and a restriction of their professional activities to midwifery only: that is, they would be unable to provide induced abortions.

Andrianakos was correct to suggest that midwives were performing abortions in 1930s Athens, as they also were in early 1940s Hermoupolis,[63] and his suggestions had in fact been the legal requirement since the 1830s, were repeated in legislation of 1912 and had been articulated as the aim of all professors of midwifery at Athens University since its creation.[64] However, unqualified midwives continued practising in most of the rural parts of the country into the 1960s, as there were simply very few qualified ones.[65] In 1924, the director of public health, Phokion Copanaris, mentioned the existence of 575 trained midwives and 58 practical ones who had undertaken a short course and qualified, a meagre number that could not cater to the needs of the country.[66] In 1925 Copanaris asserted that although the major urban centres were served only by qualified midwives, villages had almost exclusively unqualified ones.[67] At the same point that Andrianakos was setting out his argument, the Mykonos community was paying for Flora Nazou, a local young woman, to study as a midwife provided that she would work on the island for five years.[68] She almost certainly did not practice for long, however, as other, non-qualified, midwives dominated the practice on the island. Only in the early 1950s were the two unqualified midwives on the island ordered by the county chief physician (Nomiatros) of the Cyclades to stop practising because qualified practitioners had established themselves on the island.[69] At least one of the unqualified midwives continued to practise long after that date.[70] On Hios, while some qualified midwives were based on the island in the 1930s, many empirical ones continued to work there until 1970.[71] Similarly, elsewhere it was only in the late 1950s that qualified midwives arrived, practising in parallel with the unqualified midwife already established in the area, presumably until the latter retired.[72]

Andrianakos used his remarks, furthermore, to argue that the state should close down clinics run by midwives, as these constituted 'a social disgrace and a public danger'.[73] Midwives should be fully trained and, for the major cities where maternity clinics operated, Andrianakos recommended, a new type of midwife should be created, the nurse midwife, who would be the assistant of the obstetrician gynaecologist, whereas in the smaller towns and villages, municipal and community midwives, respectively, should exist and practise. And this did indeed happen exactly as prescribed by Andrianakos, though not as quickly as he would have liked. In pre-World War II Greece, midwives were mentioned as frequently as physicians as performers of abortions.[74] In 1954, although specialised physicians performed curettage, there were also plenty of 'uncouth old ladies' doing so, while women still used 'abortive medicines' obtained from the pharmacy.[75] In provincial Greece, and even where maternity clinics existed, midwives continued to routinely perform abortion in the late 1950s and early 1960s: 'The midwives … an aunt of mine had two abortions done in her house, without sedation, without anything, those times! Holy mother! And shrilled and shouted, the woman. Different times! Primitive situation!'[76] Things changed very quickly from then on, however: although most maternity clinics were in major urban centres, there were some in smaller towns too, such as Hios and Hermoupolis. In 1956, physicians attended around 39% of births and midwives attended an equal percentage. By 1969, 79% were attended by a physician and only 18% by a midwife, demonstrating the take-over of midwives' work by physicians, probably gynaecologists.[77] Danezes argued that in the 1960s virtually all induced abortions were obtained by D&C performed almost exclusively by experienced gynaecologists. A very small number, only in the provinces, were performed by general physicians, while virtually none were performed by midwives.[78] This was emphasised by an informant who had spent most of his professional life practising as a physician on Hios, though his wife (W) had mentioned earlier on an abortion performed by a midwife:

W. They would go to the maternity clinic then.

...

Q. And the abortions would take place there? In the maternity hospital?

W. And in private clinics. When later on new physicians arrived and they set up their own clinics … money, you should see!

A. … and other people [physicians] who set up clinics and of course, of course they did it as a profession then, because every abortion cost some money, cost some money and of course it presupposes great secrecy. Secrecy. Not to … But the interruption of pregnancy had always its dangers. The danger of perforating the uterus or causing damage was always there ….[79]

Thus, the abortion service previously partly provided by midwives was taken over swiftly in the 1960s by obstetrician gynaecologists. They replaced midwives at the same time that the use of abortifacients was eliminated, all responsibility henceforth resting in the hands of these newly trained professionals. This was implicitly but clearly promoted by the change in the law of 1950 which, as noted above, punished self-induced abortion with a higher sentence than one performed by a third party, while the clause which outlined a maximum sentence of ten years for the repeated performance of abortion was aimed at midwives, since the physicians could argue that they were attempting to save the life or health of the patient.[80] Non-physicians, when arrested, had no defence against the law.

One of the reasons why physicians were so eager to take over from midwives, despite the illegality of abortion, was monetary payment, as the interview quoted above indicates. The patient was paying not only for the competence of the physician in performing the procedure but also for secrecy, which was of paramount importance. These factors made abortion expensive, for many prohibitively so—although for most not as expensive as bringing up a child. Andrianakos himself emphasised in 1930 that the 'abortion industry was a lucrative one both for midwives and physicians'.[81] One can only assume that it became even more lucrative when it was transferred to the safe hands of specialised obstetrician/gynaecologists. The potential for enrichment from such a widespread practice as abortion was clear to those studying medicine in the 1960s.[82]

A. I would have never become a gynaecologist for those two reasons you mentioned … the abortions.
Q. Did you know about it while you were a student?
A. Of course! Everybody knew about it. It was not a secret, the whole world. The women would sit and chat, 'I had an abortion' she would say. Married women; single ones did not talk about it much.
Q. The married ones were saying it; they did not have any problem [talking about it]?
A. The children [should] not hear it; but we did hear it, we were children.
Q. Children? Not as students? Do you refer [to hearing it] as a child?
A. As young children and as students.
Q. So you knew about it long before you went to university?
A. Of course! It was not only me knowing it, everyone knew it. The whole world knew about it. It wasn't that I knew it, the whole world knew it. It was widespread [knowledge].
…
Q. Can I ask you where did curettages take place?
A. In the early years they took place in the private surgery. Later on in private clinics. The hospitals of course could not; in the hospitals they could not take place since these were controlled. In the private surgeries and private clinics.
Q. To what degree would you say, if you happen to know, to what degree were these safe?
A. As safe as any other gynaecological surgery that was taking place in a private clinic or surgery.[83]

Thus, the increasing availability of abortion work for gynaecologists and the potential for a good income contributed, at least in the early post-war years, to a significant increase in the number of gynaecologists, especially in the major cities. Andrianakos' vision for his profession had thoroughly materialised by the 1970s: almost all abortions and most births took place in major cities, where maternity hospitals and obstetrician gynaecologists were based, with women increasingly travelling there from the provinces to obtain their services, partly for the anonymity that places such as Athens offered.[84] Trained midwives proliferated and, indeed, became the mere assistants of the obstetrician gynaecologist. While in the 1950s some qualified midwives worked on their own in rural areas, gradually this practice was abandoned.[85] Thus, unlike the situation in the west, where anti-abortion campaigns were led by physicians against non-qualified practitioners, in Greece the 'battle' of abortion was fought in the 1930s and 1950s by the emerging specialisation of obstetrics and gynaecology against the mostly untrained midwives and the general physicians. The battle was short-lived: thoroughly backed by the state, the obstetrician gynaecologists emerged as the clear winner.

The law offered some protection to those physicians performing abortions from a very early point, particularly from 1924 onwards. At the same time, it increasingly threatened with prosecution those who performed abortions without medical qualifications. Much, if not all, of the change in the legal situation concerning abortion was driven by physicians and gynaecologists. Until the 1980s women were involved only as vessels of the pregnancy or as midwives, but in neither case did they voice their interests.

Was the 1986 law liberating after all? It was, in the sense that women could choose to have an abortion without any consultation with a physician at all, something that is still compulsory in many liberal societies, Britain among them. However, the earlier laws were very liberal towards practising physicians and had enough 'loopholes' to make abortion safe for physicians to procure. Physicians performing an abortion could argue, from 1924 onwards, that they acted in good faith and for the benefit of the pregnant woman, suggesting that her health or life was threatened. Women, having no medical training, could not argue that, and neither could midwives. Most significantly, the state was not particularly interested in pursuing those who carried out abortions, and did so extremely infrequently.

Conclusions

The law, as it stood during the first 90 years, faithfully represented the understanding of the people as to what was permissible and what not. As the majority of the women who took action did so in the very early days of a potential pregnancy they could not be accused of an offence that was not covered under the wording of the existing law. As very few women would act after the third or fourth month, hardly any cases reached the courts.[86]

The changes to the law made in 1924 and 1950, reflecting the practices and beliefs of the medical profession—which, to a degree, also reflected those of the populace—granted a privileged position to physicians to perform induced abortion for health and moral reasons. This allowed physicians to increasingly perform induced abortions, mostly in urban areas, with little fear of prosecution. Moreover, it provided physicians with the opportunity to highlight the evils of unqualified midwives and to work towards their virtual elimination by the 1960s. At the same time, gynaecology went from strength to strength, leading, very quickly, to the complete replacement of midwives in the delivery room and to their virtual exclusion from that role. Simply put, in the 1960s untrained midwives disappeared, trained midwives assumed a very limited authority and gynaecologists became the primary, if not the exclusive, providers of advice and support to women on 'women's' issues. Much of that was accomplished as a result of the provision of induced abortion through curettage and the fear that it would, otherwise, have been provided by untrained midwives.

Notes

1. Panteles D. Mpertsekas (1945) *Oi Kindynoi kai ai Epiplokai tes Amvloseos kai ta Iatrodikastika Provlemata Autes* (Athens: Euth. Hristodoulou), p. 100.
2. The original articles are available in Mpertsekas, *Oi Kindynoi*, p. 100 and also in Kostas Sofianos (1988) *To Nomiko Kathestos tes Paidikes Elikias kai tes Neotetas (1833–1900)*, 2 vols (Athens: Istoriko Arheio Ellenikes Neolaias), p. 7, 18/30 December 1833. All translations are by the author, unless otherwise stated. The original words are also given in those instances where it was felt that the translation could not be precise. *Eirkte* is the term used when imprisonment occurs as a sentence for felony. *Fylakisis* is the term used when imprisonment occurs as a sentence for a lesser offence, that of misdemeanour (*plemmelema*). Article 305 refers to cases when an abortion takes place against the mother's wishes or knowledge. As this is not something of interest in this study, this article is not explored.
3. Georgia I. Tsiomalou (2010) 'E Nomothesia peri tes Tehnetes Diakopes tes Egkymosynes: Koinoniologike proseggise' (unpublished undergraduate dissertation: Aristoteleio University Thessaloniki), p. 45, http://invenio.lib.auth.gr/, citing Elisavet Symeonide-Kastanide (1984) *E Amvlose os Provlema tou Poinikou Dikaiou* (Athens: Sakkoula), p. 75.
4. Nikolaos Kostes (1849) *Egheiridion Maieutikes* (Athens: S.K. Vlastos), pp. 81, 66. Kostes had been educated in Germany.
5. Kostes, *Egheiridion*, p. 81.
6. Kostes, *Egheiridion*, p. 81.
7. Vasileios Parlapanes (2014) 'E Iatrodikastike sten Ellada mesa apo demosieumata tou 19ou kai ton arhon tou 20ou aiona' (unpublished PhD thesis: Aristoteleio University Thessaloniki), Article 294, p. 135.
8. This contrasts the modern understanding of the word in Greek which today refers to the newborn.

9. Similar references are available in the writings of other obstetricians: Nikolaos Alex. Petsales (1902) *Peri tes ton Ymenon Episheseos. Symvole eis ten Aitiologian Auton* (Athens: Estia), p. 16; Anna Katsigra (1908) *E Maieutike en te Praxei* (Athens: Auge Athenon), p. 50.
10. See, for example, Mpertsekas, *Oi Kindynoi*. For more such references see Chap. 4.
11. N. Sp. (11 December 1901) 'E apotropaios praxis', *Empros*, 6(1841), p. 1.
12. Myle was the content of a molar pregnancy. See Chap. 4.
13. This is explicitly stated in a footnote (Konstantinos N. Kostes (1877) *Ermeneia tou en Elladi Ishyontos Poinikou Nomou*, vol. 2 (Athens: Typografeio Paliggenesias Io. Aggelopoulou), p. 405); Haralapos Tzortzopoulos, *Sholia eis ton Ishyonta Ellenikon Poinikon Nomon, Teuhos 1, Egklemata kata tes Zoes kai tou Somatos* (Athens: Athena, 1926), p. 185. Also L. Mantas (1945–60) 'Amvlosis' in *Evdomadiaia Egkyklopaidike Epitheorese O Elios*, vol. 2 (Athens: Elios), 480.
14. Konstantinos N. Kostes (1892) *Ermeneia tou en Elladi Ishyontos Poinikou Nomou*, vol. 2, 2nd edn (Athens: Anestes Konstantinides), pp. 450–1.
15. This is a point that has never been raised by the numerous legal commentators of the interwar period. Rather, some emphasised that the law indicated that abortion should be punished at all stages.
16. Kostes (1877) *Ermeneia*, vol. 2, p. 404. Kostes emphasised that the modern laws of France and Bavaria made the distinction between abortion before and after ensoulment redundant (Kostes (1877) *Ermeneia*, vol. 2, p. 403).
17. N. Momferatos (18 December 1905) 'Ar. 174(1905), Aparaiteton Stoiheion eine "na eteken e meter nekron vrefos e prooron"', *Themis Evdomadiaia Dikastike Efemeris*, 16(33), 513.
18. N. Gregorogiannes (13 May 1928) 'Ar. 708(1927), Amvlosis-vevaiotea stoiheia-emvryon zon e nekron', *Themis Evdomadiaia Dikastike Efemeris*, 39(18), 292.
19. Parlapanes, 'E Iatrodikastike', p. 121 citing the Penal Code of 1834 (*Poinikos Nomos tou Vasileiou tes Ellados 1834* (Naupleio: National Printers)); the Penal Code of 1835 (*Poinikos Nomos tou Vasileiou tes Ellados. Diatagma peri metatyposeos tou Ellenikou keimenou tou Poinikou Nomou 1835* (Athens: National Printers)); and Ioannes P. Pyrlas (1872) *Synekdemos Iatrodikastike*, vol. 2 (Athens: Passares).
20. Konstantinos N. Kostes (1871) *Ermeneia tou en Elladi Ishyontos Poinikou Nomou*, vol. 1 (Athens: Typografeio Paliggenesias Io. Aggelopoulou), pp. 349–50. Kostes clearly articulates that a caesarean was to be equated with the foetus death.
21. Kostes explicitly states that the husband and the woman's relatives were not to be asked for their opinion (Kostes (1871) *Ermeneia*, vol. 1, p. 350).

22. Kostes (1871) *Ermeneia*, vol. 1, p. 350.
23. Parlapanes, 'E Iatrodikastike', p. 125, citing Pyrlas, *Synekdemos.*
24. M. Venizelos (1881) *Maieutike* (Athens: n.p.), p. 558.
25. Venizelos, *Maieutike*, p. 558. A similar comment can be found in Th.A. Saktoures (1899) *Peri Apoxeseos tes Metras en te Maieutike kai Gynaikologia* (Athens: Sp. Kousoulinou), p. 71, suggesting that Venizelos was not exceptional.
26. Kostes (1892) *Ermeneia*, p. 453. The fact that Konstantinos Kostes, professor of law, was the son of Nikolaos Kostes, professor of obstetrics, may have made the former more sensitive and aware of issues involving child-bearing and abortion.
27. E. Symeonidou-Kastanidou (1995) *Egklemata kata tes Zoes* (Thessaloniki: Sakkoula), p. 784; Tzortzopoulos, *Sholia*, p. 212.
28. Article 282 (Tzortzopoulos, *Sholia*, p. 212).
29. V.A. Fotakes (January 1924) 'Ypo poias peristaseis dikaiologetai e iatrike amvlosis', *Iatrike Proodos*, 39(1), 4.
30. Symeonidou-Kastanidou, *Egklemata*, pp. 784–5.
31. Mpertsekas, *Oi Kindynoi*, pp. 100–1.
32. G.K. Lameras (August 1929) 'Endeixeis diakopes tes kyeseos epi kakoethon emeton', *O Praktikos Iatros*, (8), 315.
33. Anonymous (1930) 'Allelografia tou Praktikou iatrou. 3e erotesis', *Ellenike Iatrike*, 4(4), 435.
34. Kerameus Thessaloniki (1930) 'Eis to 3on erotema. Emmetoi egkyon', *Ellenike Iatrike*, 4(4), 546.
35. Tsiomalou, *E Nomothesia*, p. 46. Paxson suggests that abortion became illegal as a result of the 1950 law. However, the new 1950 penal code simply incorporated and clearly rearticulated what was already in practice through draft laws, interpretations of the law and 'justifications' for performing abortion (Heather Paxson (2004) *Making Modern Mothers: Ethics and Family Planning in Urban Greece* (Berkeley: University of California Press), p. 52).
36. Tsiomalou, *E Nomothesia*, p. 47.
37. Mpertsekas, *Oi Kindunoi*, p. 88.
38. Konstantinos Metropoulos (1954) *Ygieine tes Egkyou. Enas Polytimos Odegos gia ten Ygieine Diaviose tes Egkyou* (Athens: Papademetriou), p. 139.
39. Tsiomalou, *E Nomothesia*, pp. 43–4.
40. Konstantinos I. Roukas (1979) *Genetesiai Sheseis kai Prokletai Ektroseis eis Spoudastikon Plethysmo ton Athenon* (Athens: n.p.), p. 30.
41. Symeonidou-Kastanidou, *Egklemata*, p. 785.
42. Giannes Lexouriotes (1986) *Oi Koinonikes kai Nomikes Antilepseis gia to Paidi ton Proto Aiona tou Neoellenikou Kratous* (Athens: Dodone), pp. 272–3.

43. Tryfon K. Kontos (1883) *Peri Examvloseos e Amvloseos* (Athens: Enosis), p. 7; Timoleon Kardaras (1894) *Praktike Iatrike ton Oikogeneion* (Athens: Georgiou Fexe), 2nd edn, p. 47; Tryfon K. Andrianakos (1 May 1930) 'Organosis tes Proleptikes Iatrikes pros Katapolemesin tes Tehnetes Ektroseos kai Prostasian tes Teknogonias kai tes Metrotetos (Anakoinosis en to A Panellenion Synedrion Ygieines)', *Ellenike Iatrike*, 4(10), 1026.
44. Andrianakos, 'Organosis', 1026.
45. Hristodoulos Ant. Kampoures (1933) *Therapeutikai kai Koinonikai Endeikseis tes Tehnetes Ektroseos* (Athens: Georgiou Vasileiou), p. 32.
46. See, for example, I. Hatzesarantos (1 March 1920–28 February 1921) 'Ar. 295(1919), 'Systasis e synautourgia', *Themis Evdomadiaia Dikastike Efemeris*, 31(66); V. Tampakopoulos (1 March 1921–28 February 1922) 'Ar. 211(1921), 'Apopeira amvloseos para thelesin metros', *Themis Evdomadiaia Dikastike Efemeris*, 32, 259.
47. Mpertsekas, *Oi Kindynoi*, p. 100. The draft law became official law in 1951.
48. Metropoulos, *Ygieine*, p. 138.
49. F. Kavvadias (1 April 1967) 'Symperasmata apo ten syzetese tes Ellen. Etairias Eugonikes. Zetountai ... apogonoi', *Eleutheria*, 23(6917), 3; Ioannes M. Danezes (1969) 'E Tehnete Ektrosis os Diethnes kai Ellenikon Provlema', *Iatrike*, 15(3), 200, referring to a 1967 round table discussion on 'the problem of abortion'.
50. Vasilios Valaoras, A. Polychronopoulou, D. Trichopoulos (1969) 'Greece: Postwar abortion experience', *Studies in Family Planning*, 1(46), 14.
51. Roukas, *Genetesiai*, p. 30.
52. Symeonidou-Kastanidou, *Egklemata*, p. 38.
53. Marilyn El-Shahawi, 'Greece: Abortion Policy', www.un.org/esa/population/publications/abortion/doc/greece.doc (accessed 2 May 2013) giving as a source of information 'The Population Policy Data Bank maintained by the Population Division of the Department for Economic and Social Affairs of the United Nations Secretariat'.
54. Symeonidou-Kastanidou, *Egklemata*, p. 38.
55. Fabrice Cahen (2011) 'The "effectiveness" of public policies: The fight against "criminal" abortion in France, 1890–1950', *Revue d'Histoire Moderne & Contemporaine*, 58(3), i–xxvii.
56. This exact point—that the mother's life and health takes precedence over that of the foetus—was made in the Greek parliament in 1986 by the socialist PASOK MP Athanassios Filoppoulos when arguing for the full legalisation of abortion (Paxson, *Making*, p. 187).
57. Andrianakos, 'Organosis', 1025.
58. Andrianakos, 'Organosis', 1029.
59. Andrianakos, 'Organosis', 1030. The various adverts of physicians in the press certainly support his position.

60. Andrianakos, 'Organosis', 1030–1. In 1929 there was one gynaecology and obstetrics hospital in the country, with ninety-six beds, and four maternity hospitals with 220 beds (NSSG, *Statistical Yearbook of Greece 1930*, p. 445).
61. Andrianakos, 'Organosis', 1033.
62. Andrianakos, 'Organosis', 1033.
63. See No. 24, Mykonos, who had a 'midwife' perform her first abortion because she would cost less than a physician; however, the informant had major health problems subsequently. No. 5 Syros.
64. Tryfon K. Andrianakos (1937) 'Exelixis kai Proodoi tes Maieutikes kai Gynaikologias en te Neotera Elladi', *Ellenike Iatrike*, 11, special issue, 41–54 outlining the history of the constant attempts to 'educate the midwives so that the country will gradually get rid of the empirical ones'; Phokion Copanaris (1925) 'Greece' in *International Health Year-book 1924. Reports of the public health progress of twenty two countries* (Geneva: League of Nations), p. 202, referring to the 'Law of 1912 regulating the practice of the Medical profession'.
65. No. 23 Mykonos, herself an empirical midwife, argued, referring to unqualified midwives, that some were 'like a physician, she was like a physician, very good'. Interestingly, the same informant, when referring to the death of her father in the early twentieth century, remarked 'we did not have good physicians here'. Blum and Blum refer to the empirical midwife who served the mainland populations they studied in the late 1950s–early 1960s (Richard Blum and Eva Blum, *Health and Healing in Rural Greece* (Stanford, CA: Stanford University Press, 1965), pp. 150–1).
66. Copanaris, 'Greece', p. 212.
67. Phokion Copanaris (1933) *Demosia Ygeia kai Koinonike Iatrike* (Athens: Hr. Hronopoulou), p. 485.
68. *E Mykonos*, 20 December 1934.
69. *Nea Mykonos*, April 1954; *Nea Mykonos*, February 1957.
70. No. 23 Mykonos.
71. Sevaste Haviara-Karahaliou, *E Laike Iatrike tes Hiou* (Athens: Gasci-Hellas), pp. 462–3.
72. Blum and Blum, *Health and Healing*, pp. 150–5.
73. Andrianakos, 'Organosis', 1033.
74. No. 2 Hios. Significantly, the informant herself refused to have an abortion because of the danger involved. No. 10, Hios. No. 7D, wife of physician.
75. Metropoulos, *Ygieine*, pp. 138–42.
76. No. 7D. It was the wife of the informant who commented on my question concerning abortions in the community. The wife originated from the island. Blum and Blum also discuss the case of the empiric midwife based in rural mainland Greece who also worked in an Athens clinic where she

would see clients from the village and offer them her services, including the performance of caesarean sections to five-month-pregnant single women (*Health and Healing*, p. 50).

77. *Movement Naturel de la Population de la Grèce en 1961* (1963) (Athens: National Printers), p. xv; *Movement Naturel de la Population de la Grèce en 1969* (1971) (Athens: National Printers), p. xv.
78. Danezes, 'E Tehnete Ektrosis', 200.
79. No. 7D, informant and his wife.
80. Even the 1986 abortion law punishes self-abortion with a sentence of a maximum of one year's imprisonment (Symeonidou-Kastanidou, *Egklemata*, p. 786).
81. Andrianakos, 'Organosis', 1026.
82. No. 5D, graduated from medical school in 1968.
83. No. 6D, graduated from the Athens medical school in 1965. He was born in 1941. See also further discussion in Chap. 10.
84. In the early 1980s and beyond women had to make 'considerable efforts to obtain an induced abortion. These included the inconvenience of going to a doctor in the main town (40 miles away) and incurring travel costs as well as the cost of the operation, which is currently about 10,000 drachmas', not an insignificant amount for the time (H. Lovel and C. Bakoula (1985) 'Lack of family planning leading to induced abortion in rural Greece', *International Planned Parenthood Federation Medical Bulletin*, 19(3), 1).
85. For a number of such examples of unqualified midwives who practised beyond 1950 see N.X. Razes et al. (2008) *Anadrome. Gynaikeies Morfes tou Parelthontos me Prosfora ston Elleniko Ygeionomiko Horo* (Athens: Diktynna). This centrally based battle of gynaecology against the untrained midwives was not necessarily replicated in smaller localities, where, in many cases, physicians and untrained midwives not only harmoniously co-existed but in many cases collaborated (See, for example, Evaggelia Kamme (May 1992), 'Mikra ethografika meletemata tou topou mas. Tropos zoes-Prosopa. Oi gynaikes tes Mykonou. E Margarita e Mamme', *O Mykoniates*; No. 23 Mykonos, untrained midwife). See also Blum and Blum, whose study of population in rural mainland Greece revealed how local women preferred to consult—and pay—the empiric midwife, rather than see the educated one, who was paid by the state and therefore did not require further payment (*Health and Healing*, pp. 150–6).
86. However, as Cahen has pointed out, this does not necessarily mean that the anti-abortion policy was 'ineffective', as it would have had other social implications (Cahen, 'The "effectiveness"', p. xxv).

CHAPTER 7

The Ethics of Abortion: Poverty and Stigma

The Physicians

The twentieth-century references to abortion that appear in medical writings, in literature and in the press were, in general, short, but usually heavy with disapproval. And occasionally, mostly away from the public arena, individuals would express their opposition to abortion in stronger terms. So, in 1925 the physician Michael Iliou, in an article published in the medical journal *Ygeia*, argued for much tougher legislation against the 'crimes that parents commit against their own guts' so that punishment could be meted out to both parents and their collaborators—midwives and physicians who undertook such tasks, according to Iliou, for 'quick enrichment'. He presented a strong moral position, based upon his Christian beliefs, and encouraged the state to intervene in order to preserve the 'vitality of our race'.[1] An almost identical position was taken the subsequent year by the gynaecologist Haralampos Tzortzopoulos, who argued that abolishing punishment for abortion 'could bring social upheaval[, as] is obvious from the fact that such abolishing was included in the program of those political parties that are hostile towards [our] current social regime'—meaning the Soviet Union and Communism.[2] In 1930 the gynaecologist Tryfon K. Andrianakos, speaking at the first conference of hygiene, lamented that the existing strict laws on abortion were very rarely enforced.[3] He too saw this induced abortion 'industry' as a

V. Hionidou, *Abortion and Contraception in Modern Greece, 1830–1967*, Medicine and Biomedical Sciences in Modern History,
https://doi.org/10.1007/978-3-030-41490-0_7

source of enrichment for midwives and physicians but also viewed it as responsible for the decline in society's morals.[4]

In 1928 the Socialist Association of Women (Socialistikos Omilos Gynaikon) published its 'program', which included the right to abortion 'in those cases where it is performed by a physician and in order to save the life or health of the pregnant [woman]'.[5] The draft law of 1924 contained provisions relating to abortion performed not only to save the woman's life but also when major health effects were involved, suggesting that the Socialist Association of Women demanded little over and above what was already being proposed: their requests supported the change in the law, rather than demanding much more from it.

The 1930s, however, signalled a radical shift in the way abortion appeared in print: abortion was not only mentioned in the press but also extensively discussed. The origins of such discussions can be traced partly to the 1924 draft law but mainly to events outside Greece. In late 1930 Apostolos Doxiadis, a paediatrician who also served as Minister of Health (1922–1924) and Deputy Minister of Hygiene (1928–1929) in the Liberal government of Venizelos, published a series of articles, inspired by the Lambeth Conference that took place in the summer of that year at which the Anglican Church essentially accepted birth control, in the liberal newspaper *Eleutheron Vema*, in which he discussed the restriction of population and the various facets of the problem.[6] He stressed that 'even today abortions are much more common than anyone may think'—although physicians such as himself were well aware of the situation[7]—and explained the different experiences of the affluent, who could afford a safe, discreet abortion, and the poor, who would 'pay' for abortion with imprisonment or even their own life.[8] Although comparatively brief, Doxiadis' references to abortion attracted reactions such as that of the physician D. Saratses, who wrote in the pages of the same newspaper that he wished to see abortion legalised.[9] Doxiadis' articles also brought a strong reaction in the form of an anonymous article in the Church-sponsored journal *Ekklesia* ('Church').[10] Interestingly, this referred to abortion only once and in response to Saratses' proposal, which it viewed as representing the efforts of 'many from the "leading class" steering towards the extreme Bolshevik anarchy'.[11] This public comment, articulated in the strongly anti-Communist political climate of the time, would have felt threatening for individual physicians who dared to express such a liberal point of view. This was a recurrent tactic in 1930s Greece, as the owner of the *Eleutheron Vema* commented at a different point in time: 'by hurling this deliberately vague word [communism] at anything they find displeasing and against all their ideological or personal rivals they hope—and sometimes manage—to obscure the simple truth'.[12] In 1929 the Liberal Venizelist government had voted through the infamous *Idionymon* law, 'for the protection of the social status quo' by means of an initial six-month imprisonment for those who 'aimed at the implementation of ideas leading to the forcible overthrow of the prevailing social order'.[13] The law was liberally used to suppress communism and 'alleged' communists in the 40 years that followed. No wonder that even the official newspaper of the Greek Communist Party, *Rizospastes*, had carefully avoided discussion of abortion, referring to it for the first time in 1931 when discussing German efforts to amend the restrictive abortion law there.[14]

The discussion of contraception and pro-abortion events in Weimar Germany encouraged a mainstream liberal newspaper, *Makedonia*, to publish an editorial in late 1931 addressing the 'social issue' of abortion and inviting individuals to offer their opinion.[15] As many Greek gynaecologists and physicians were trained in Germany, they would certainly have been following the events there in relation to abortion closely. In response to the editorial, in late 1931 and early 1932 a series of articles appeared in the paper, written by a variety of experts, most of them physicians of different specialisations, each one examining the issue from a different angle. Though there were points of disagreement among the authors, there were also areas of nearly universal agreement, including the necessity of legally permitted, induced abortion when the mother's life was in danger or when the pregnancy was a result of rape. In terms of the mother's life, abortion had already been legally available since 1924 provided that the mother had received the approval of three physicians who had discussed the case.[16] Such provisos, nevertheless, made abortion, even when the mother's life was in danger, accessible to only a few—namely, the very affluent and urbanites—hence the requests for a relaxation of the restrictions of the existing law.[17] Indeed, even authors who rejected abortion wholesale accepted that it should be made legally available for those pregnant as a result of rape.[18]

Somewhat surprisingly, the majority of authors in the 1930s recommended the legalisation of abortion for unwed women in order to prevent the birth of illegitimate children, and all that this brought to Greek society.[19] The arguments presented by these writers were virtually identical, irrespective of the ideological background of the author: both a married woman who carried the child of someone other than her husband or a girl who had fallen 'victim' to a man who promised to marry her but refused to do so were considered by society to be dishonoured, were scorned by parents, relatives and friends and eventually were divorced by the husband or disinherited by the parents, respectively. Such a pregnancy, all authors agreed, could and on many occasions did lead to murder (mostly of the lover by the husband or the brother).[20] All of the above destroys the civil order, authors argued. Removing the pregnancy, which was ultimately responsible for the disturbance of civil order, would therefore help to maintain the social balance and was the only humane resolution to the situation.[21] Essentially, the effects of an illegitimate birth upon Greek society were felt to be so enormous, complicated and unbearable for all those involved and those around them that it was infinitely preferable, despite any ethical problems related to the foetus, to perform an abortion.[22] It was a 'chimera and utopia', Panteles Mpertsekas argued in 1945, for anyone to hope that the penal code alone would ever be able to prevent such abortions from taking place.[23] Reversing the argument, he apportioned responsibility to the state, for expecting young women to bear illegitimate children when the state itself did not offer any protection to the child or the mother in such cases.[24] Similarly, a decade earlier, both Mpertsekas and Hristodoulos Kampoures had strongly recommended that the state should legislate to recognise illegitimate children and offer them protection; provide financial help to the pregnant mother of an illegitimate child; and enforce marriage between the expectant mother and the father, when possible. Although support for the foetus was unambiguously expressed, the language used by these authors on the necessity to abort illegitimate foetuses was uncompromising:

> what is preferable and more legitimate? To sustain and keep alive an incomplete existence or to forestall so many adverse and multiple consequences at the expense of an existing and active mother? Without doubt every logical person is obliged to choose the mother to be saved rather than for the unborn foetus to live off her.[25]

Mpertsekas in 1945, like Kampoures in 1933 and the host of physicians and others who participated in the *Makedonia* exchange, focused on the inadequacies of the Greek state, in terms of both legislation and finance, and on the questionable way Greek society reacted to the 'deceived' women.[26] None of the authors apportioned responsibility to the 'deceived' women, not only because 'it is only human to be deceived' but also because the single girl 'surrenders' herself only when truly in love.[27] This liberal approach to abortion, typical of many physicians in the 1930s and 1940s, did see some opposition:[28] a few writers argued against abortion in moral terms, suggesting that if it were to become legal, very quickly the moral basis of traditional Greek society would collapse;[29] others suggested that the purpose of marriage was to have children and thus couples should use means to avoid childbearing if they could not afford more children, rather than resorting to abortion.[30] Nevertheless, many commentators of the time articulated very strong arguments in support of prolific mothers whose poverty made more children impractical.[31] Mpertsekas and others highlighted the very difficult economic situation that obliged many married women to seek employment outside the home, becoming, for example, servants or washer-women. A pregnancy would, Mpertsekas argued, curtail the ability of such women to work, and thus further impoverish their families and existing children.[32] He believed the penal code punishing abortion in such cases to be punitive and suggested ironically that a law should be introduced 'abolishing the financial impoverishment of people' and imposing strict marriage prohibitions among the poor. For humanitarian reasons, Mpertsekas argued, the law should permit impoverished women to undertake induced abortion, as 'the very strong and early developed emotion of motherhood never forgives her for the destruction of the life of her own child', and these emotions were the most severe punishment possible for a mother who could not afford more children. Moreover, aborting mothers were further emotionally punished by the performance of abortion itself.[33] As noted above, one of Mpertsekas' suggestions was that the state should follow the lead of other countries and offer financial help and support to the poor in society, rather than punish them when they attempted, through abortion, to prevent a further worsening of their situation. In this regard his attitude to the state and the church, who effectively demanded that impoverished couples bear children, was somewhat caustic: '[the state] providing only the severity of the penal code and [the church] its elevated perceptions; they do nothing but ignore the reality and oppose the poor who at the end they [the state and the church] push towards abortion from non-scientific hands, with grave consequences for the poor.'[34] Even physicians who stood against abortion believed that the improvement of the financial situation of poor mothers would substantially reduce the incidence of abortion.[35] As early as 1932 the anonymous author of an article published in *Socialist Life*, presumably a socialist feminist, had also argued for the right of poor women to determine the number of their children through the availability of legal abortion.[36]

Mpertsekas also dealt with a third, numerically significant group that resorted regularly to abortion, namely those women among the affluent and the aristocracy who saw pregnancy as an obstacle to their social life. He cited estimates that such women had on average 1.5 children, whereas poorer Athenians had on average 3.0.[37] Although some authors argued that even the affluent were under severe financial pressures that obliged them to resort to abortion, Mpertsekas saw their choice to restrict procreation as individualistic and essentially selfish.[38] Moreover, he argued that such trends were also seen among the educated in rural areas and that a significant reason for this behaviour was that women wanted to retain as far as possible their youth and beauty by avoiding childbearing through the use of contraception and abortion. This trend Mpertsekas vehemently opposed, and he strongly recommended that physicians not perform abortions in such cases. In such cases he wanted to see strict enforcement of the law as well as the reinforcement of values of religion and homeland 'as inexhaustible sources of strong ideological and human uplifting'.[39] Similarly, Konstantinos Metropoulos, writing in the early 1950s, recommended that abortions should be permitted only if the woman had three live children.[40] And, although supportive of abortion for women carrying illegitimate pregnancies, he proposed that this should be restricted to one per woman, presumably believing that two 'mistakes' by the same woman indicated loosened morals rather than simple errors.[41] Some continued to argue against abortion and the moral decline that it would bring, referring in many cases to the needs of the nation.[42]

The liberal discourse supporting induced abortion thus seems to have been waning in the 1950s—or, at least, those who were of this view became silent. A eugenics society set up in Greece in 1953 engaged obstetricians, paediatricians and population experts (all physicians) in a public meeting and discussion on abortion on March 29, 1967, at which the results of two investigations on abortion, funded by the American Population Council and the International Planned Parenthood Federation, were presented and discussed.[43] The principal investigator was V. Valaoras, who emphasised the 'extreme decline' of fertility in Greece and argued that the purpose of the 'state, the Church and the science in Greece is to teach potential parents today to avoid those terrible homicides, which is what abortions are'.[44] This event enjoyed wide coverage in the national press, although once the Colonels' dictatorship came to power in April

1967 further public discussion of the issue effectively ceased. The issues of abortion and low population growth came to the fore again after 1974—that is, after the re-establishment of a democratic regime.[45] Silence in fact characterised much of the public discourse of the 1950s and 1960s in relation to induced abortion. Reports on abortion did appear in the press throughout this period, but as something that occurred elsewhere.[46] For example, in an article reporting on abortion among advanced societies and entitled 'Is induced abortion a crime?' the introduction comments that

> [i]t is no secret to anyone that hundreds and thousands of human beings never manage to see the daylight due to induced abortions. Illicit or married couples, who do not wish to take on the responsibility of a child, resort to this method, to bring to a stop the annoying pregnancy. Is this act an irretrievable right or do they commit the offence of homicide?[47]

The article reported widely on the practices and laws in many advanced countries but refrained from making any direct links to or mentions of Greece. In an earlier issue of the same newspaper, a translated article discussed Alfred Kinsey's work in the USA and included a brief reference to induced abortion.[48] However, it was also in the 1960s that Valaoras and his collaborators undertook a number of major surveys on abortion and widely publicised their results, though mostly within academic circles.[49]

The Church

What is glaring in all these contemporary discussions is the absence of the Greek Orthodox Church and references to its teachings. As early as 1924 the Archimandrite Danielides, in his *Life of the Young People*, condemned the 'spirit of hedonism' that led women to avoid childbearing, using various methods to destroy their foetuses and occasionally murdering themselves too in the process.[50] In the exchange of opinions in *Makedonia*, mentioned above, the only Christian contribution came in the form of a translated article by A. Herbert Gray.[51] Regrettably, this proved to be focused on birth control rather than abortion, reflecting the interests of his society at the time. The Greek Church seemed to have little to contribute to the discussion on abortion. Only in 1933 did the Archimandrite Seraphim Papakostas, leader of the Christian organisation *Zoë*, deal with the issue of childbearing from the Greek Orthodox point of view.[52] In recent times this book has been assessed as representing quite accurately the concerns of the Greek Church at the time.[53] Nevertheless, and despite the full endorsement of the book by the Church from 1937 onwards, it did not originate with the Church but with an organisation that was created as a private initiative 'as a result of the inefficacy of the official church to fulfil the religious needs of its flock'.[54] In short, Papakostas was attempting to fill the gap created by the Church's lack of interest in and unwillingness to deal with social issues such as birth control and abortion.

Papakostas's book discussed abortion explicitly, but the focus was much more on contraception and its use. His view of abortion was that it was the second worst method of individuals averting themselves from the responsibility of children, the most egregious being the abandoning of an infant by its married mother.[55] He emphasised that the foetus is alive from the moment of its conception, in accordance with medical writings,[56] and, despite the fact that abortion 'in our time is hugely popular', he blamed physicians and midwives for performing what he equated with an act of murder.[57] Although in this first decisive movement of the Church, as well as in subsequent articulations of its position, the timing of ensoulment is fixed, in the past Dionysios Pyrros o Thettalos, a senior physician and cleric in early nineteenth-century Greece, was much more ambivalent.[58] His conclusion in 1831 was that knowledge on the issue was limited and only God had the definitive answer. He himself saw a very close link between ensoulment and quickening:

> The soul therefore ... enters the human after his conception and creation in the womb of the woman. When and after how many days [the soul] establishes itself (diorizetai) no one knows except for God, [the soul's] creator .... This is the rational (logike) soul that puts into motion the foetus in the mother's womb.[59]

His position on ensoulment, it might be assumed, did not contradict the teachings of the Church at the time. Papakostas, writing a century later in support of the argument that ensoulment occurs at conception, quoted both the Greek physician K.N. Louros, who was firmly against *any* induced abortion, and the existing legislation of the early 1930s,[60] as well as making use of foreign publications, such as that by Charles Gore, bishop of Oxford.[61] Interestingly, Papakostas rejected the argument put forward by Marie Stopes, Margaret Sanger and some Greek physicians that the availability and knowledge of contraception would reduce the need and practice of abortion. Instead, he asserted, 'what we observe is that the number of abortions increases as the use of contraceptives increases', a situation he attributed to the inefficiency of the available methods.[62]

The Church's first decisive move in articulating its position on the issue of childbearing—and indirectly of abortion—came in the first encyclical of the Greek Church on childbearing in 1937, which was overseen by Archbishop Hrysostomos Papadopoulos and strongly condemned abortion.[63] It remained the central text on this issue, with simple reiterations of its message taking place in 1958 and 1972. In a further encyclical issued in 1968 by Bishop Meletios of Kythera, he declared, after summarising the evidence on the extensive practice of abortion, that the Holy Synod had decided that declining fertility was a result of the loosening of morals.[64] In the same year another encyclical reiterated previous ones while further declaring that life is present in the sperm and that 'at every stage of the pregnancy it enjoys the rights of life of a personality'.[65] The mother, the physician and the midwife—but, tellingly, not the father—were all criminals responsible for a murder when an abortion was performed. Yet a different encyclical, published also in 1968, very soon after the previous, and focused specifically on abortion, became known as the encyclical of abortions.[66] This started by calling abortion an act of perversion.[67] The author listed the 'usual' reasons for abortion as eugenics, morality—referring mainly to illegitimate pregnancies—and the health of the mother. These, the author declared, were not issues for any human to decide upon; even physicians should not be allowed to make decisions that relegate the life of the foetus to an inferior position to that of the mother. The choice was a clear one between the ephemeral, temporal life and the spiritual life.[68] In 1971 a Church committee set up to investigate the 'Population problem' of Greece remained active for much of the following decade.[69] A further encyclical issued in 1978 saw the Church standing by its earlier position on abortion and encouraging the state not to proceed to the legalisation of abortion; physicians not to perform it; and confessors to keep to their instructions.[70] Again, this was a reaction to the legal discussions taking place at the time—discussions that led to a further liberalisation of the law in that same year.

The position of the Church can be readily summarised as a constant and unmoving one in opposition to abortion in virtually all circumstances. What is fascinating to observe is the Church's timing in officially expressing its position: it did so not when the rest of society was publicly discussing the issue; rather, it made its announcements at times when wider discussion was muted, as in 1937, during the Metaxas dictatorship,[71] and in 1968 and 1969, during the Colonels' dictatorship. At these times public dialogue on such social issues was silenced as a result of the nationalistic and ultra-conservative political situation, especially regarding women and their role in society, and the Church felt comfortable enough to express its position, secure in the knowledge that there would be no untoward reaction from the public, physicians or, indeed, anyone else.

The Women

Women used emmenagogues as such throughout the nineteenth and twentieth centuries. The switch that occurred to the use of these or similar substances as abortifacients—or, for that matter, women beginning to seek curettage—involves a moral leap on the part of an individual because in the latter case a foetus may be involved. The decisions made by women were shaped by their understanding of the form and attributes of early pregnancy, and oral evidence suggests that laypersons' understanding of ensoulment, along with that of the lower ranks of the priesthood, was much closer to Pyrros' position than to the Church's. Even among physicians there was no one unified position regarding the timing of ensoulment. In any case, whatever an individual physician's position on ensoulment, it did not appear to determine their position on abortion.[72] Even the position of the Church—or, more precisely, its practitioners—was not a completely unmoving one. This divergence in beliefs is evident even beyond 1950,[73] although the degree to which popular beliefs influenced Greek physicians or vice versa remains to be examined in the future. An example of a rather ambiguous stance towards 'bringing on the menses' is shown in responses of a woman from Mykonos, who was in a similar situation to the informant from Rhodes discussed in Chap. 4, speaking of her experiences in the 1950s:

> I said to the midwife I am pregnant, I am ten days overdue, I think I am pregnant. She says 'have hot baths every night and climb on a tub and jump' .... I am 10 days [late], it would not be murder. But I did not do anything .... I thought to myself, leave it. If something were to happen to me? What if I do commit murder? If the child is formed (demeno)? No, no ... I thought what if something happens to my kidneys, if I get a haemorrhage and I will end up dying too? And I did not do anything, never [for none of her pregnancies] .... The midwife, an old woman, told me a 'traditional method' (praktiko), she thought ten days is early. If it was longer, she

> would not have told me. Ten days is nothing, just with the hot bath, it would start [the period]. But I did not do anything, I was afraid.[74]

The early days following a missed period were, as discussed in Chap. 4, a time of ambiguity for physicians, untrained midwives and women. Although this informant did not follow her midwife's advice because of her fear of the possible effects on her health and life, she did also consider the possibility that the child may have already been 'formed', and refers twice to the possibility of committing murder. This informant was not desperate to avoid the pregnancy and so did not proceed, which may partly explain her expression of her ethical qualms during the interview. For other individuals, with stronger incentives to avoid a birth, the existing ambiguity around the issue of when the child was formed would have provided the moral space required to take the necessary decision and not consider the action as abortion.

It is perhaps significant, however, that this same informant, despite her anxiety about the possibility of 'committing a murder', did not associate what had been suggested to her by the midwife with what I referred to when I mentioned abortion:

Q. Have you ever heard from other women that they … had abortions? Getting rid of the baby?
A. No, not in my time, they did not do those things. But now [they do] …. Did they not know then? Were they scared? Who knows?'[75]

It appears, then, that for this informant the actions the midwife suggested she take after ten days of menstrual delay bore no relation to abortion as it was performed at the time of the interview, in the 1990s, or to curettage performed by physicians at the time of her dilemma in the 1950s. She viewed her situation simply as a matter of bringing her menses back.

Other informants, who did brave the suggestions offered to them, often found the tried methods inefficient:

Q. You had seven children. Would you have liked more?
A. [Laughs] Of course [not], even those we had … we did not want them. But since god sent them, we did not want to break/destroy them (halasoume).
Q. To destroy them? How would you destroy them?
A. Don't they? Do they not?

Q. Did they do this at that time? Do you mean abortion?
A. They did! Of course they did!
Q. So, you knew that you could … ?
A. Oh no, I never did …
Q. No, I mean that if you wanted to do it, you could have done it! Did you not want or did you not know that you could destroy them?
A. Listen, I had a child, we said it was my Katina [born] in 1939 and Giorgos [born] in 1940. How old was Katina [when I fell pregnant with the next one]? For goodness sake! They would say, do this, do that. And I drank many times drinks, supposedly they would do … but they didn't.
Q. Who was giving you those drinks? What kind of drinks were those?
A. How can I remember now?
Q. Were these from a physician? A midwife?
A. From female friends.
Q. Did you know what it was?
A. They told me. This vegetable, boil it.
Q. And the child will fall?
A. But it did not fall![76]

At about the same time—that is, in the 1930s and 1940s—some women from Mykonos had undergone curettage abortions in Athens/Piraeus while living there. Though these were 'modern', that is performed by midwives and physicians, ethical questions remained vivid in the mind of the women:

Q. Did you have a miscarriage?
A. Me? I am a murderer.
Q. After the third?
A. It was the first. And after my son Kostas, two abortions. Because my husband insisted. My husband did not want us to have any children.
Q. And the first one, did you … ?
A. In the first one I went through a lot. I was very lucky to survive it.[77]

The informant suffered major health problems following her first abortion, which had been performed by a 'midwife' chosen by her husband in preference to a physician to reduce the cost. Similarly, an informant from Syros admitted that his wife had 'two or three' abortions during the occupation years (1941–1944), as there was an ongoing famine there. The abortions were 'easy to arrange', as there were a couple of midwives on the island who were happy to perform them.[78] This informant did not express any moral qualms, possibly because he was a man but also probably because the famine, he felt, fully justified the couple's decision to abort. Thus, those seeking abortion in towns and cities seem to have been well served from the 1930s onwards, and in rural Greece things were beginning to change as well: by the 1950s, rural women were employing the whole array of terminology and methods, usually starting with traditional methods and proceeding to modern ones, with moral questions being present to different degree depending on the methods used:

A. Lots of worries. Putting my feet in limewater, jumping off walls …
Q. Why did you put your feet in limewater?
A. For my period to come. Traditional methods (praktika). I prepared limewater and put my feet in. What did I not put [inside me] from below! I forget what it was called, permanganate? No, no. I was in danger of being poisoned, so that the period would come.[79]

When the methods mentioned failed and she reached the second month of pregnancy, this informant sought advice from the local physician, whom she and her husband knew well in a professional capacity.

> I went there with a purpose, *there weren't then abortions* but I said, I am 27 years old and have 5 children! What will happen? And he tapped my shoulder and he said to be careful. Because I was upset and I thought, me a mother to kill my child? And I became sad and stopped and I kept it.[80]

Thus, the first stage for this informant in the 1950s was an attempt to 'bring on her period', a course of action about which she had no moral qualms or concerns for her own welfare. During the second stage, she consumed 'drinks' and inserted objects inside herself, again in an attempt to bring the period on; however, these methods gave rise to concerns about her health. All these attempts occurred early on, in the first month of the pregnancy. During the second month the visit to the physician took place hoping for an end to the pregnancy, despite her statement that abortions were not then available. However, the informant's visit to the physician gave rise to her use of language such as 'child' and 'killing', possibly utilising the terminology employed by the counselling physician and suggesting that she was experiencing moral qualms about the consequences of the procedure.

It is in the interviews from Mykonos—that is, among the oldest women I discussed abortion with—that the strongest ethical stance is revealed, in, for example, their reluctance to name the action, let alone perform it. This was especially the case for those who spent their whole life away from major urban centres.

Q. So, you did not know [how to have fewer children]?
A. No, I did not … not even to have a child and to …
Q. Get rid of it (rixei)?
A. Oh no, no, no. God help (alimono)!
Q. God help? Did you not know about such things on Mykonos then?
A. No, no, no.[81]

Those informants who were aware of abortion, or who were prepared to acknowledge that they were aware of it, had nevertheless discarded the idea of employing abortion themselves despite declaring that they would have liked fewer children:

Q. Could you have done it [abortion] here?
A. No, but I did not want to … for any of the children. I had them all strong [healthy] children.
Q. Had you heard of instances of other women who went to Athens?
A. Er, yes, they did, yes. I don't know who but I had heard that they were going.
Q. So it was known.
A. I did not want [to do] that.[82]

One strong reason for rejecting the notion of terminating a pregnancy was the fear of committing a sin, although, interestingly, the origins of this feeling did not come directly from the church or the priest:

> I was scared of the sin. Sometimes there were some women and … they destroyed them. I did not like that. Whatever God wants … with God's fate they grew up, none of them got ever ill …. There were also the old women, old [thinking] women and they would say, my dear it is a pity/sin and every child is born with its own fate. So I was fearful too.[83]

The fear of undertaking an unethical deed was evidently present in the thinking of other informants too:

Q. So, were they not careful?
A. Whatever came, came [whatever came was accepted]. They did not do then what they are doing these days.
Q. Why? Did they not know?
A. I don't know. They feared in case they did something bad.
Q. What kind of bad thing? To whom?
A. Misdeed (kako). That the thing they would destroy (halasoune) ….[84]

It is noteworthy that these women articulated their unease about abortion as stemming not from its illegality and the possibility of punishment by law but rather from the ethical problems surrounding it.

Women and men who had spent time in Athens seemed more prepared to undertake abortion, even when they acknowledged that it was not an ethical course of action.[85] An informant from Mykonos, for example, had three abortions while residing in Athens.[86] Her husband, who was instrumental in the decision-making, was a sailor and had wide experience of life outside Greece. However, it is possible that the main reason for this particular informant's ready admission of her abortions was that they had not been her choice; rather, they had been imposed on her. Informants who were the sole decision-makers in undertaking an abortion were much more reluctant to acknowledge that they had one. One informant, for example, initially denied that she had had an abortion and, even though she acknowledged that she had not wanted any more children, she initially presented her loss of a pregnancy as a miscarriage. Only later on did she interrupt me to explain why and how she undertook the abortion in the very early stages of the pregnancy, concluding that 'this is my sin. You are the first one that I said it to. I have not told even the confessor.'[87] Such an extreme concealment is understandable on three levels, those of the individual, the family and wider society: the informant, who had her own qualms about the procedure, had misled her husband into believing that she had suffered a miscarriage, while living within an island society whose ethical code condemned abortion. While concealment addressed the last two problems, it could not address the first. Nevertheless, the informant had not regretted her decision, and her family circumstances had allowed her to overcome her own ethical concerns. She clearly articulated right from the start, even before she mentioned the 'miscarriage', that she had not wanted more children because she was very busy in the family business which, she felt, she ran on her own, while the husband failed to shoulder his share of the responsibilities. The importance of the business and the improvement of her family's financial situation were prominent throughout the interview and the informant was proud of her own achievements. These factors, along with the informant's familiarity with Athens and the easy access to abortion it offered, meant that an abortion was the obvious course for her. However, the attitudes to abortion prevalent in her own community meant that she never felt able to trust the local confessor sufficiently to ask for forgiveness.

Once again, the absence of the church and the priests from the informants' discourse is palpable. Despite the ethical qualms that many of the women articulated, neither the Church nor priests were ever mentioned as possible bastions of ethical law. It seems that 'old ladies' and some physicians were foremost among those influencing the ethical decisions of the women.[88] As Herzfeld argued, there are two separate concepts of sin in Greek society: the societal, as expressed by the informants quoted above, and the ecclesiastical.[89] The local priests, who could and frequently did marry, led lives very similar to those of their flock. It is not surprising, therefore, that they seem to have themselves embraced birth control, though not necessarily abortion. Averof, for example, in his survey of the late 1930s, reported that two priests who were questioned declared that they supported birth control: one had only three children after 13 years of marriage, the other had four after 14 years.[90] Blum and Blum reported a similar situation in the areas they studied in the late 1950s and early 1960s.[91] Even a Catholic priest on Syros, when a parishioner sought advice as to whether he was permitted to restrict his fertility, was not discouraging, but advised the informant to follow his own conscience.[92] Eugenia Georges' informants demonstrated that the Church's instructions had little bearing either on aborting women in the 1990s or on the two confessors who readily offered forgiveness to the two informants who confessed their abortions.[93] Similarly, one of my Athenian informants stated that her confessor responded by saying that abortion was sinful and advising her not to have any more, but did not admonish her for her actions.[94] This implicit forgiveness that some confessors offered to aborting women does not seem to be exceptional despite being contrary to the explicit instructions of the Church, which in 1978 felt it necessary to reiterate to the confessors in no uncertain terms that they were 'instructed by the Synod to say the same thing to all and not to transgress from the [official] line', something that seems to have been happening often enough.[95] Whether women were offered forgiveness or not, they seem to have confided to their priest quite often about undertaking abortions: Blum and

Blum's best estimates of abortion levels in the rural communities they studied came from their 'knowledgeable priest'; indeed, this was knowledge that physicians and others either did not have or did not want to share.[96] The tacit acceptance and unofficial forgiveness of abortion by—at least some of—the lower echelons of the Church allowed women to continue doing what their own consciences and, frequently, those of older advising women guided them in doing. The hope of forgiveness made it possible for women to have abortions without feeling obliged to forfeit their links to the Church. The majority of women did seriously consider the ethical aspects of abortion but, still, many continued with the procedure. The complex relationship and interactions between the Church and popular religiosity have been very competently discussed by Nikos Kokosalakis. Through the principle of 'economy' (Oikonomia), which essentially means that the institution of the Church makes compromises in accepting transgressive popular practices—including, here, abortion—the harmonious co-existence of the two is sustained.[97]

Conclusions

This discussion has outlined the general disconnect of the state from the abortion discourse and the influence of the political situation on the fate of such a discourse. Although the effects of politics on abortion discourse are well known in the contemporary USA, for example, where funding to certain organisations associated with abortion depends on the stance of the government of the day, this was never thought, previously, to have been the case for Greece. Here we observe a juxtaposition between state, Church, physicians and population in which Church and state, for much of the observed period, were opposed to abortion, whereas physicians and the population were discreetly engaged in it whenever individuals deemed it necessary. Many physicians supported abortion as a social necessity, each seeing it as justified under some—not always the same—circumstances. Few rejected it outright. It appears that physicians had a virtually exclusive right, by virtue of their profession, to engage in such a discourse. But a free discourse was not always possible; during dictatorships and nationalist or socially conservative governments the climate did not favour a liberal discussion and there was silence about the issue from all except the Church, which would become most vocal in its opposition to abortion at exactly those times. Public discourse would occur only when the political climate was right. Considering both the polarisation of the discourse on abortion and the wider adoption of birth control in the 1930s an extensive public engagement with birth control might be expected. Nothing, however, could be less true.

Notes

1. Michael Eliou (15 September 1925) 'E Enishysis tes Zotikotetos tes Fyles mas', *Ygeia*, 2(18), 262. However, the author makes it clear that abortion was not the only reason for the very small number of children that some couples had.
2. Haralampos Tzortzopoulos (1926) *Sholia eis ton Ishyonta Ellenikon Poinikon Nomon, Teuhos 1, Egklemata kata tes Zoes kai tou Somatos* (Athens: Athena), p. 179.
3. Tryfon K. Andrianakos (1 May 1930) 'Organosis tes proleptikes iatrikes pros katapolemesin tes tehnetes ektroseos kai prostasian tes teknogonias kai tes metrotetos (anakoinosis en to A Panellenion Synedrion Ygieines)', *Ellenike Iatrike*, 4(10), 1026.
4. Andrianakos, 'Organosis', 1026.
5. Anonymous (3/4 December 1928) 'To programma tou S.O.G', *Sosialistike Zoe*, cited in Iris Aude-Kalkane (1997) *Mia antartissa tes Poles sten taragmene Athena. Athena Gaitanou-Gianniou 1880–1952* (Athens: ELIA), p. 60. S.O.G was created in October 1919 and represented the female expression of the Greek socialist movement. It became a significant part of the feminist movement, one that focused not only on the vote but more significantly on social issues that affected women's everyday lives (Anonymous, 'To programma', pp. 54–65).
6. Richard Allen Soloway (1982) *Birth Control and the Population Question in England, 1877–1930* (Chapel Hill: The University of North Carolina Press), p. 316.
7. Apostolos Doxiadis (12 September 1930) 'E These tes Gynaikos', *Eleutheron Vema*, pp. 1–2.
8. Doxiadis, 'E These', 1–2.
9. D. Saratses (3 February 1931) 'E Anthropotes ekfylizetai?', *Eleutheron Vema*, p. 3.
10. Anonymous (4 October 1930) 'E prolepsis ton Genneseon', *Ekklesia*, 40, 325.
11. Anonymous, 'E prolepsis', 325.
12. Mark Mazower (1997) 'Policing the Anti-Communist state in Greece, 1922–1974' in Mark Mazower (ed.) *The policing of politics in the twentieth century* (Providence: Berghahn), p. 138, citing D. Livieratos (1987) *Koinonikoi agones sten Ellada (1927–1931)* (Athens: n.p.), p. 29.

13. Mazower, 'Policing', pp. 138–9.
14. Anonymous (27 March 1931) 'Apergia peines Germanidos iatrou', *Rizospastes*, 14(6854), p. 2. The same newspaper at later dates discussed the liberal law on abortion in Soviet Union and subsequently its restriction (Anonymous (31 December 1932) 'The issue of abortions', *O Neos Rizospastes*, 2(462), p. 1; Anonymous (12 August 1935) 'Sovietikes apanteseis sta erotimata ton ergaton olou tou kosmou', *Rizospastes*, 5(450/7885), p. 2; Anonymous (30 May 1936), 'Ste Sovietike Enose: Zoeres syzeteseis gia to Zetema tes ektroses', *Rizospastes*, 6(669/9013), p. 2). In both occasions, the presentation of the Soviet situation was shaped to respond to the Greek readership rather than 'trouping' Soviet progressiveness. If anything, there was much more space dedicated in this newspaper on the revoking of the liberal abortion policy in the late 1930s. There were, for example, articles on *Rizospastes* on the 30 May 1936, 9 June 1936, 18 June 1936, 23, June 1936 and 28 June 1936.
15. Cornelia Usborn (2007) *Cultures of Abortion in Weimar Germany* (New York: Berghahn), p. 3. Anonymous (16 March 1931) 'Ta ethe tes epohes mas. E polekrotos ypothesis tou Dros Volf. Eine dikaioma tes gynaikas e ektrosis?', *E Proia*, pp. 1, 5.
16. Georgios K. Zouraris (24 December 1931) 'Einai Egklema e Ektrosis e Apeleutherotikon Kinema?', *Makedonia*, 22(6955), p. 1. Zouraris was a physician and sexologist.
17. Zouraris, 'Einai Egklema', pp. 1, 5.
18. See, for example, N. Garakes (29 December 1931) 'Einai Egklema e Ektrosis?', *Makedonia*, 22(6959), p. 1. Garakes was a physician.
19. Emm. Perres (15 January 1932) 'E ektrosis os koinonike anagke', *Makedonia*, 23(6974), p. 3 (Perres was a physician); Th. P. Theofylaktos (4 January 1932) 'Prepei na ekteleitai e ektrosis?', *Makedonia*, 23(6963), p. 1; Hristodoulos A. Kampoures (1933) *Therapeutikai kai Koinonikai Endeikseis tes Tehnetes Ektroseos* (Athens: Georgiou Vasileiou), p. 6.
20. On a description of such a situation in fiction see the chilling short story 'To pistoma' (Konstantinos Theotokes (1982) *Diegemata (Korfiatikes istories)* (Athens: Kimena), originaly published in 1898). Plenty of real life stories in the newspapers also described such situations. See, for example, Efi Avdella (2002) *Dia Logous Times. Via, Synaisthemata kai Axies se mia Metemfyliake Ellada* (Athens: Nefeli), though this monograph focuses on the 1950s and honour killings. Newspapers were full of reports of such honour killings in inter-war and post-war Greece. See, for example, Anonymous (16 March 1931) 'Fonos dia logous times eis ton Peiraia', *E Proia*, p. 5.
21. See, for example, Kampoures, *Therapeutikai*, pp. 6–7, 28–9; Theofylaktos, 'Prepei', p. 1.

22. This position remained in force at least until the end of the 1970s and seems to have been widely—though not by all—accepted and consistently practiced irrespective of the law since rates of illegitimacy remained extremely low throughout the twentieth century in Greece. See also Demetres Siatopoulos (1949) *E Gynaika kai ta Koinonika tes Zetemata kato apo to Fos tes Aletheias* (Athens: Maurides), pp. 13–31 and Konstantinos Metropoulos (1954) *Ygieine tes Egkuou* (Athens: Papademetriou), p. 137 expressing similar sentiments though the later clarifying that no more than one 'mistake' should be permitted to each unmarried woman. Perres, 'E ektrosis, p. 3; I. Pontikopoulou (10 January 1932) 'E ektrosis einai egklema?', *Makedonia*, 23(6969), p. 1; Theofylaktos, 'Prepei', p. 1.
23. Panteles D. Mpertsekas (1945) *Oi Kindynoi kai ai Epiplokai tes Amvloseos kai ta Iatrodikastika Provlemata Autes* (Athens: Euth. Hristodoulou), pp. 66–7.
24. Mpertsekas, *Oi Kindynoi*, pp. 70–1.
25. Kampoures, *Therapeutikai*, p. 28.
26. Kampoures, *Therapeutikai*, p. 27.
27. Kampoures, *Therapeutikai*, p. 28.
28. Andrianakos, 'Organosis', pp. 1025–34; Jacques D. Zancarol (1934) *L'evolution des Idées sur l'avortement Provoque. Etude Morale et Juridique* (Paris: Librairie Lipschutz). In the 1960s see N. Louros (1967) 'L'Influence des Avortements sur le Problème Demographique de la Grèce', *Academy of Athens*, 42.
29. Garakes, 'Einai Egklema e Ektrosis?', p. 1.
30. Perres, 'E ektrosis', p. 3.
31. Anonymous (23 December 1931) 'Einai Egklema e Ektrosis e Apeleutherotikon Kinema? Dyo Endiaferonta Arthra', *Makedonia*, 22(6954), p. 1; Zouraris (24 December 1931) 'Einai Egklema', p. 1; Georgios K. Zouraris (28 December 1931) 'Einai Egklema e Ektrosis e Apeleutherotikon Kinema?', *Makedonia*, 22(6958), p. 1; Hr. Papatheofilou (6 January 1932) 'Einai Egklema e Ektrosis? E Gnome tou Hr. Papatheofilou', *Makedonia*, 23(6965), p. 1 (the author was a gynaecologist); Kampoures, *Therapeutikai*, p. 6.
32. Kampoures, *Therapeutikai*, pp. 24–6; Mpertsekas, *Oi Kindynoi*, p. 72; Zouraris (24 December 1931) 'Einai Egklema e Ektrosis?', p. 1.
33. Mpertsekas, *Oi Kindynoi*, pp. 77–8. Similarly, Kampoures acknowledges the strength of maternal instinct in all women, whether they chose to abort or not (Kampoures, *Therapeutikai*, p. 26).
34. Mpertsekas, *Oi Kindynoi*, p. 83.
35. N.S. Louros (21 June 1930) 'E prostasia tes teknogonias', *Ergasia*, 1(24), 15–16.

36. S.Z. (January 1932) 'Nomimes ektroseis—to dikaioma ton ptohon na men kanoun paidia', *Socialistike Zoe*, 4(39), cited in Aude-Kalkane, *Mia antartissa*, p. 113.
37. Mpertsekas, *Oi Kindynoi*, pp. 83–4, citing Doxiadis but without providing the full reference.
38. Anonymous (23 December 1931) 'Einai Egklema e Ektrosis?', 1; Zouraris (24 December 1931) 'Einai Egklema', p. 1; Zouraris (28 December 1931) 'Einai Egklema', p. 1; Hr. Papatheofilou (6 January 1932) 'Is abortion a crime? The opinion of Hr. Papatheofilou', *Makedonia*, 23(6965), p. 1 (the author was a gynaecologist); Kampoures, *Therapeutikai*, p. 6.
39. Mpertsekas, *Oi Kindynoi*, p. 86.
40. Metropoulos, *Ygieine*, p. 138.
41. Metropoulos, *Ygieine*, p. 138.
42. I. Zagkarolas (1951) 'To Egklema tes amvloseos eis ton neon Poinikon Kodika', *Poinika Hronika*, 1(1), 495, cited in E. Symeonidou-Kastanidou (1995) *Egklemata kata tes Zoes* (Thessalonike: Sakkoula), p. 764.
43. Vasilios Valaoras, A. Polychronopoulou and D. Trichopoulos (1965) 'Control of Family Size in Greece (The Results of a Field Survey)', *Population Studies*, 18(3), 269; Vasilios Valaoras, A. Polychronopoulou and D. Trichopoulos (1969) 'Greece: Postwar Abortion Experience', *Studies in Family Planning*, 1(46), 10–16.
44. F. Kavvadias (1 April 1967) 'Symperasmata apo ten syzetese tes Ellen. Etairias Eugonikes. Zetountai … apogonoi', *Eleutheria*, 23(6917), p. 3.
45. Alexandra Barmpouti (2015) 'Eugenics and Induced abortion in post-war Greece', *ACTAE historiae, medicinae, stomatologiae, pharmaciae, medecinae veterinariae*, 34(1), 46–7.
46. Anonymous (28 January 1967) 'Ekatomyria paidia den erhontai ste zoe. H Germania egklematei … ', *Empros*, 9(4), p. 7.
47. Anonymous (18 April 1964) 'Ena akome provlema tes epohes mas. E amvlosis einai egklema? Yparhoun hores opou o nomos ten anehetai e ten epitrepi ypo orous', *Empros*, 70(16), p. 10.
48. Kan Parman (3 May 1958) 'Ai "statistikai" Kinsey', *Empros*, 63(229), p. 3; Anonymous (25 February 1958) '"Egkymosyne, gennesis, ektrosis". Apokalyptike ekthesis tou Institoutou Kinsey dia tas Amerikanidas', *Makedonia*, 47(15313), p. 3.
49. See, for example, Valaoras et al., 'Greece', 10–16; Valaoras et al., 'Control', 265–78.
50. Athanas. Vettou Danielides (1924) *E Zoe ton Neon* (Athens: Paraskeua Leone), p. 171.
51. A. Herbert Gray (31 December 1931) 'Abortions or fertility regulation', *Makedonia*, 22(6971), p. 1.

52. Serafeim Papakostas (1947) *To Zetema tes teknogonias (To demografiko provlema apo hristianikes apopseos)* 2nd edn (Athens: Adelfotes theologon 'E Zoe'). Subsequent editions were published in 1957 and 1969.
53. Alexandros Stauropoulos (1981) *Demografiko Provlema, Oikogeneiakos Programmatismos kai Ektroseis. Theologike Proseggise* (Athens: n.p.), p. 9.
54. The author refers not only to *Zoë* when he makes the above comment, but he notes that *Zoë* was the most widely known organisation of this kind (Vasilios N. Makrides (2004) 'Orthodoxy in the service of anticommunism: The religious organization Zoë during the Greek Civil War' in Philip Carabott and Thanasis D. Sfikas (eds), *The Greek Civil War. Essays on a conflict of exceptionalism and silences* (Aldershot: Ashgate), p. 159).
55. Papakosta, *To Zetema*, pp. 8–9.
56. Papakosta, *To Zetema*, pp. 11–12, 59, quoting the teachings of Megas Vasileios. Interestingly, the physicians were not unified: a healthy discourse ensued and variation in opinions was expressed as to when ensoulment takes place. See also Epifanios Theodoropoulos (1986) *Progamiaies Sheseis, Politikos Gamos, Amvloseis* (Athens: Orthodoxos Typos), p. 65, citing the fact that the Greek Church celebrates the conception of, among others, the Virgin Mary exactly because it strongly believes that the human person exists from the moment of its conception.
57. Papakosta, *To Zetema*, pp. 9–11.
58. Dionysios Pyrros o Thettalos (1840) *Egkolpion ton Iatron Etoi Praktike Iatrike, Periehousa ten Ylen tes Iatrikes, ten Farmakopoiian, ten Ygieinen*, vol. 1, 1st edn 1831 (Athens: Aggelou Aggelidou), p. 241.
59. Pyrros, *Egkolpion*, vol. 2, p. 241. Interestingly, Pyrros brings into the discussion the conception of Christ by Virgin Mary as supporting evidence for his position, exactly as Theodoropoulos did in 1986, supporting the opposite view (Pyrros, *Egkolpion*, vol. 2, p. 242; Theodoropoulos, *Progamiaies Sheseis*, p. 65).
60. Papakosta, *To Zetema*, pp. 11–13. The same year that Papakostas published his book, Kampoures also published a volume on induced abortion, declaring from the start that ensoulment occurs upon conception (Kampoures, *Therapeutikai*, p. 4). Other physicians were advocating that, according to biology, the foetus 'was not a human but rather a pile of cells' (Zouraris (24 December 1931) 'Einai Egklema', p. 1).
61. Papakostas uses an exceptional number of references, almost all non-Greek and therefore perceived as modern (for example, Charles Gore (1930) *The Prevention of Conception Commonly Called Birth Control*, 3rd edn (London: A.R. Mowbray); Encyclical of Pious XI Gasti Connubii 1931).
62. Papakosta, *To Zetema*, p. 17.
63. Stauropoulos, *Demografiko provlema*, pp. 9–10.

64. Meletios Galanopoulos Metropolites Kytheron (1969) *Egkyklioi 537–680* (Kythera: n.p.), Egkyklios 660 (27 September 1968).
65. Galanopoulos Metropolites Kytheron, *Egkyklioi*, Egkyklios 664 (26 October 1968).
66. Stauropoulos, *Demografiko Provlema*, p. 10.
67. Galanopoulos Metropolites Kytheron, *Egkyklioi*, Egkyklios 665 (1 November 1968).
68. Galanopoulos Metropolites Kytheron, *Egkyklioi*, Egkyklios 666 (7 November 1968).
69. Stavropoulos, *Demografiko Provlema*, p. 10.
70. E Ierarhia tes Ekklesias tes Ellados (1978) *Synodike Egkyklios tes Ierarhias tes Ekklesias tes Ellados* (Athens: Typografeio tes Apostolikes Diakonias), pp. 4–6.
71. *Rizospastes*, for example, discusses abortion in 1935–36 but in relation only to other places, not to Greece (Spain, Germany and the Soviet Union). After 1936 and until 1950 there are no references to abortion. In the 1950s there are a few references to abortion, and more in the 1960s; the newspaper *Eleutheria* regularly discussed abortion outside Greece: Michel Real (11 March 1967) 'Roumania 1967: Mia mikre Politistike Epanastase', *Eleutheria*, 23(6900), p. 3, referring to Rumania; Emerson Chapin (18 April 1964) 'Ta Demografika Provlemata eis ten Iaponian', *Eleutheria*, 20(6013), p. 3, referring to Japan; Anonymous (29 October 1960) 'Auxethesan poly ai Ektroseis eis ten Ouggarian', *Eleutheria*, 16(4936), p. 3, referring to Hungary.
72. Kampoures, *Therapeutikai*, p. 4; 'We cannot refuse that according to science the embryo is not a human but a pile of cells' (N. Garakes (29 December 1931) 'Einai Egklema e Ektrosis?', *Makedonia*, 22(6959), p. 1); I. Pontikopoulou (10 January 1932) 'Einai Egklema e Ektrosis?', *Makedonia*, 22(6969), p. 3.
73. John Riddle (1998) *Eve's Herbs: A History of Contraception and Abortion in the West* (London; Cambridge, MA: Harvard University Press), p. 222; Metropoulos, *Ygieine*, p. 143.
74. No. 2 Mykonos.
75. No. 2 Mykonos.
76. No. 27 Mykonos, born 1906.
77. No. 24 Mykonos.
78. No. 5 Syros.
79. No. 22 rural Syros. The informant probably referred to potassium permanganate, which at the time seems to have been in use in Britain, France and the USA (J.C. Miller (10 March 1951) 'Potassium Permanganate as abortifacient', *British Medical Journal*, 4705(1), 526). This was apparently an inefficient abortifacient, as it proved to be for the informant too.

80. No. 22 Syros, author's emphasis.
81. No. 15 Mykonos.
82. No. 1 Mykonos.
83. No. 13 Mykonos, married in 1926.
84. No. 26 Mykonos. A similar expression was used in a 1901 article when discussing a woman who found herself facing a dilemma because she was 'unable to feed what was conceived in her womb' and thus had to decide whether to 'make it miserable [i.e. bring up a child in poverty] or to destroy it before it is born' (N.Sp. (11 December 1901) 'E apotropaios praxis', *Empros*, 6(1841), p. 1).
85. No. 24 Mykonos.
86. No. 24 Mykonos.
87. No. 20 Mykonos.
88. See interview No. 22 Syros, in which the informant was dissuaded having an abortion by the physician, though she did not express this herself. She went to see the physician to discuss abortion, but came out of the meeting saying that 'me a mother, to kill my child!'
89. Michael Herzfeld (1985) *The Poetics of Manhood. Contest and Identity in a Cretan Mountain Village* (Princeton, NJ: Princeton University Press), Chap. 7.
90. Evaggelos Averof (1939) *Symvole eis ten Ereunan tou Plythesmiakou Provlematos tes Ellados* (Athens: n.p.), p. 81.
91. Richard Blum and Eva Blum (1965) *Health and Healing in Rural Greece* (Stanford, CA: Stanford University Press), p. 76.
92. No. 9 Syros.
93. E. Georges (2008) *Bodies of Knowledge: The Medicalisation of Reproduction in Greece* (Nashville: Vanderbuilt University Press), pp. 266–9.
94. No. 12 Athens.
95. E Ierarhia tes Ekklesias tes Ellados, *Synodike*, p. 6. In contrast, Barmpouti argues that the Greek Orthodox Church, in its 'economy', condemns the act and not the agent and therefore any woman returning to the Church with a petition would be excused (Barmpouti, 'Eugenics', 42).
96. Blum and Blum, *Health and Healing*, p. 76.
97. Nikos Kokosalakis (1987) 'The Political Significance of Popular Religion in Greece', *Archives des Sciences Sociales des Religions*, 64(1), 41. See also Heather Paxson (2004) *Making Modern Mothers: Ethics and Family Planning in Urban Greece* (Berkeley: University of California Press), pp. 60–2.

CHAPTER 8

Contraception and Its Methods, I: Natural Methods

One of Ansley Coale's preconditions for a 'major fall' in fertility to occur was that 'effective techniques of fertility reduction must be available'.[1] This links also to the question of whether the transition of fertility from high to low levels was an adjustment to changing socio-economic circumstances or an innovation in birth control methods.[2] Gösta Carlsson asked whether birth control was in fact practised within marriage 'on a considerable scale' before the secular decline of fertility. This in turn begs the question whether—or implicitly assumes that—there were methods available for couples to readily employ before the decline and, consequently, whenever they decided to control their fertility. Or did couples and individuals decide to control their fertility but had to subsequently find methods or maybe think of some of the methods for themselves (such as withdrawal)? Such a scenario implies that couples would have had to innovate meaning that some individuals and groups would lag behind others who had more knowledge of methods. This is, in very simple terms, the argument put forward by Gigi Santow, who suggested that coitus interruptus was the kind of method that might be 'invented' multiple times, as each couple discovered it for themselves when they needed a method to control their fertility.[3]

This and the next chapter, following an introduction to the publications referring or alluding to birth control methods, will investigate what users did actually know and employ. Sources such as letters to women's

V. Hionidou, *Abortion and Contraception in Modern Greece, 1830–1967*, Medicine and Biomedical Sciences in Modern History,
https://doi.org/10.1007/978-3-030-41490-0_8

magazines and oral interviews provide us with an understanding of the methods couples actually used and what women and sometimes men thought of them. In the rest of this chapter, each of the most widely employed natural methods in Greece is examined, namely breastfeeding and coitus interruptus, but also abstinence. The rest of the methods employed by Greek couples, namely appliance methods and the Pill, are examined in Chap. 9.

Writing About Contraception

Books were an important source of knowledge of contraceptive methods, at least for the educated. In Greece, the published books related to or referring to birth control amount to no more than two per decade between 1860 and 1920. Translations of foreign texts also circulated, although these were not numerous either. Those written by Greek authors and published in the nineteenth century refer not at all or only very briefly and in passing to birth control, even in conveying information on, for example, condoms. The earliest, written by Georgios Kyriakides, first published in 1865 in Athens, focuses on the sexuality of married men and women.[4] His emphasis was on the importance of procreation, and sex was treated as its necessary prerequisite. Though male onanism in the presence of a woman was explicitly described, this was done in order to explain the principles of conception rather than how to avoid it. In the late nineteenth century others, such as K.P. Kardamates, discussed and condemned (neo-) Malthusian ideas as being against God's wishes.[5] In 1889 the Greek obstetrician Antonios Kindynes addressed sterility and its cure, touching in the process on Neo-Malthusian principles, coitus interruptus and douching.[6] At the turn of the century yet another publication advocated complete abstinence and no masturbation prior to marriage because of its 'negative effects'.[7]

Barely a handful of publications, therefore, explicitly referred to methods of birth control in nineteenth-century Greece, and the first two decades of the twentieth were not significantly more informative, except for the translation of Jean Marestan's *L'Éducation Sexuelle*, first published in Greece in 1920.[8] To counter Marestan's outspoken and liberal publication, which referred to all known-to-date contraceptive methods, others, such as the 1924 publication of Hrestos Euaggelou, recommended to young single men abstinence and condoms in order to address the dangers of venereal diseases.[9] However, from 1925 to 1938 a good number of Greek-authored books were published that referred explicitly to contraception. Following M. Moyseides' first publication,[10] more followed by him and others in the late 1920s and the 1930s: these works, invariably authored by physicians, would refer to all or merely to some of the then-available methods, always indicating that contraceptive methods were harmful to the users' health but also usually recommending to the reader one or two methods that were the 'least harmful'.[11]

The 1950s and 1960s differed significantly from earlier times, in that almost all publications acknowledged that couples controlled their fertility and usually mentioned and described in varying detail the contraceptive methods used. Interestingly, virtually all publications targeted young married couples, aiming to inform them about the sexual aspects of marriage, one of which was contraception.[12] As in the 1930s, most contraceptive methods were listed, with emphasis placed on douches, coitus interruptus, suppositories, pessaries and condoms.[13] By now, explicit advertisements on the necessary equipment for douching also appeared in women's magazines. Despite mention of all the methods available, it appears that not all were equally used; for example, we learn from Konstantinos Metropoulos that vaginal caps were expensive and therefore virtually never used in Greece.[14] All the methods were declared inefficient and dangerous to varying but significant degrees, with long and alarming lists given of the potential mental and physical health effects of their use:[15] the worst of these, for women, was eventual sterility.[16] However, it was universally agreed that the use of contraceptives was acceptable, even compulsory, when diseases such as syphilis or other conditions affecting the mother were present.[17] Tsakires recommended in such cases that 'the least dangerous [contraceptive] method should be used along with the Ogino-Knaus' method, and that, if accidents were to happen, the couples should 'resort to abortion which in such circumstances is legal'.[18] Women did worry that the long-term use of contraception would damage their fertility, and the written works of gynaecologists reinforced this fear at every opportunity.[19] The implicit assumption in all discussions was that all couples would eventually have children and none would remain childless unless they were unlucky enough to suffer from sterility.

In the 1950s the availability of detailed information on methods was becoming normal in urban centres, appearing in publications other than simply those relating to sexuality. For example, the respectable *Encyclopaedia of the Greek Woman*, authored by a group of physicians and published in 1954, reproduced two sections on contraception from one of the two books that detailed all then-known contraceptive methods.[20]

These sections, amidst advice on nutrition and family health, were entitled 'Childbearing at will' and 'Contraceptive methods against pregnancy'.[21] In the equally widely accessible 1956 edition of the *Great Greek Encyclopaedia*, under various terms related to sexual urges (Genetesios orme) and marriage (Gamos), continence, douches, coitus interruptus, anal sex and oral sex were discussed, and it was indicated that although the last three were reprehensible they were not perversions.[22] It is even more significant that such discussions were taking place at least since 1950 in the advice columns of popular magazines. In the popular women's magazine *E Gynaika* ('The Woman'), published from 1950, the column 'The gynaecologist answers' listed a variety of methods in response to the queries of readers. To those readers who were clearly ignorant, the following answer, for example, presented virtually all the available and acceptable methods:

> Again about the same matter. It seems that you do not pay attention to the answers. There are many methods of prophylaxis, with elastic condom, with various suppositories, douches with acidic content, citric acid, vinegar, alumina, peroxide of hydrogen, etc. And the method Ogino-Knaus .... If you are careful, you should not become pregnant. All these make sense both theoretically and practically, of course there are exceptions to all rules. Let us hope you will not be the exception.[23]

At other times the gynaecologist, presumably tailoring his answer to the specific question, would refer only to those methods favoured by most Greek medical writers:

> As to the prophylaxis, this is safe only with the usual protection of the rubbers [condoms]. Also, the Ogino-Knaus method exists, that is, being careful during the ovulation days, that is from the 11th to the 18th, starting from the first day of period. At least in theory, I believe this is the best and the most successful [method].[24]

Another response stressed that '[e]ffective medicine does not exist. Douches with vinegar, one [vinegar] to three water, before and after, create an acidic environment and prevent fertilisation'.[25] At all times, they emphasised the lack of full effectiveness of any of the methods, and occasionally suggested the combination of two different methods: 'In relation to what you are asking, there is no effective method. The method you use is not good. It is preferable [to use] condoms and to pay great attention to the ovulation day.'[26] Moreover, they were acquiescent of emmenagogues, especially when mentioned by the correspondent: 'Effective method against conception does not exist. The most effective and less harmful is that of the rubber condom. *Emagol* does not harm but does not prevent.'[27] All in all, condoms, douches and the Ogino-Knaus method seemed to have been those methods favoured—or, more correctly, tolerated—by physicians, and which they would recommend to interested couples.

What, then, were the methods that people actually used? This is much more difficult to ascertain, as sources on such personal issues are very scarce, reflecting the reticence of people writing about such personal experiences. However, the oral history interviews conducted on Mykonos in 1994 provide us with some answers to this question. Since then, additional interviews conducted in subsequent years around different themes also provide glimpses of people's knowledge of contraception practices. Having briefly outlined above what had been written in Greece on contraception, I now turn to a discussion of individual methods that were of some significance in Greece, juxtaposing the literature regarding those methods—from not only Greece, but also Britain and the USA—with the actual understanding, perception and use of the practices among the wider Greek population.

Using Contraception: The Users' View

Breastfeeding

Breastfeeding is a natural method that can delay conception, as was well known among elderly informants. This was the only method that the informants did not hesitate to mention, and all were happy to explain how it worked. And, interestingly, both women and men were happy to discuss breastfeeding both in general and specifically as a 'contraceptive'. Men were so unwilling to discuss other forms of contraception with me, a young and educated woman, that I soon stopped interviewing men on Mykonos altogether. However, for men breastfeeding was not linked in any way to sexuality, and therefore they had no inhibitions in discussing it freely. One of the informants, a 90-year-old man from rural Hios, explained how he heard about it as a young boy during one of the evening outdoor gatherings of old women—gatherings at which children were also present.[28] Such unguarded conversations in front of children never took place on topics involving sexuality.

Q. Did your wife breastfeed your child?
A. Yes …
Q. How long did she breastfeed, can you remember?
A. One a year, another less, another more. Some who did not want to have children they would breastfeed them because if you breastfeed them, they say, you don't have children [don't become pregnant].
Q. Really?
A. Yes. They extended the breastfeeding [period].
Q. Did many know that?
A. They knew.
Q. Where did you get to hear about it? From your mother?
A. Those days we used to go to houses in the evenings and we would sit and we learned, your grandma would talk to you, your mother would talk to you. They told you there and you put [what they said] in your mind.[29]

Breastfeeding was almost universal in rural Greece, but less prevalent in urban areas.[30] Its duration, however, differed from place to place, with a minimum of around eight months and a maximum of around two years.[31] The 1920s and 1930s saw a campaign on the part of those physicians who were concerned with levels of infant mortality, especially in urban centres, encouraging women to breastfeed more. This targeted primarily urban working-class women who were in employment, but also the upper classes who employed wet nurses for their children.[32] In the mid-1940s P. Paulides referred to weaning happening at 'the earliest 14 months after the delivery'.[33] Even in the urban centres of Athens and Thessaloniki in the 1960s the rates of breastfeeding were high: 90% of women reported having breastfed their children, with 65% having breastfed them for at least 15 months.[34]

When mothers wanted to delay the arrival of the next conception and birth, they would breastfeed the child beyond the time expected in that locality. As an informant from Mykonos explains, her sister breastfed her child to the age of 'two years, two and a half years', whereas the usual duration on Mykonos was 'one, one and a half year, depending' on the individual circumstances:

Q. How long did you breastfeed [your children]?
A. It was my sister; she would take her child to the seaside and when they returned [he would say to her] 'come, give me a drop, give me

a drop, I will bring the small stool for you to sit', so that he [the child] would stand … two years, two and a half years.[35]

Q. Were all children breastfed that long?

A. They had a flaw here [on the island]. When they breastfed, they did not see their menses [they did not menstruate] and they did not have children soon. And so they were forced to breastfeed them in order not to give birth one after the other [in close proximity] and have the children.[36]

Another example comes from Rhodes in the late 1920s, where a mother breastfed her son up to the age of five because, as he heard his mother explain to others, if she kept nursing 'she wouldn't get pregnant again'.[37] Women and men had an excellent understanding of the timing and the sequence of events, even though they were not aware of the 'scientific' reasoning behind them:

Q. You said you were breastfeeding the children up to the age of two years. Did you ever get pregnant while you were breastfeeding?

A. No. As soon as the 'mystery' [menstruation] appeared, two or three months, four [months] would pass and then I would 'catch' a child [become pregnant]. I did not have a child.

Q. Oh, so while you were breastfeeding …

A. Yes, I did not have a child. It would come after two years.

Q. After two! That long?

A. Three, four months would pass [after the arrival of the period] and then I was again ready [to conceive].[38]

In later years, some women introduced contraception only after their period returned, following prolonged breastfeeding: 'Because I was breastfeeding I did not have period. When it returned, I was taking precautions.'[39] Not only had they a thorough understanding of the effects of prolonged breastfeeding on their own body, they were also aware that its effects differed from woman to woman: 'It works for some but not for others.'[40] Furthermore, in some places the practice had a name. For example, on Mykonos a woman whose ovulation was visibly delayed through breastfeeding was referred to as one that 'kratovyzietai'.[41]

This knowledge was passed from the older to the younger generation freely. Midwives may have discussed it with women; physicians, in contrast, were certainly not the source of such information. First, working-class women residing outside urban areas up to the late 1920s or even the 1930s would have rarely visited a physician.[42] Moreover, this was a 'method' not discussed by the vast majority of writers on this subject matter. However, Nikolaos Kostes and Moyseides did discuss it: Kostes explained that while the woman 'produces milk there are no menses and neither does she conceive in most cases, while she breastfeeds',[43] while Moyseides, writing about 'natural' methods, referred to the 'extending of breastfeeding in order to avoid pregnancy'.[44] He added that this was a method that was 'rather often used, especially among the working classes', but that it was neither safe nor without dangers. However, it is not clear whether he had knowledge of the use of the method among the Greek working classes or whether he was simply quoting Dutch writer Th. Van de Velde, who had stated in his own work that a danger of employing this method was the atrophy of the woman's reproductive organs.[45] After Moyseides' discussion, there are no further references to this method by physicians. It would have been female empirical practitioners, advising women on issues of child rearing, including breastfeeding, who may have had an input on such a topic.[46]

References to the effect that prolonged breastfeeding had on individual women's fecundity do exist in the international historiography. For example, in England, George Drysdale indicated in 1861 that 'in some lactation prevents conception, in others it does not'.[47] Breastfeeding had been used in early twentieth-century England for its contraceptive properties[48] and a number of publications in German and English at around this time went as far as to advise readers that the contraceptive effects of breastfeeding could be prolonged after the child's weaning by the husband breastfeeding.[49] However, repudiation was quick. Iwan Bloch rejected the method since the desired effect would occur only exceptionally. Moreover, protracted breastfeeding would be 'extremely harmful' to the mother, just as 'an excessive protraction of lactation after normal delivery is known to be deleterious'.[50] In 1922, the English physician Courtenay Beale also rejected the method for similar reasons: its unreliability, and the possibility that it would be injurious to the child and to the mother if breastfeeding were to be prolonged 'beyond the period when her milk is of real nutritive value'.[51] Margaret Sanger referred to the method in her 1915 *Family Limitation*, tactfully introducing the method with '[T]here is also the knowledge that nursing after childbirth prevents the return of the menstrual flow',[52] and warning merely that women should not 'depend upon this too much, especially after the fifth or sixth month'. However, by

1931, and possibly as early as 1926, Sanger was referring to it as a 'superstition' only.[53] By this time, this was not a method recommended by Sanger or any other proponent of contraception. Neither did Stopes recommend this as a possible method. She introduced the link between breastfeeding and postponed conception with the unambiguous phrase 'a common impression', and simply explained that that link did not exist: 'it is absolutely untrue that suckling in itself affords a safe or even tolerably secure method of contraception'.[54] In her *Letter to Working Mothers* she not only indicates that this is not a 'good' method but also frames it as failing the breastfed child.[55]

Oral and interview evidence is available from Turkey, Norway and Finland, as well as for Greece, for the use of breastfeeding in postponing conception. A Turkish informant, who started her childbearing around 1950, decided after her second birth that she did not want more children: 'First, my milk protected me. Then I protected myself.'[56] Much later, in the early 1990s, a young Turkish woman breastfed her second child and did not have her period for nine months. Her first child hardly breastfed, and she used the Pill immediately after the realisation that she had no milk, suggesting that she had been expecting to rely on the breastfeeding method, and demonstrating her strong trust in it.[57] The first survey of Finnish professionals concerning contraception, in 1914, included only three questions, one of which was whether breastfeeding was used to 'avoid conception'.[58] The responses confirmed that this was indeed the case.[59] In Norway, as early as 1866, there were reports of the 'popular belief' among 'ordinary women' linking prolonged breastfeeding with delayed conception, leading to a research project undertaken by physicians that examined the validity of the belief.[60] When elderly Norwegian women and men were interviewed in 1981, two of the respondents mentioned that their mother and aunt had employed that method, though the informants themselves questioned its validity.[61] They had been born in the period 1891–1911 and this was presumably the approximate period in which the method was employed.[62] Similarly, German folklore accounts from the 1890s mention prolonged nursing to age three as a way of hindering conception.[63]

Although a significant number of the Greek informants referred to the use of breastfeeding to delay conception, all, with the exception of an informant from Mykonos and another from Syros,[64] referred to their mother's generation rather than their own. This seems to have also been the case in Norway.[65] This method constituted for these informants the primitive past, at least in comparison to the efficacy of the measures they themselves employed, and they expressed pity for the ignorance of those who used it: 'They knew this [method] and they would use this trick. Well, this was the only trick they used. They didn't know anything else, poor women.'[66] The period that these informants were discussing was presumably the 1910s and earlier—a time when knowledge of other methods was very limited, at least among the working classes, but the need for such knowledge was already there:

Q. You said you had two children because you brought up your mother's children. Did your mother want to have nine children? Did she ever tell you she would have preferred to have fewer?
A. Yes, of course she would have preferred.
Q. Did she tell you that?
A. Of course she did not want the children. She would be upset whenever she became pregnant.
Q. Why did she have them then?
A. Because there were no means, there were no [contraceptive] means.
Q. Did she not know anything?
A. She did not know anything. She was an innocent woman.
Q. Did you discuss that with her and she told you that?
A. Yes, of course. I was grown up then [when we discussed it]. She was saying 'how do the other women take precautions?' She did not know anything.[67]

The reason breastfeeding has been little discussed as a contraceptive method among demographers becomes clear when reading a 1960s *Manual of Contraceptive Practice* that introduces the topic of breastfeeding as a contraceptive method with the statement '[a]ccording to old wives' tales, nursing mothers cannot conceive'.[68] The three-paragraph piece concludes with the advice that 'effective measures of control' should be employed before the first post-partum menses to cover the 5% risk of pregnancy during the postpartum amenorrhoeic period.[69] With the 1988 Bellagio Consensus, however, breastfeeding acquired the scientific stamp of approval that enabled its inclusion ever since in official family planning manuals, on an equal footing with appliance and hormonal methods.[70]

Breastfeeding was a natural method under the control of women and one that was fully accepted within their role as good mothers. Moreover, it was not associated with sexuality, and therefore knowledge of it was freely passed to all. Its pitfalls were also well known. The medicalisation of family planning from the 1930s in the USA and Britain and after World War II elsewhere, however, meant that this method was either ignored or dismissed as an unscientific 'old women's tale'. This was, to a degree, the case even in Greece among those informants who reported the method as one that their mother used in the absence of better, more modern methods.

Abstinence: Sex and Knowledge

Much has been written about the significance of abstinence in Victorian England, both prior to and within marriage, in terms of its importance in regulating fertility.[71] With the increasing influence of 'purity literature' during the nineteenth century, female passivity was encouraged, sex was narrowly linked to procreation and, in the absence of acceptable or fool-proof contraceptives, sexual abstinence was seen by some as the secure way of achieving freedom from excessive childbearing.[72] The paramount importance of abstinence as a way of controlling childbearing in England has been emphasised by some, Simon Szreter particularly emphatically, although he concedes that for most couples abstinence would have been a hit-and-miss affair more akin to 'coital spacing'.[73] This argument has been put forward most strongly for England, although in reference to the period from 1930 Szreter and Kate Fisher refer only to 'partial or temporary abstinence'.[74]

Though much ink has been spent in the past on discussing continence, much of the discussion was focused on the pre-marital period. Malthus was probably one of the first to explicitly connect abstinence with a reduced number of children in a population, although even he referred to the postponement of marriage and pre-marital abstinence rather than abstinence within marriage.[75] He also referred to the difficulty in sustaining such a preventive measure, which often resulted in sexual relationships outside the marriage and the birth of illegitimate children: 'These considerations are calculated to prevent, and certainly do prevent, a very great number in all civilized nations from pursuing the dictate of nature in an early attachment to one woman. And this restraint almost necessarily, though not absolutely so, produces vice.'[76]

Attitudes and expectations in Greece in the late nineteenth century and the first half of the twentieth seem in line with Victorian thinking in terms of pre-marital sexuality. Single women *had* to be innocent, both in terms of knowledge but also in practice.[77] The material representation of such innocence in Greek society at that time was the hymen, which was much discussed and studied.[78] Such proclaimed 'innocence' and virginity, while perhaps not universal, represented the reality for the overwhelming majority of single women throughout the study period:

Q. May I ask you, since you mentioned your cousins [in relation to menstruation]? Did you discuss such issues often?
A. Well, as girls/young women we did discuss, yes. We had the curiosity but, sweetheart, we did not know much. I remember being 16 years old ..., there were two cousins, an auntie, and two cousins of my mum's, who were pregnant. And one would say she was three months pregnant, the other seven months. How on earth do they know that they are seven and eight? I wanted to ask my mother but I was ashamed/shy .... One day I said 'Mum, how do they know that one is three and the other four, for example'? 'The menses stop and so they know', she told me. That was her answer then. Even when I got married, my mum did not say to me even five, ten words. Despite the fact that I was out [in the public], I was [dealing] with men, illegal [communist party] gatherings, various things, I had been in prison and when I got married she did not say anything to me. To tell me 'you know, you are getting married, the a or the b'. They were not very [vocal] those years, parents those years. I don't know, was it only my [mother]? I don't know.
Q. May I ask where did you find out? At the end, where did you find out the basic things that you had to know [sexual knowledge]?
A. My husband.
Q. Your husband. And being in prison and in the gatherings?
A. No I did not [learn there]. Maybe we have had platonic love affairs, for example for him to see me, me to see him, etc. but I did not have [sexual relationships]. I got married ... I say things that ... I got married and I was a virgin the day I got married, my husband respected that. I was scared of it [sex]; I perceived it as something bad. And most women were [virgins at marriage]. Now, that [virginity] is of no importance ... I tell them [her children] sometimes [how it used to be] and they say 'Where do you think you are/live?' And I say 'My son, where am I? I don't know!' My husband used to say sometimes 'it took me two years to get you around [in terms of sexuality]'. Do you understand? I was not stupid. Not only I was not stupid but I was very [outgoing]; they used to see me talk, laugh, to get out, to

> joke, to say [things]. But those things [sex], I was careful. I was scared of it.[79]

This informant got married at an advanced age and was unusual in enjoying freedom of movement and having access to political gatherings; such freedoms were certainly not available to women pre-1940 and to only a few rural women in the 1950s and even the 1960s. However, she lacked very basic sexual knowledge and was therefore scared of its consequences, which made her unwilling to engage in pre-marital sexual relationships. This was exactly what societal silence on those matters aimed to achieve, and it seems to have achieved it to a very large degree.[80]

The need to maintain the 'innocence' of 'girls' (that is, unmarried women) was made very clear during my interviews, when invariably my elderly female informants, after my first question about sexuality or contraception, would stop and stare at my fingers to see whether I was married or not. Marriage, not age—at the time, I was in my early 30s—was the enabling factor in allowing such discussions to take place even in 1994, the year I was conducting the interviews on Mykonos. As I was not married at the time, and therefore not wearing a ring, I had to explain on each occasion that I was engaged and aware of sexual matters. Only then would they answer my questions.[81]

Ignorance on sexual matters was therefore very extensive. Equally extensive, however, was that concerning childbearing, even when informants had older, married sisters with children with whom they were on good terms:

Q. When your sister gave birth, did she give birth in your house?
A. She gave birth in her own house.
Q. Who helped her? Did she give birth on her own? Did she give birth with a midwife?
A. With a midwife.
Q. Were you in there? Did you help her?
A. No, old women. They did not allow young women to get in there. Especially unmarried girls. Old women would go and they were sitting with the midwife.
Q. Did you know what was happening in there?
A. Oh well, she had tummy pains but we would not enter. They would not let us. The old women were there, they would pray.
Q. With your friends, did you talk about those things?

A. No, [not] about such [things], [not] about obscene [things]. We were busy with embroidery.
Q. For example, what is a baby, how is it made?
A. No, nothing of the sort, we never discussed, never. Not what happens or what it is, never.
Q. Did your mother ever say anything to you?
A. No, no, no, she was a serious woman, strict.
Q. Someone else? Mayne your grandmother?
A. No. My grandma Maria? She only sung.
Q. No one talked to you, said anything to you? What will happen when you get married, how children are born?
A. We did not discuss such things .... My sister, only after she got married, she got pregnant. I did not know that only if I got married I would get pregnant [laughter]. How do you expect us to know? We did not know them. Neither were these things commented on somewhere else. No one. Not even our [female] friends. Our friends were concerned with what dresses we would make, how we will get dressed at Easter, what embroidery we will make and nothing more.[82]

This informant emphasised the discrete, impervious worlds of single and married women. Even though the married sister and her children lived for many years in the parental house along with the informant, who was single, there were no conversations to be had that would allow the unmarried sister to acquire the knowledge that was afforded, discreetly, to married women. It was marital status that determined the kind of knowledge that a female could have access to. Conversations touching on sexuality, including contraception, between mothers and daughters would occur after the daughter was married, although as time passed that began to change:

Q. Did your mother know what you knew? Did she know about contraception, this and that?
A. She did not say anything in front of us. And I did not ever discuss in front of my children [about such things]! Compare that to today. My ... daughter, would talk when she was married with [her] children. She said 'like you, who would not let us listen! When you wanted to talk to a woman [female friend] you would say [to us] "Go to the windmill to see if a boat is coming"'?
Q. So, when you wanted to talk [with other married women] you would get the children out?

A. They would get out so that we could talk.
Q. As single girls, did you talk about such things?
A. If it was ... when married we did talk about such things. But not much.[83]

By the 1950s and within the urban setting there were various possible sources of information on sexual matters, such as magazine articles and agony aunts' or gynaecologists' columns.[84] Books written by sexologists or family encyclopaedias would also provide such information, again, exclusively to urban readers. Rural residents would only exceptionally have access to these types of publication, especially prior to 1940:

Q. Did you know that if he wanted [to prevent a pregnancy] he could?
A. Yes! How would we know? Did we know any of that?! Did we read books [with incredulity]? We graduated from primary school with millions of difficulties in the great poverty of Asia Minor [as refugees on Hios]. We finished the primary school, we used to go to school and I had the pencil hanging around my neck so that the lead would not break because I could not afford another one.[85]

Preventing girls from acquiring sexual knowledge aimed to 'protect' them from getting involved, or seeking to get involved, in pre-marital sexual relationships. This was to a large degree achieved, and women, at least in some mainland rural areas, had to display the evidence of their virginity on the morning after the wedding.[86] However, while continence for women prior to marriage was an unquestionable social necessity, for men it was not: although abstinence was recommended to Greek men prior to marriage, it was understood that transgressions would occur, especially in the cities.[87] The justification for such a disparity was to be found, we are told by experts of the time, in the distinct sexual instincts of men and women. That of men was 'constantly vigorous', whereas for women it was non-existent, 'except when the presence of a man will awaken' her sexual instinct,[88] or 'coquetry'.[89] This absence of sexual instinct in the woman, one author suggested, explained why men could not abstain from sex, while women could.[90] Thus, men were entitled to pre-marital sex; indeed, for them it was an 'organic necessity'.[91] Men in rural areas may not have had any such relationships prior to marriage, but that would have been the result of a lack of opportunities, rather than societal expectations. Urbanite men would rarely have been virgins at marriage, most of them having experienced pre-marital sex with a prostitute in one of the legal brothels that operated in towns and cities.[92] However, to an extent in the 1930s and certainly after World War II a discernible change could be seen in Greece, again in urban areas. Although generally meeting with strong social disapproval, single men and women would enter into romantic and sometimes sexual relationships. Most of those ended in a marriage, but it was those that did not that we know most about, as in a number of cases they ended in the honour killing of one of the two partners and, inevitably attracted a large amount of publicity.[93]

The societal expectations of sexual behaviour prior to marriage were thus clear to all, despite some variation from place to place and over time. Equally clear were the expectations of the nature of marital relationships after marriage. Marriage was built around the sexual relationship of the husband and wife, and the absence of it, whether voluntary or involuntary, was a reason for divorce. Church teachings on this were emphatically clear. Conjugal 'rights' referred to both men and women. As Moyseides argued, within marriage permanent abstinence 'for physiological and biological reasons is both unacceptable and inapplicable' and would lead marital life into 'ruinous ascetism from a hygienic point of view'.[94] N.N. Drakoulides, in an article entitled 'Sexual abnormalities', prescribed that abstinence up to the age of 21 for men and 28 for women was normal; however, beyond those ages, he cautioned, it causes 'serious disturbances to both sexes', leading to psychological problems and psychogenic impotence.[95] Thus, complete abstinence within marriage was inconceivable for healthy individuals. In situations when a further birth was feared or was simply undesirable, there was thus no suggestion or discussion of abstinence, but, rather, other solutions would be suggested. In one case the mother-in-law suggested to her daughter-in-law that she remove herself from her family and become a servant while the mother-in-law, who was working as a servant at the time, volunteered to look after her son's family: 'My mother-in-law messaged me "Come, don't stay there to have [more] children". Many children, I had six children. "Come to work and I will come to look after the children."'[96]

However, some of my informants did indicate that they would avoid, to a degree, sexual contact:

A. I was careful too, I could see the situations/times, I could see the poverty; my husband was rather old [more than 20 years older than the informant].

Q. Were you careful or was it your husband?
A. If a third [child] came along, that would have been ok. Since it didn't, we moved on.
Q. How were you careful? Can I ask you how you were careful?
A. Well, you avoid a little bit.
Q. You?
A. Yeah, sure, you avoid. What can you do, dear?[97]

While avoiding sex 'a little bit' was acceptable, especially when the age gap between the partners was large, refusing it altogether was not, even to those who were not keen themselves:

> He is not a man who … every night like others. Let me say, apologies for saying it, once a week and if it happens. He was working too, such people get tired, do you understand? It depends on the person too. I see others, god save, can you put up with someone like that [sexually demanding]? I am not, I don't like it so much. But since I am his wife, I cannot deny it to him, not completely. Now we are of age, it should not [happen], those things are not allowed.[98]

As the same informant indicated earlier, her husband 'was not a difficult person. You said no to him, [it meant] no. He was easy to communicate with.' Such was not always the case, however, and neither were all accepting of a curtailment of their 'rights'.[99] Mihael Kaires refers to exhausted working-class women with many children, who 'avoided or did not seek' the conjugal 'chore'.[100] His advice to them was that their 'duty was never to complain for their husband's eagerness, not to repel him and not to distance him from her, not to deprive him of the conjugal embraces, but rather to be flattered for the vivacity which she had inspired'.[101]

While the cultural rejection by all—authors and informants—of the concept of *complete* abstinence within marriage is significant, and informants reported that it was an idea alien to them, nevertheless, the restriction of coitus on religious and culturally prescribed days was socially acceptable and 'enforceable', even if husbands were not keen on such a disruption to their sexual activities:

> Listen, we guarded … do you want me to tell you? … The first year that I was with my husband, he was like a mule. We are not animals. We observed [abstained on] Wednesdays, we observed Fridays, we observed Saturday

> evenings, we observed the festive days, we observed the Lent. I had three children, I did not want; I declared to my husband 'Unless 40 days [after birth have passed], there is none [no sex]. That is the logic. How many women became pregnant before the 40 days? That is what we did.[102]

Similar references to refraining from intercourse during 'fasting' periods or days were made by an older informant who had observed this while living with her own grandparents for some years as a child.[103] She recalled that on such days her grandmother would make herself less 'attractive' to the grandfather by, for example, not wearing earrings, thereby signalling that intercourse was not on the agenda.[104] This amounted to a regulation of coital frequency, but not to abstinence, which refers rather to a prolonged period of time or even a permanent situation.[105]

While up to around 1920 there were some authors who advocated premarital continence for men, Georgios Kyriakides, writing in the mid-nineteenth century, argued that it could cause impotence.[106] After 1920 many more authors, all physicians, argued against continence for the same reason.[107] Some offered a theoretically prescribed number of coital acts per week for 'healthy' men, with abstinence prescribed only in cases of serious illnesses, during menstruation and for those aged 70 and over.[108] Drakoulides suggested that the reduced use of the genital glands would have a number of effects, including memory loss, headaches, stress, trembling of the extremities and dullness.[109] He instructed that an adult man should have sex twice a week, as abstinence could result in any of the following: ejaculation, spermatorrhoea, impotence, obesity or various psychoneuroses.[110] Along similar lines in the mid-1940s, Paulides was arguing that 'no human force can resist the invincible urge of eros/sex and if it could, life would lose its main attraction'.[111] However, the Archimadrite Serafeim Papakostas retorted, arguing that the power of the human will is superior to the power of sexual desire, at least until the time of marriage, for most people.[112] Others, such as Anastasios Antonopoulos, articulated their pro-continence arguments in a more forceful way even in the 1950s, declaring that 'the damages of continence are imaginary and hypothetical'.[113] His arguments moved between religious, military and medical ideas of continence, refuting all those arguments against continence and exhorting its usefulness.[114] However, his book—dedicated to army officers—was explicitly addressing the needs of 'young' men and thus had no bearing on continence within marriage.[115] Nonetheless, Antonopoulos and Papakostas, representing the military conservative Right and the vocal, visible representation of the Church, were by that stage the exceptions.

From the 1920s onwards therefore, and in the face of such arguments, abstinence within marriage was unthinkable and was not practised as a way of avoiding childbearing. However, the sexual norms of society continued to enforce an embargo on knowledge for single women about all things sexual and relevant to childbearing, in contrast both to men and to married women, who were able to access such information.

Coitus Interruptus or Withdrawal

Coitus interruptus is probably the method on which most has been written, and that most widely practised in the twentieth century. It is described in detail in the Bible, where it is called the act of Onan.[116] There are very few, if any, marriage manuals in the nineteenth- and twentieth-century international bibliography that do not mention this method, even if only to condemn it. Francis Place refers to withdrawal in his first published handbill as the method that could be used as an alternative to his recommended sponge,[117] but any reference to it disappeared from subsequent handbills. Shortly after this, however, withdrawal took centre stage in Robert Dale Owen's *Moral Physiology*. He stressed that this was the method employed by the 'cultivated classes' in France, Italy and, he believed, also in Germany and Spain.[118] Whether this was true or simply a means of promoting the method remains to be judged. Owen believed the method to have been 'in all cases, effectual', with the advantage of being without any side effects.[119] Charles Knowlton's *Fruits of Philosophy* also discussed the method and recommended it, without referring to any side effects.[120] George Drysdale cited Owen extensively in his discussion of the method and referred to the wide use of the method by the French.[121] However, beyond contraception advocates, physicians were scathing on the side effects of this method, which were seen as troubling for both men and women. For men, the imperfect and/or incomplete ejaculation would 'tease his organs' and leave him unsatisfied. The wife was prevented from the benefits that the semen would bestow on her uterus, leading in the long term to a host of medical conditions, including hysteria.[122] A handful of physicians did challenge such assertions, arguing that there was no evidence to support such conclusions,[123] but the majority of authors referring to the method listed a number of harmful consequences and advised their readers to avoid its use. Even physicians such as H.A. Allbutt, who did recommend the method, if not to all, mentioned that it was 'hurtful to the nervous system in many persons'.[124] Curiously, though, he went on to add that withdrawal was 'advocated by many eminent physicians'.[125]

Both Stopes and Sanger in the 1910s and 1920s admitted that withdrawal was widely used but nevertheless opposed it; in 1914 Sanger declared that while it was 'a perfectly safe method' and one that was not 'so dangerous to the man as some authorities have formerly viewed', she nevertheless recommended that it should not be used due to the 'injure' it caused woman, leaving her in a dissatisfied state.[126] Within three years she had changed her mind, however, arguing that it was the 'ignorance of scientific means of preventing conception' that led women to be involved 'in harmful practices', the most common being coitus interruptus.[127] Sanger cited no fewer than seven physicians on the harmful consequences of the method, which included chronic metritis and, most importantly, neurasthenia. Stopes, meanwhile, rejected the method as one that had done 'an incredible amount of harm' to the men and women who practised it.[128] Courtenay Beale, a physician and contemporary of Stopes, articulated a similar message about coitus interruptus: it greatly affected women owing to the lack of sexual satisfaction they experienced, and led them to neurasthenia; all in all, it was 'gravely injurious to women's nervous organisation'.[129] It seems that the relatively lengthy and repetitious discussion of withdrawal that Beale afforded in her book was due to its apparent popularity.[130] Ettie Rout, in the same year, described the method as widely practised, 'unromantic', 'nerve-racking' and 'objectionable'.[131] Konikow too, one of the first American female physicians to publish on contraception, rejected the method as 'unsafe, abnormal and unhealthy' both in 1923 and in 1931.[132]

One possible reason for writers' negative attitude to the method is its early association with onanism, with some authors, such as Bergeret, naming it 'conjugal onanism'. Although he also included oral sex within this term, a reading of his book *The Preventive Obstacle, or, Conjugal onanism* indicates that he considered the prime activity under the heading conjugal onanism to be coitus interruptus. Any association with onanism would be highly negative, considering the 'moral panic' that had resulted from the definition and discussion of onanism towards the end of the eighteenth century. Bergeret outlined the negative effects of the method. For women these included metritis, leucorrhoea, menorrhagia, metrorrhagia, tumours, uterine hyperesthesia, hysteralgia, uterine colics and neuroses, neuralgias, mammary congestion, uterine cancer and diseases of the ovaries. For the man, urethritis and diseases of the prostate were the two ailments they could expect to suffer from. Ultimately, the most dreaded effects were sterility for women and impotence for men.[133] The translator P. De Marmon 'was struck by the number of diseases and moral troubles caused by that unnatural practice entitled congeal onanism', and went on, essentially, to attribute all the cases of 'female disorders' he had come across and for which he had been unable to identify a cause to 'conjugal onanism'.[134] Stopes also used the term *onanismus conjugalis* in 1923, although her list of side effects was much shorter than Bergeret's.[135] Just like Marmon, however, Greek physicians were quick to adopt Bergeret's list of side effects and, while not all were mentioned in every publication, Greek physicians collectively mentioned all of them at some point.

K.P. Kardamates, who explicitly discussed and defined conjugal onanism in the late nineteenth century, included coitus interruptus within it.[136] In 1927 writers were still using the term onanism: Sygkelakes placed it first on his list of contraceptive methods, defining it as 'the partial/half-finished coitus. At the moment of ejaculation the husband suitably withdraws'.[137] Stefanou, writing in the same year, referred to onanism as an act 'against nature'—that is, 'undertaken solitary or in combination of two or more people with body-parts or foreign appliances or movements'.[138] He lamented that even married people were engaged in such activities in an attempt to avoid procreation.[139] The prolific writer Moyseides, writing in the 1930s, classified the method under 'perversions and deviant coital practices' and stated that it was a 'un-natural' practice.[140] While such associations with onanism and other 'perversions' ceased to be mentioned beyond 1932, these earlier associations in both Greek and European/American literature may help to explain the long lists of the method's perceived side effects, most of which also applied to masturbation.

According to Kardamates, one of the effects of the method was metritis, while children conceived despite its practice would be eugenically compromised.[141] Sygkelakes warned that the method not only 'destroys the health' of those practising coitus interruptus but also results in their erotic frigidity. Moreover, he added, it led to permanent sterility, as over time the uterus would get 'used to be[ing] sterile'.[142] Yioel, writing in the late 1930s, argued that the use of coitus interruptus had negative effects for women, who would suffer from the lack of sperm absorption and from reduced or irregular menstruation, congestion of the reproductive organs, diseases of the ovaries and leucorrhoea.[143] As far as men were concerned, the method could result in 'melancholy, marasmus and neurasthenia'.[144]

Moyseides, while conceding that it was certainly harmful, argued, however, that the extent of the effects depended on the individual's 'physical and mental endurance and temperament'.[145] In the early 1950s, women's queries in magazine columns also indicate that the method was used by them but opposed by the responding gynaecologists. One stated 'The prophylactic method that your husband uses is not the right one. He is harming himself and you too', while in another case only the harm to the husband was mentioned.[146] Such advice was consistent, as can be seen in an earlier quote from the same magazine in which all known methods were mentioned and recommended in the gynaecologist's response, except for coitus interruptus.[147] These views of coitus interruptus were central in making the Ogino-Knaus method one of the most frequently recommended, especially after World War II, as, we are told, at least for some of the days in the month 'the liquids that the man deposits in her vagina, so useful for women's bodies' would remain there and benefit the woman.[148] Greek authors thus consistently and without exception both listed coitus interruptus among the existing and practised methods and firmly rejected it, citing a varied but very long list of potential side effects that rendered the method unusable to those who wanted to safeguard their health.[149]

Considering physicians' negativity towards coitus interruptus, the degree to which the populace relied on the method is baffling. The same authors who rejected the method mentioned that it was the most widely used method among all social groups because it was so simple.[150] It could also be pointed out that it was also free. So, even Yioel, who rejected coitus interruptus and recommended the condom, nevertheless admitted that in 1938 it was the 'most commonly used method and it was employed by all classes because it is simple and it is considered the safest'.[151] Zouraris made similar comments in the 1950s. In Valaoras' study of a sample of the population in 1962–1963 withdrawal was found to have been the method that was practised most widely, its use varying from 65% to 72% in rural areas and between 30% and 48% in urban areas, depending on the age of the wife in both cases.[152] While the percentages of couples practising withdrawal in rural areas did not present any pattern, a larger proportion of younger urbanites were practising withdrawal than were older urbanites.[153] The youngest urbanites showed an almost equal preference for withdrawal and condoms.

However, the oral histories, which capture the testimonies of many of those who were early in controlling their fertility, do not suggest that coitus interruptus was the most commonly used method. There are some possible reasons for this. To start with, the language used to describe coitus interruptus is imprecise. While the terms referring, for example, to condoms or sponges are clear-cut, coitus interruptus can be described in a number of ways, only one of which is the straightforward 'pulling out'. It could be and has been argued that, because of its naturalness, informants forget to mention it, favouring the reporting of appliance methods. However, I believe that this is not the case among the Greek informants, who were willing and eager to mention, for example, breastfeeding as a contraception method, an equally natural method and one that I did not mention to them explicitly, unlike coitus interruptus. Nevertheless, coitus interruptus was indeed used by some of the interviewed couples:

A. I got married in 1936 … and it took 7 years and [then] I had Stefanos.
Q. How did you manage that?
A. Well, I don't know. I did not have any abortions; I did not take any medicines, no nothing. The husband was careful.
Q. May I ask how he was careful?
A. Are you married?
Q. I am engaged.
A. He was pulling out.
Q. Only that? Nothing else?
A. Nothing else.
Q. Did you know anything else [other methods] if you happened to want to use something else?
A. I, for my part, I don't know what they do now a days. I did not do anything. I did not do abortions, I did not do miscarriage, I did not take pills, neither did I ever go to a physician to ask.
Q. When you got married, did you know anything about those things?
A. I did not know, poor me, but my husband was telling me.
Q. Did he tell you right from the start that he did not want to have many children?
A. Yes, he did not want [children].
Q. And was he taking care from the beginning [of the marriage]?
A. He was taking care from the start. How did I catch Stefanos, I don't know. How did I catch him! When I told him [the husband], he almost killed me.
Q. Did he want only one then?
A. …. He did not want *any*, but you get fooled.[154]

This female informant, from rural Mykonos, describes a situation in which the husband unilaterally took the decision to have no children, informed her right from the start of the marriage and proceeded to practise withdrawal. His extremely efficient application of coitus interruptus resulted only in two pregnancies, with the first coming after seven years of marriage. This is an unusual case, in that the husband took the full initiative and responsibility in carrying out his decision, which happened to be much against the wife's wishes, although she never dared voice them. Within another couple, too, the husband willingly practised the method following the birth of three children, only two of whom survived infancy:

Q. How come you had only three children?
A. Because I was working a lot in the coffee shop, I was working a lot.
Q. And you decided that you did not want any more?
A. Yes. I was working a lot in the coffee shop and it was hard. What should I do? The children that my mother had [ten]? What will I be looking after? The children or the work?
Q. Did your husband agree [with this]?
A. Eh, yes.
Q. Were there many families like yours that had few children as you did?
A. Yes. Now even more so. More than three!
Q. Now [yes, it is uncommon to have more than three], but I refer to your time [1930s].
A. They had started to have fewer [at the time].
Q. Had they started then?
A. There is a man [living] nearby. He is not alive anymore. He had two wives. His wife died and he remarried. He had twenty-five children with the two wives. Can you believe that?
Q. When was that? Your time or your mother's time?
A. His daughter is still alive.
Q. Were people saying anything about it?
A. What could they say? And another one with more than twenty-five children, but with two wives.
Q. Do you believe those couples wanted to have those ten children or did they have them because they did not know?
A. They did not know. They did not know.
Q. But you did know?
A. [Laughter]
Q. Where did you learn [about the methods]? In Athens?

A. Eh yes, one [woman] with the other ... they started waking up [being informed]. They said, they had children, my mother had so [many] children. To make some money [instead, they thought]. I did not even learn any letters [I was not educated]. I didn't even learn to sign my name. Well. Was all that good? Was it all that good?
Q. Where did you learn about those things? Did you learn them in Athens [where she was a servant in the 1920s until 1927] or did you learn them on Mykonos?
A. Eh, with life, there and here.
Q. The first time, do you remember? Where did you hear about those things? Where did you find out you can have as many children as you want?
A. One with the other, we [women] spoke.
Q. Can I ask how [you took precautions], with what way [what way did you use]?
A. Eh he was careful (fylagontane).
Q. And did your husband want to?
A. Of course! If he did not want to ... [it would not have been possible].[155]

This was a strong-minded woman who was determined to move away from the poverty of her parental family, and she was very successful in doing so. She laid out the reasons why she wanted to have significantly fewer children than her mother had had, and defended her position by asking me—someone working in a university—whether it was acceptable that her family could not even send her to school. Having given her reasons for having only three (two surviving) children, she indicated that the method used was coitus interruptus, a method that required the co-operation of the husband because 'If he did not want to', it would not have been possible to practise it. However, this was not a woman who would have been constrained by her husband, whom she considered as 'someone who did not work much ... he used to go fishing for fun. And he drank wine.' When eventually she became pregnant, despite using coitus interruptus, she wanted to have an abortion in Athens, but he did not: 'so many years we did not have a child, let's have one now.' The informant had different ideas, but did not contest his view. Instead she pretended to be unwell, went to Athens to consult a physician and there had an abortion. On returning home, she told her husband that she had had a miscarriage while away. This was a determined woman with a very clear and unwavering view of her priorities. She did discuss the issues with her husband following her first three pregnancies, which happened each year after her marriage. She must have had convinced her husband to be 'cautious' after the three births; she did discuss her fourth pregnancy with him but when she failed to convince him about having an abortion she proceeded to fulfil her plans anyway in secrecy.

However, not all were willing to adopt withdrawal, and some were not willing to adopt any method at all. For example, another informant on Mykonos mentioned towards the end of her interview that 'I, apart from withdrawal [which I used] a couple of times, and I did not use it again. I don't want [precautions]. Whatever God sends, He will send, I said.' However, the informant had children in 1920, 1923, 1925 and 1928, and, after a gap of seven years, during which she did not use contraception, she had another one. By then the family was in Athens and when she next became pregnant she had an abortion. Following that, because of menorrhagia, she was advised to have a hysterectomy, which she did. In a lengthy discussion she explained that men were not accepting of withdrawal even when they knew of it as a method, just as she never used sponges, a method she had known about since she was young, after she was married:

Q. Did you know then what prophylaxis was? Did you know, in case you wanted [to use it]?
A. No. We did not know then. Then I … for the man to pull away.
Q. Did you know that though?
A. We knew that. Men were getting sick. They would say 'now, you cannot have that'.
Q. Did they not want to? Do women know about [this method]? Did you know about it but men did not want [to practise] it?
A. Yes, I did not have many [den kaloekana]; I did not have many children. All the women I know, they had ten or more children.
Q. Why did they not have fewer?
A. Peasants.
Q. Did they want to have so many?
A. They had children: poverty, hunger and many children.
Q. Why did they not have fewer children since it was such poverty?
A. They did not know how to take precautions.
Q. They did not know how to take precautions. The peasant women (horianes). Did the town inhabitants know?

A. They did not use [contraception]; in the beginning, no one did … because they did not have anything else. That was their cinema, that was their celebration/part, that was their laughter, that was … love. They did not have anything else. When the woman did not fancy the man, men would whinge. 'Oh you, leave us alone you and all that' [women would say]. And I was little then. And they [men] said, 'we have a little thing and we are not even in charge of it'. And, what is more, they whinged.
Q. So women did not want [to have sex] or did they not want to have children?
A. I am telling you, there was nothing else [but sex]. One brought the other [sex brought the children].
Q. Where did you learn about taking precautions? From your female friends? Who told you about precautions? Did everyone know?
A. [No]. We did not have discussions like that!
Q. With your husband? Would you talk [about that]?
A. No. My husband when I married him, he was nine years older than me. And when I told him that I would have a child, he said 'How do you know you will have a child?' He did not know that the period stops.
Q. Did he know about precautions?
A. Even if he did [know], he did not want to because [he did not like the idea]…[156]

Thus, despite having some knowledge of contraceptive methods, the informant and her husband hardly ever used them. What is also interesting to note here is the informant's first-person reference to coitus interruptus: 'I did not use it again.' This to someone brought up in late twentieth-century Greece sounds odd, as coitus interruptus is understood to be *the* male method of contraception. In my early interpretation of the interviews I assumed this to be a slip of the tongue and simply ignored it.[157] However, another informant used similar expressions too:

Q. Did you take care or was it your husband who did?
A. Anyway, he did and I did too.
Q. Did you find out from your husband [how to take care]?
A. No, they did not know things like that. As much as I could, I was taking care.
…

Q. Can I ask you again how you were taking care?
A. We can't be saying that!
Q. Withdrawal? Sponge?
A. Pulling away, whatever way we could. I did not want any more children. I couldn't anymore. I had only one kidney.
Q. Did you have an operation?
A. Yes, I had one kidney. And still I had so many children.
Q. Did the physician tell you not to have [any more] children? … Did the physician tell you …
A. He told us, yes, to be careful because we did not know if the one kidney would hold on. But it did.
Q. Did he tell you how to be careful?
A. He could not tell us! Whatever [way] we knew/understood. What should the physician tell me? The physician told me 'be careful because we do not know whether the kidney will last'.
Q. And you said you were careful.
A. I was careful, I was careful.
Q. Did you go and purchase something from the pharmacy?
A. We did something. We did purchase.
Q. Condoms?
A. Whatever we could.
Q. Was it easy to buy them?
A. Yes.
Q. Was it not a problem? Was it not shameful? Were you ashamed?
A. To a degree. I never had an abortion.
Q. Did your husband buy them or did you buy them?
A. Ah, does he know now? What does he know! Those people don't know.
Q. So you were making sure …
A. A woman told me that other women were using the condom. The men that is. Other women were using the sponge. I don't know.
Q. You don't know of those [methods]. What did you use?
A. I was taking care any way I understood, whatever [way] I could.
Q. Did you use douches?
A. Neither did I use douches. Nothing. That is, I was taking care in whatever way I could.
Q. Did you make sure you did not have contact [coitus]?

A. Contact? I took care and I was pulling away; he was pulling away; sometimes we put on a condom; sometimes we did not put on [a condom].[158]

Just as a man could pull away, a woman could do the same. And both the previous informants suggested that this was what they did, although at times the man would pull away too. Both this informant and the one quoted previously also mocked their husbands' lack of knowledge, suggesting that men were, at times, as ignorant as their wives in these matters, if not more so. Another informant, this time from Hios, describes a comparable situation:

A. God wanted them [the children], I praise and thank Him, I had six children …
Q. Would you have liked more children?
A. Pardon?
Q. Did you want to have had more children?
A. Mm, there was someone in our village who had twelve, and [someone else had] nine.
Q. How come you had only six then?
A. Eh, now they tell me 'Why did you have [many] children? How did you have them? Ee, what should we do with them? To get rid of them [to abort them]? We did not get rid of them [we did not abort them]! (E, ti na kanoume? Na ta rixoume? Den ta rihname!).
Q. Could you get rid of them if you wanted?
A. Of course, if we wanted didn't we go to the physician and get rid of them?
Q. To whom? In Volissos or in Hios Town?
A. No, in Volissos.
Q. In Volissos too then?
A. The physician from Volissos was coming to the village regularly.
Q. Oh, so he could do it [the abortion] at home too? You knew that even then?
A. God forbid, I did not get rid of [abort any] (den erixa).
Q. Have you heard …
A. Only a miscarriage I had, how it happened, I did not even realise … And I praise God, I thank him, and the way I gave birth to my other children, this happened too [the same way].

Q. Can I ask you? Were you careful (prosehate) and you had only six or did it just happen [by chance]?
A. What would I be careful of?
Q. I don't know. No?
A. To be careful of my husband, that is?
Q. Yes.
A. What can I say, my daughter? I am even ashamed to say it. But my husband, many a times I was fooling him (ton ekoroideua) and I would say to him, no, no, it is dust, it is dust. [As a way to distract him]. He would ask, what dust? He would pull out. Nothing else … [I did not use anything else].[159]

This informant had her children in the 1920s, 1930s and 1940s and, despite not having had any abortions, she was extremely well informed about the possibility of doing so and how it could be achieved. In terms of contraception, rather than directly mocking her husband's lack of knowledge, she declared that she 'was fooling him' into practising coitus interruptus. Whether this female-controlled withdrawal was more widespread than this sample of three women suggests is not necessarily the issue here, although, interestingly, Jane and Peter Schneider also reported its practice in Sicily among couples married in the 1950s and 1960s.[160] The significant point to be made is that it *did* occur and that some women were better informed than their husbands;[161] they sometimes informed them, though at other times they did not, and sometimes they practised withdrawal despite the husband. The advice and encouragement the informant quoted above received from her mother-in-law in becoming a servant in Istanbul in order to avoid further childbearing further points to women's initiative with contraception at a time when, at least some, husbands seemed to have been the more ignorant member of the couple.

Yet another informant revealed that even when two sisters were aware of the method, depending on whether there was or not co-operation between wife and husband, the outcome was very different. This informant, from rural Mykonos, moved to Athens and soon afterwards, in 1929, was married to a fellow Mykonian. When discussing her own siblings, the last one of which was born in 1928, she indicated that her last two sisters 'happened unexpectedly', explaining to me that the parents were taking precautions:

Q. How did they take precautions? What did they know?
A. Do you not know how they were taking precautions? Those years they would pull out.
Q. Was that all?
A. Eh yes, they did not have [anything else] then. Especially here on Mykonos, that was it all. They did not know any other method.[162]

When the discussion came to her own sister, with whom she was close and would discuss everything, including contraception, the informant explained that her sister's husband 'did not want to take any precautions ... he did not like it. He went to wherever it went, for as long as it went', despite her sister not wanting to have many children. Her sister had six children. The informant herself had a child in 1929, who died aged 2, two more in 1932 and 1934 and a miscarriage in 1935. Subsequently she moved back to Mykonos and had no further children, having practised control with the full co-operation of her husband:

A. Yes, I did not have another child. *I did not want* to have another child.
Q. You were taking care, weren't you?
A. Eh yes, of course. You take your measures and you say [to yourself], hold on. That's how it is. Life, my dear, has many difficult paths (aponerides). We, the peasants, those years suffered a lot, a lot. Because you would ask your mother for a piece of clothing, a cardigan, you asked for a cardigan ... and my mother would say to me: go and gather brushwood ... and I went and gathered eighteen loads (gomaria) of brushwood—one load is six armfuls—and I would carry them [on my back] and bring them down [from the countryside to the town] in order to get a cardigan. All that in 1924, 1925. Those years, we, single women, suffered here....
Q. Would you have liked more children?
A. I would have liked one child with the second husband. Once I gave up [hope] he made my child his [adopted her child], and it was the same, if not better.
Q. Did you not take precautions then?
A. I never did with him [the second].
Q. And the first one?
A. With the first one, yes, I did.[163]

Thus, while coitus interruptus was a simple method, its acceptance by the population was incremental and its practice, in the early days, was not sex-specific. In the Greek setting women did not pretend ignorance of the method, although such knowledge, for them, as I have argued elsewhere, sometimes came after marriage. Similarly, Turkish women interviewed in the 1990s Istanbul did not pretend ignorance and negotiated with their husbands over its use.[164]

Coitus interruptus thus needs to be re-evaluated as *not* an exclusively male method but still as one of the easiest and most convenient methods and one that was employed at the earliest stages of fertility control. These women were certainly not the first ones to practice coitus interruptus: Aetios, a Greek physician of the fourth century AD, described how 'during coitus, when the man is about to ejaculate, the woman ought to hold her breath and withdraw a little in order that the sperm might not penetrate the uterine cavity'.[165]

Its full acceptance and widespread use as a male method in the 1950s and 1960s Greece, and in later decades, when men took pride in their ability to 'control' their flow, appears to have been very different from the situation among the first groups of contraceptors in the late 1920s and the 1930s. Moreover, the population seems to have completely ignored the advice of the writings of physicians not to use this method, which was seen by gynaecologists as a perversion that had deleterious effects for men and women, as the advice given in 1950s popular women's magazines, and cited above, suggests:[166]

> The method you are using is easy but not only it is not the best but it is also the most harmful. Therefore you have to abandon it immediately even if you suffer a lot. It is only your age that allows that method, but it should not continue.[167]

> You are not under any danger except for vaginal slackness (halarosi) and perversion. Your husband is under threat of greatest dangers and so you need to avoid it.[168]

Interestingly, coitus interruptus seems to have been the only method that these magazine readers appeared to have knowledge of, along with emmenagogues. Despite the advice given to them by the magazines, as well as by all the relevant literature, this was the main method in use for avoiding conception in the 1950s 'because it is simple, easy and can be used at every opportunity without other complementary instruments and means'.[169]

In the 1960s much of what we know comes from the work of Valaoras and his associates. In 1962–1963 they interviewed a significant number of women, and subsequently their husbands, from urban and rural areas.[170] The sample involved only couples who at the time had a young child, and covered women who were born from 1910 onwards, although the majority were born after 1925.[171] Therefore, the urban sample did not cover the early contraceptors but rather the second generation of urban contraceptors. The informants were asked explicitly whether they had attempted to limit family size and whether they had used specific methods.[172]

During the 1950s authors outside Greece put forward a different interpretation of the method from that of the contraception radicals of early decades of the twentieth century, focusing on the efficacy of the method, the reasons behind its failures and a psychological interpretation of such failures. The Swede Elisabet Sjövall, chair of the National League for Sex Education of Sweden, explained in a short piece on coitus interruptus that for around half of the men practising the method it had proved 'an effective method of contraception'.[173] For the other half its failure was largely attributable to patterns of ejaculation and/or the control the individual was able to exert. Sjövall assessed the efficacy of the method on a retrospective basis, judging it to be effective when, following '5 to 10 years' of use, no pregnancies have resulted,[174] and discusses the effects of the method on men through the concept of virility and the association of the method with impotence. Rather than blame coitus interruptus for causing impotence, she explains how this method may not be suitable for all men, in that its application might cause some men psychological difficulties that in turn would lead to impotence.[175] Those men, she suggested, should seek different methods. For women too, the psychological effects of coitus interruptus could result in frigidity. Sjövall does not, therefore, list the 'usual' host of physical (and some psychological) illnesses that Greek and other physicians did at the time. A later publication mentions no side effects other than the possibility of 'sexual frustration in both partners',[176] adding that it is 'difficult to estimate' the effectiveness of the method and providing a failure rate of ten pregnancies per 100 women years. However, Rogow and Horowitz in 1995 and Santow in 1993 questioned its assumed inefficiency, revealing the almost complete lack of scientific studies of the method and questioning the discrediting of coitus interruptus by family planning researchers.[177] By 2000 the WHO guide to contraceptive methods mentions no side effects of any kind in relation to coitus interruptus, while explaining in its introduction that 'current policies and health care practices in some countries are based … on long-standing theoretical concerns that have never been substantiated'.[178] One can only assume that the authors were referring to coitus interruptus and the writings of many physicians both in the West and in Greece. Just as the working-class British informants of Fisher and Szreter ignored 'the putative psychological effect' mentioned in the British guides and embraced the method, the Greek working class also embraced it, and continued to do so for decades even after the Pill became available, ignoring the warnings of physicians.[179] However, judging from the high levels of its use even in the 1950s and 1960s, the Greek middle class employed the method too in the earlier stages of the fertility decline. One reason behind this opposition of writings and practice may well have been the inaccessibility of such writings to the wider population. More importantly, there were no advertisements for or public discussions of *any* methods, with the exception of condoms and to a lesser degree of douching. Thus, the wider population had to rely on trial and error and a self-evaluation of whatever methods they happened to find out about. Those for whom the method worked well had no reason to change, as the new information they would need to do so would have to be actively sought. The only product permitted to be advertised, as intimated above, was condoms and by the early 1960s urban couples that were exposed to such advertising were favouring condoms more than rural couples, possibly also suggesting that the middle class, concentrated in urban areas, was moving slowly away from coitus interruptus.[180]

There is no indication that withdrawal was an intuitive method for individuals or couples or that it was easy to become skilled in its use. This is evident in that the number of users of withdrawal among the early contraceptors was rather small. Importantly, among earlier contraceptor couples, women seemed to have been using the method, at least among the oral history sample, as often as men. Husbands of the earlier cohort were not consistently better informed than women, either. Importantly, we should cease to think of coitus interruptus as a male method: either partner can withdraw. It seems that only among the second generation of controllers—that is, at a time when information on contraception was more casually passed from person to person—did coitus interruptus become an exclusively male method, with information being much more available within male networks. This seems to have been the case in the British case, too, with women in the second half of Britain's fertility decline leaving the responsibility for contraception almost entirely to men.[181]

Yet another natural method, that of the rhythm or Ogino-Knaus as it was referred to, appears to have been employed rarely by anyone despite the favourable and sometimes emphatic mention it received by physicians in the late 1930s and 1940s and in the early 1950s.[182] However, even the physicians who were referring to or recommending this method as *the* method in their publications, did not have much faith in it.[183] Some, like Zouraris, passionately recommended the method in 1947, disguised within a book referring to sterility, only because that was the only way he could publish his work on contraception amidst an ultra-right government that eventually prosecuted him for his work on masturbation.[184] The reason the Ogino-Knaus method was discussed and recommended by physicians was its widespread acceptance—at the time—in the West and by the Catholic Church specifically. This was not the position of the Greek Orthodox Church. Archimandrite Seraphim Papakostas, the most prolific author on the subject, rejected all methods of contraception in 1947.[185] Thus, the frequent favourable mention of this method by physicians was mostly dictated by political reasons. There is no evidence that the population ever favoured or used the method.

In the next chapter all other methods employed by the Greek population are discussed, that is, appliance methods such as the douche, sponge, plugs and pessaries, condoms but also the Pill which appeared in the market in 1963.

Notes

1. A.J. Coale (1973) 'The demographic transition reconsidered', in *International Union for Scientific Study of Population, International Population Conference: Liege*, 1973, vol. 1 (Liege: IUSSP), p. 65.
2. Gösta Carlsson (1966) 'The Decline of Fertility: Innovation or Adjustment Process', *Population Studies*, 20(2), 149–74.
3. Gigi Santow (1995) 'Coitus Interruptus and the Control of Natural Fertility', *Population Studies*, 49(1), 19–43.
4. Georgios N. Kyriakides (1882) *Ta Mysteria tou Syzygikou Erotos etoi Fysiologia kai Ygieine kata tas Axiologous tes Zoes Epohas ton Syzygon*, 1st edn 1865 (Athens: Io. Kostopoulos).
5. K.P. Kardamates (1886) *Peri Aunanismou, ton Apotelesmaton kai Therapeias Autou* (Athens: n.p.), pp. 10–11.
6. Antonios I. Kindynes (1889) *E Steirosis para te Gynaiki kai Therapeia Autes* (Athens: Vlastos Varvaregos), pp. 142–5.

7. Markos Komnenos (1900) *Ygieine tes Genetesiou Ormes* (Athens: Anastasios D. Fexes); Antones Kallivokas (1923) *Ygieine tes Genetesiou Ormes*, translated from the French original (Athens: Hrestos D. Fexes), pp. 26–8.
8. Jean Marestan (1920) *To Vivlio tes Agapes. E Ygieine tou Gamou*, translated by P. Paulides from the 110th edn, 1st edn 1910 (Thessalonike: P. Paulides). The title of the edition translated by P. Paulides was Jean Marestan (1910) *L'Éducation Sexuelle* (Paris: Édition de la Guerre sociale). Jean Marestan was the pseudonym of Gaston Havard. The Greek translation was reissued again in 1928 and 1945. The 1945 edition had the title *Sexoualike Diapedagogise e to Vivlio tes Agapes* ('Sex Education or the Book of Love') and was published in Athens rather than in Thessaloniki, indicating the wider interest in the book.
9. Hrestos Euaggelou (1924) *O Kindynos ton Afrodision Noson. Praktikai Symvoulai pros Profylaxin* (Athens: n.p.).
10. M. Moyseides (1925) *E Gyne: Ygieine tou Gamou kai tes Eggamou Gynaikos* (Alexandria: A. Kasigone).
11. See, for example, A. Sygkelakes (1927) *E Apokryfe Ygieine tes Gynaikas* (Alexandria: Grammata); M. Moyseides (1932) *Malthousianismos Allote kai Nyn. Eleghos Genneseon kai Aposteirosis* (Athens: Gerardon Bros); Anna Katsigra (1932) *Proetoimasia tou Koritsiou sta Genetesia Zetemata* (Athens: A.V. Pasha).
12. In the early 1950s some authors argued that the poor continued to procreate uncontrollably, as did those of lower mental capacity (Pope Speliotopoulou-Mpazinou (1951) 'Eugonia', *Alkyonides. Deltio tes Panelleniou Enoseos Dianooumenon Gynaikon* 1(6), 4–8). The author, using the examples of the USA and Sweden, expresses her anxieties about the addition of dysgenic individuals to the population and urges individuals to behave responsibly towards society and their descendants.
13. For example, Alexandros Tsakires (1954) *Megale Sexologia. Anikanotes, Steirosis kai e Syghrone Therapeia ton*, 3rd edn, 1st edn 1947 (Athens: n.p.), p. 535.
14. Konstantinos Metropoulos (1954) *Ygieine tes Egkyou. Enas Polytimos Odegos gia ten Ygieine Diaviose tes Egkyou* (Athens: Papademetriou), p. 147.
15. Metropoulos, *Ygieine*, p. 145.
16. Tsakires, *Megale Sexologia*, p. 536.
17. Tsakires, *Megale Sexologia*, p. 537.
18. Tsakires, *Megale Sexologia*, p. 537. This is essentially the rhythm method, as articulated independently by Hermann Knaus and Kyusaku Ogino.
19. See, for example, Anonymous (20 June 1951) 'O Gynaikologos Apanta: Reply to Mia Poly Eroteumene', *E Gynaika*, 2(37), p. 49; Anonymous (7 February 1951) 'O Gynaikologos Apanta: Reply to Mia Dystehismenen

Syzygo pm', *E Gynaika*, 2(27), p. 49; Anonymous (29 November 1950) 'O Gynaikologos Apanta: Reply to SAPFO', *E Gynaika*, 1(22), p. 61.

20. Anonymous (1954) *Egkyklopaideia tes Ellenidos. Iatrike ton Oikogeneion, Diaitetike, Gynaikeia Provlemata, Kallone, Symperifora* (Athens: Papademetriou).
21. Anonymous, *Egkyklopaideia tes Ellenidos*, pp. 306–7.
22. Paulos Drandakes (ed.) (1956) *Megale Ellenike Egkyklopaideia*, vol. 8, 2nd edn (Athens: Phoenix), pp. 126–7, 184–5, 187, 605.
23. Anonymous (21 March 1951) 'O Gynaikologos Apanta: Reply to Agnoia', *E Gynaika*, 2(30), p. 49.
24. Anonymous (27 February 1952) 'O Gynaikologos Apanta: Reply to Mikre Afrikana', *E Gynaika*, 3(55), p. 60.
25. Anonymous (13 December 1950) 'O Gynaikologos Apanta: Reply to D.I.M.O.', *E Gynaika*, 1(23), p. 19.
26. Anonymous (7 February 1951) 'O Gynaikologos Apanta: Reply to Peirasmos', *E Gynaika*, 2(27), p. 49.
27. Anonymous (13 December 1950) 'O Gynaikologos Apanta: Reply to Mnestera [male]', *E Gynaika*, 1(23), p. 19.
28. No. 3 Hios, born in 1909.
29. No. 3 Hios. See also Violetta Hionidou (1998) 'The Adoption of Fertility Control on Mykonos, 1879–1959: Stopping, Spacing or Both?' *Population Studies*, 52(1), 78. Also similar comments by No. 20 Mykonos; No. 28 Mykonos; No. 22 rural Syros.
30. Georgios N. Makkas (1911) *E Thnesimotes tes Paidikes Elekias en Elladi. Aitia kai Mesa pros Peristolen* (Athens: Nikolaos Hiotes); Solon Veras (14 June 1930) 'E Prostasia tes Teknogonias', *Ergasia*, 1(23), 19–20. See also Violetta Hionidou (1993) 'The Demography of a Greek island, Mykonos 1859–1959: A Family Reconstitution Study' (unpublished PhD thesis: University of Liverpool), pp. 136–7, for references to nineteenth-century Greece, and Michalis Raftakis (2019) 'Mortality change in Hermoupolis, Greece (1859–1940)' (unpublished PhD thesis: Newcastle University), for references to the early twentieth century.
31. K.A. Alexandropoulos (1960) *O Thelasmos en te Ellenike kai Xene Laografia* (Athens: n.p.); Nikolaos Haliores (1931) *Ydreika Laografika* (Peiraeus: Sorotou); Hionidou, 'The Adoption', 78–9, referring to Mykonos. See also, for example, No. 10 Hios, who breastfed her children for around two years; No. 10 Syros; No. 11 Syros mentioned that children would be breastfed to the ages of 3–4 years. No. 4 Mykonos mentioned that the infants would be usually breastfed for a year or a year and a half. Richard Blum and Eva Blum (1965) *Health and Healing in Rural Greece* (Stanford, CA: Stanford University Press), p. 153; E. Georges (2008) *Bodies of Knowledge: The Medicalisation of Reproduction in Greece*

(Nashville, TN: Vanderbuilt UP), p. 145; Vaios F. Kaminiotes (2016) *Magisses kai Mageirisses. Diatrofe, Mageia kai Gynaikeia Exousia stous Karagkounedes tes Dytikes Thessalias* (Athens: Erodotos), p. 458.

32. L.D. Hrestovitz (1891) *Tittheia e Thelasis kai Diatrofe ton Vrefon* (Athens: Nikolaos I. Kazases), pointing to the benefits of breastfeeding but discussing wet nursing extensively; Apostolos Doxiadis (1926) *Grammata pros Meteres* (Athens: Greka); No. 1, female, Syros, born 1902; No. 23, female, Mykonos, born 1907; On upper-class women employing wet-nurses see Anonymous (15 March 1860) 'Kanones pros Eklogen Katallelou Tithes (Vyzastras)', *O Iatros tou Laou*, 1(6), 85–9; Raftakis, 'Mortality', Chap. 7.
33. P. Paulides (1945) *Teknopoiese Thelematike sten Katallele Epohe kai se Peristase Eunoike* (Athens: privately printed), p. 4.
34. G. Vassiliou and V. Vassiliou (1970) 'On Aspects of Child Rearing in Greece' in E.J. Anthony and C. Koupernik (eds) *The Child in his Family*, The International Yearbook for Child Psychiatry and Allied Disciplines, vol. 1 (New York: Wiley-Interscience), pp. 433–4.
35. The same practice is noted for England by Marie Stopes (1923) *Contraception (Birth Control): Its Theory, History and Practice* (London: John Bale), pp. 66–7, quoting Allen Davenport (25 August 1826) 'Letter on the Poor Laws', *Republican Magazine*, XIV(7).
36. No. 4 Mykonos.
37. Georges, *Bodies*, p. 81. Also from Rhodes is another case observed by a British physician when he was serving in the local hospital in 1945: he noted that he observed 'children being suckled at the age of three and a half years' explicitly for that reason (A. Raymond Mills (1948) 'Peasant Remedies from the Greek Islands', *Bulletin of the History of Medicine*, 22, 447).
38. No. 12, female, Mykonos, born in 1913.
39. No. 22, rural Syros, married in 1945.
40. No. 4, female, Mykonos, born in 1902.
41. No. 13, female, Mykonos, born in 1906, referring to her stepmother.
42. Violetta Hionidou (2009) '"It Was a Bridge from Life to Death": Hospitals during the Food Crisis, Greece 1941–1944', *Social History of Medicine*, 22(2), 361–85; Violetta Hionidou (2016) 'Popular Medicine and Empirics in Greece, 1900–1950: An Oral History Approach', *Medical History*, 60(4), 492–513.
43. Nikolaos Kostes (1849) *Egxeiridion Maieutikes* (Athens: S.K. Vlastos), p. 176. Similarly, in nineteenth-century England a doctor and nurse advised a wife that she would not conceive while breastfeeding, only for that to happen immediately (Stopes, *Contraception*, p. 66).

44. Moyseides, *Malthousianismos*, p. 45.
45. Moyseides, *Malthousianismos*, p. 45 citing Th. H. Van de Velde (1929) *Die Fruchtbarkeit in der Ehe* (Leipzig: Müller Verlag), p. 331.
46. For example, No. 3 Mykonos sought and received extensive advice on how to feed and wean her child on Mykonos in the 1930s from one such practitioner she called a 'giatrissa' (female doctor).
47. George Drysdale (1864) *The Elements of Social Science; or, Physical, Sexual, and Natural Religion, by a Graduate of Medicine*, 4th edn, 1st edn 1861 (London: E. Truelove), p. 487.
48. Wally Seccombe (1992) 'Men's "Marital Rights" and women's "Wifely Duties": Changing conjugal relations in the fertility decline' in John R. Gillis, Louise A. Tilly and David Levine (eds) *The European Experience of Declining Fertility. A quiet revolution 1850–1970* (Cambridge, MA: Blackwell), p. 83; Elizabeth Roberts (1995) *Women and families: An oral history, 1940–1970* (Oxford: Blackwell), p. 99.
49. Karl Buttenstedt (1904) *Happiness in Marriage (Revelation in Women): A Nature Study*, 3rd edn, 1st edn 1900 in German (Friedrichshagen: n.p.); Richard E. Funcke (1906) *A New Revelation in Nature. A Secret of Sexual Life. No More Prostitution* (Hanover: n.p.), p. 70. Both cited in John S. Haller and Robin M. Haller (1974) *The Physician and Sexuality in Victorian America* (Urbana: University of Illinois Press), pp. 120–1.
50. Iwan Bloch (1909) *The sexual life of our time in its relations to modern civilisation*, translated from the 6th German edn by M. Eden Paul (London: Rebman), p. 701.
51. Courtenay Beale (1922) *Wise Wedlock. The Complete Treatise on Birth Control & Marriage* (London: Health Promotion), p. 130.
52. Margaret Sanger (1915) *Family Limitation* (New York: n.p.), p. 6.
53. Margaret Sanger (1931) *Happiness in Marriage*, 10th edn, 1st edn 1926 (Cornwall, NY: Cornwall Press), p. 210.
54. Stopes, *Contraception*, pp. 64–5.
55. Marie Stopes (1925) *A Letter to Working Mothers or How to have Healthy Children and avoid Weakening Pregnancies* (London: Mothers' Clinic for Constructive Birth Control), p. 6.
56. Zeynep Angin and Frederic C. Shorter (1998) 'Negotiating reproduction and gender during the fertility decline in Turkey', *Social Science Medicine*, 47(5), 559.
57. Angin and Shorter, 'Negotiating reproduction', 560.
58. Kari Pitkänen (2003) 'Contraception in Late Nineteenth- and Early Twentieth-Century Finland', *The Journal of Interdisciplinary History*, 34(2), 199.
59. Pitkänen, 'Contraception', 200–1.

60. Sølvi Sogner (2003) 'Abortion, Birth Control, and Contraception: Fertility Decline in Norway', *The Journal of Interdisciplinary History*, 34(2), 224.
61. Sogner, 'Abortion', 225.
62. Sogner, 'Abortion', 219. In Norway the 10 per cent decline had been achieved by 1908. For Finland it was 1910 (Sogner, 'Abortion', 212).
63. R.P. Neuman (1978) 'Working Class Birth Control in Wilhelmine Germany', *Comparative Studies in Society and History*, 20(3), 416.
64. No. 12 Mykonos and No. 22 Syros.
65. Sogner, 'Abortion', 224–5.
66. No. 7 Mykonos, male, born in 1905.
67. No. 10 Mykonos, female, born 1916. See also Hionidou, 'The Adoption', 79–81.
68. Christopher Tietze (1964) 'Lactation' in Mary S. Calderone (ed.), *Manual of Contraceptive Practice* (Baltimore, MD: The Williams & Wilkins Company), pp. 230–1. However, see M. Livi Bacci (1977) *A History of Italian Fertility During the Last Two Centuries* (Princeton, NJ: Princeton University Press), p. 256; Hionidou, 'The Adoption'; and, subsequently, Simon Szreter, R. Nye and F. Van Poppel (2003) 'Fertility and Contraception during the Demographic Transition: Qualitative and Quantitative Approaches', *The Journal of Interdisciplinary History*, 34(2), 141–54; and the collection of essays in the same issue.
69. Tietze, 'Lactation', pp. 230–1.
70. Anonymous, 'Lactational Amenorrhea Method (LAM)', *Contraceptive Technology and Reproductive Health Series*, https://www.fhi360.org/sites/default/files/webpages/Modules/LAM/s1pg14.htm (accessed 17 December 2018); World Health Organization (2000) *Improving access to quality care in family planning: Medical eligibility criteria for contraceptive use* (Geneva: WHO), p. 1.
71. See Szreter, who has been the most vocal supporter and discussant of this (Simon Szreter (1996) *Fertility, Class and Gender in Britain, 1860–1940* (Cambridge: Cambridge University Press), pp. 389–441).
72. Haller and Haller, *The Physician and Sexuality*, p. 102. Lucy Bland (1986) 'Marriage laid bare: Middle-class women and marital sex 1880s–1914' in Jane Lewis (ed.) *Labour and Love. Women's Experience of Home and Family, 1850–1940* (Oxford: Basil Blackwell), pp. 128–9; Szreter, *Fertility*, pp. 389–441.
73. Szreter, *Fertility*, p. 394.
74. Simon Szreter and Kate Fisher (2010) '"We weren't the sort that wanted intimacy every night": birth control and abstinence in England, c.1930–1960', *The History of the Family*, 15(2), 152–3. Others have also discussed abstinence, but this has rarely been interpreted as significant.

However, it seems that it may have been important among physicians in the Netherlands in the late nineteenth century (F.W.A. Van Poppel and Hugo Röling (2003) 'Physicians and Fertility Control in the Netherlands', *Journal of Interdisciplinary History*, 34(2), 164, 184).

75. However, this was not the understanding of most, who believed that Malthus advocated abstinence within marriage. See, for example, Marestan, *To Vivlio*, p. 133. Marestan found the method 'inappropriate but also inhumane', as it made love prohibitive to the poor.
76. Thomas Malthus (1798) *An Essay on the Principle of Population* (London: Printed for J. Johnson, in St. Paul's Church-Yard), p. 9, http://www.esp.org/books/malthus/population/malthus.pdf (accessed 9 January 2019). Beyond the first edition, he referred to 'moral restraint', meaning the postponement of marriage until the couple could afford to support a family (T.R. Malthus (1993) *An Essay on the Principle of Population*, edited by Geoffrey Gilbert (Oxford: Oxford University Press), p. xviii).
77. Maria Kyriakidou (2003) 'Female Bodies, Sexuality and Leftist Feminism: The "Personal as Political" in interwar Greece', Past and Present of Radical Sexual Politics conference, University of Amsterdam, 3–4 October 2003, http://www.iisg.nl/womhist/radsexpol.html (last accessed 14 January 2019).
78. See, for example, the recounting by Louros—an eminent obstetrician—of an incident that occurred in the 1940s, entitled 'Caesarean and virginity' (N.K. Louros and K.N. Alivizatos (1979) *Dyo Giatroi Thymountai* (Athens: Filippote), pp. 71–2); D. Diamantopoulos (1957) *Iatrike Egkyklopaideia tes Gynaikas* (Athens: Gerolympou), pp. 28–34; also the reply to a reader's letter by the gynaecologist who emphasised in his reply 'the existing social perceptions about the virginal hymen' (Anonymous (29 November 1950) 'O Gynaikologos Apanta: Reply to SAPFO', *E Gynaika*, 1(22), p. 61).
79. No. 22 Hios, urbanite, female, married in 1955 at the age of 30.
80. This is also described by Kaires with reference to parents (Mihael Nik. Kaires (1939), *Akindynos Erotas. E Ygieine ton Neon Syzygon kai e Ygieine Profylaxis ton Neon* (Athens: Anatole), p. 70).
81. See No. 16 Mykonos later in the text when asking explicitly whether I was married or not. Similarly, Arnold reported that in the early 1980s, when she attempted to discuss birth control and abortion with 'childless women', they acted as though embarrassed and claimed to 'know nothing' (Marlene Sue Arnold (1985) 'Childbirth among Rural Greek Women in Crete: Use of Popular, Folk and Cosmopolitan Medical Systems' (unpublished PhD thesis: University of Pennsylvania), p. 267).
82. No. 18 Mykonos, female, middle-class urbanite.
83. No. 4 Mykonos.

84. The bi-weekly women's magazine *E Gynaika* was replete with articles referring to love and sex. See, for example, Emma Drake (4 October 1950) 'Ti Prepei na Xerei e Nea Gynaika?', *E Gynaika*, 1(18), pp. 12–14, where one of the sections is entitled 'Conjugal relationships'; Anonymous (18 October 1950) 'To Thauma tou Eautou sas', *E Gynaika*, 1(19), pp. 14–15, where one of the sections was entitled 'Your sexual life'; Nikoletsopoulos (4 April 1952) 'Erotas & Sexoualismos', *E Gynaika*, 2(31), p. 28. See, for the concerns of the women about their virginal hymen, Anonymous (21 March 1951) 'O Gynaikologos Apanta: Reply to Ktypemene I.A.H.', *E Gynaika*, 2(30), p. 49, where the reader is advised that her illness could not have affected her hymen. In another case the gynaecologist discusses the possibility of a broken hymen, suggesting that, since there was no blood, the hymen was not broken (Anonymous (18 April 1951) 'O Gynaikologos Apanta: Reply to Arapina Konstantinoupolen', *E Gynaika*, 2(32), p. 52).
85. No. 5 Hios.
86. See, for example, K.V-Th.P.-N.D. (1956) 'O Gamos' in Paulos Drandakes (ed.) *Megale Ellenike Egkyklopaideia*, vol. 8, 2nd edn (Athens: Phoenix), pp. 127–31.
87. Moyseides, *Malthousianismos*, p. 42.
88. N.N. Drakoulides (1956) 'Genetesion Enstikton' in Paulos Drandakes (ed.) *Megale Ellenike Egkyklopaideia*, vol. 8, 2nd edn (Athens: Phoenix), pp. 184–5.
89. Anna Katsigra (1932) *Proetoimasia tou Koritsiou sta Genetesia Zetemata* (Athens: A.V. Pasha), p. 98.
90. Female desire was confined to the necessity for 'love, affection, support in life, children' (Katsigra, *Proetoimasia*, p. 99).
91. Drakoulides indicated that this was necessary only after the age of 20 (N.N. Drakoulides (1956) 'Genetesios Apohe' in Paulos Drandakes (ed.) *Megale Ellenike Egkyklopaideia*, vol. 8, 2nd edn (Athens: Phoenix), p. 186); Nikolaos Gyras (1939) *Prin kai Meta ton Gamo*, 4th edn (Athena: G. Vallianatou), p. 39.
92. Kaires, *Akindynos Erotas*, p. 68.
93. Efi Avdella (2002) *Dia Logous times. Via, Synaisthemata kai Axies ste Metemfyliake Ellada* (Athens: Nefele); Anonymous (5 January 1929) 'Ethelese na ten Foneusei dia Logous Times', *Skrip*, 32(9218), p. 4; Anonymous (8 May1959) 'Paredothesan oi Adelfoi foneis oi katakreourgesantes ton stratioten', *Makedonia*, 48(15635), p. 3.
94. Moyseides, *Malthousianismos*, p. 42.
95. N.N. Drakoulides (1959) *Sexoualikes Anomalies (Apohe-aneparkeia-anikanotes-anafrodisia)* (Athens: Neotate Iatrike Egkyklopaideia), p. 1.

96. No. 10 Hios. In the 1930s she spent approximately two years away working in Turkey while in her early 40s and by the time she returned she was going through menopause.
97. No. 4 Hios.
98. No. 19 Mykonos.
99. No. 4 Mykonos.
100. Kaires, *Akindynos Erotas*, p. 78.
101. Kaires, *Akindynos Erotas*, p. 79.
102. No. 21 Mykonos. During the forty days following labour women were expected not to leave their house and not to have sexual relationships. During the same period, the woman and the infant were considered particularly vulnerable, especially because of the presence of evil spirits (xotika) and fairies (neraides). On these, see Charles Stewart (1991) *Demons and the Devil. Moral Imagination in the Modern Greek Culture* (Princeton, NJ: Princeton University Press).
103. No. 4 Mykonos. This was prescribed by the Orthodox Church, in addition to abstinence on Saturday and Sunday (Anna Matthaiou (2006) 'Syzygikes Sheseis kai Sexoualikoteta sta Hronia tes Othomanikes Kyriarhias: Kanones, Protypa, Sympsefismoi', *Ta Istorika*, 23(44), 149). Similarly, when a woman was to offer the communion bread (prosforo) to the church she had to abstain for three days before starting the preparations of the bread (Kaminiotes, *Magisses*, pp. 450–1).
104. For a similar point, linking the wearing of jewellery with a declaration of sexual availability, see Persake's short story 'To koritsi', situated on the island of Aegina in the first half of the twentieth century (Ioulia Persake (2016) *Katohe kai Peina. Istories tes kathe meras* (Athens: Estia), pp. 59–76).
105. See, for example, Stopes, who strongly condemned 'abstinence' but encouraged, rather, infrequent sex, in order to maximise attraction and ultimately satisfaction (Marie Stopes (2004) *Married Love*, edited by Ross McKibbin (Oxford: Oxford University Press), pp. 74–7, 48–51).
106. Kyriakides, *Ta Mysteria*, p. 159.
107. Moyseides, *E Gyne*, p. 88; M. Moyseides (1927) *Aunanismos Kindynoi-Profylaxis-Therapia* (Athens: Gerardon Bros); Tsakires, *Megale Sexologia*, pp. 667–73; Antonios Gregoriades (1949) *Afrodisia Nosemata kai Anikanotes. Ygieina Paraggelmata kai Profylaxis ton Neon* (Athens: n.p.), pp. 20–1, 56–8; Georgios K. Zouraris (1947) *Sexoualike Zoe: Apohe, Egkrateia, Akolasia kai e Exasthenisis tes Ormes*, 3rd edn (Athens: n.p.), pp. 54–5. Outside Greece at the same time—and earlier—a wide range of authors was also arguing against continence. See, for example, Sanger, who listed continence under 'Harmful methods' (Margaret H. Sanger (1917) *The Case for Birth Control. A Supplementary Brief and Statement*

of Facts (New York: Modern Art Printing Co.), Chap. 6, http://www.gutenberg.org/files/54599/54599-h/54599-h.htm, accessed 20 December 2018); and Marestan, *To Vivlio*, p. 60.
108. Moyseides, *E Gyne*, pp. 80–3.
109. N.N. Drakoulides (1931) *E Sexoualike Egkrateia kata ton Polemon os Syntelestes tes Metapolemikes Psyhosyntheseos* (Athens: n.p.), p. 6.
110. Drakoulides, *E Sexoualike egkrateia*, p. 6.
111. Paulides, *Teknopoiese*, p. 7.
112. Serafeim Papakostas (1961) *Agnotes Gamos Gynaika* (Athens: Adelfotes Theologon 'E Zoe'), 2nd edn, pp. 19–20. This particular chapter, entitled 'Purity', was a reproduction of an earlier publication that was published in the Christian journal *Aktines* in April 1946.
113. Anastasios V. Antonopoulos (1953) *E Sexoualike Diafotesis ton Neon* (Patras: Synadinou Bros), p. 28.
114. Antonopoulos, *E sexoualike*, p. 28.
115. Antonopoulos, *E sexoualike*, Introduction.
116. Genesis 38:9. However, Onanism came to mean masturbation.
117. Francis Place (1823) *Contraceptive Handbill: To the married of both sexes*, Form A and Form B, cited in Norman Edwin Himes (1936) *Medical History of Contraception* (London: G. Allen & Unwin), pp. 214, 217–8.
118. Robert Dale Owen (1831) *Moral Physiology*, 2nd edn (New York: Wright & Owen), p. 6.
119. Owen, *Moral Physiology*, pp. 80–2.
120. Charles Knowlton (1877) *Fruits of Philosophy. A Treatise on the Population Question, edited by Charles Bradlaugh and Annie Besant*, 1st edn 1832 (London: Freethought Publishing Co), p. 81, https://archive.org/details/fruitsphilosoph00knogoog/page/n10 (accessed 30 March 2019).
121. Drysdale, *The Elements of Social Science*, pp. 473–5. Bergeret subsequently clarified that the French working classes employed this method widely, while the wealthier used condoms (L.F.E. Bergeret (1870) *The Preventive Obstacle, or, Conjugal Onanism*, translated by P. De Marmon from the 3rd French edn (New York: Turner & Mignard), p. 5, https://play.google.com/books/reader?id=N1RMB5FxX8MC&hl=en_GB&pg=GBS.PA12, accessed 28 December 2018).
122. Haller and Haller, *The Physician and Sexuality*, pp. 114–5, citing among others S.G. Moses, 'Marital masturbations', *St Louis Courier of Medicine*, VIII (1882), 168–73.
123. Haller and Haller, *The Physician and Sexuality*, p. 115, citing Jacques Bertillon (1874) 'Mariage Démographie Hygiène Matrimoniale', in Dechambre (ed.) *Dictionnaire Encyclopédique des Sciences Médicales*, 2nd series, vol. 5, pp. 7–83; Ely Van de Warker (1884) 'A gynecological study

of the Oneida community', *American Journal of Obstetrics and Diseases of Women and Children*, XVIL(8), 785–810; and Anonymous (1884) 'Does male copulation without emission injure female health?' *Medical News*, XLV, 240–1.

124. H. Arthur Allbutt (1894) *The Wife's Handbook. How a woman should order herself during pregnancy, in the Lying-in Room, and after Delivery with hints on Management of the baby and on other matters of importancy, necessary to be known by married women*, 1st edn 1886[?] (London: R. Forder), p. 48.
125. Allbutt, *The Wife's Handbook*, p. 48.
126. Sanger, *Family Limitation*, 1st edn, pp. 6–7.
127. Sanger, *The Case For Birth Control*, pp. 185–6.
128. Marie Stopes (1918) *Wise Parenthood. A Sequel to 'Married Love'* (London: n.p.), pp. 24–5; Stopes, *Married Love*, pp. 58–9; Marie Stopes (1923) *Contraception (Birth Control): Its Theory, History and Practice* (London: John Bale), pp. 69–82. Similar claims against the methods continued to be made in the 1970s and even the 1980s, as Rogow and Horowitz eloquently showed (Deborah Rogow and Sonya Horowitz (1995) 'Withdrawal: A Review of the Literature and an Agenda for Research', *Studies in Family Planning*, 26(3), 144–5).
129. Beale, *Wise Wedlock*, pp. 121, 80.
130. Beale, *Wise Wedlock*, p. 121.
131. Ettie A. Rout (1922) *Safe Marriage: A Return to Sanity* (London: William Heinemann (Medical Books) Ltd), http://www.gutenberg.org/files/16135/16135-h/16135-h.htm.
132. Antoinette F. Konikow (1923) *Voluntary Motherhood: A Study of the Physiology and Hygiene of Prevention of Conception* (n.p.), p. 18, https://archive.org/details/23KonikowVoluntarymotherhood/ (accessed 31 March 2019), pp. 10–11; Antoinette F. Konikow (1931) *Physician's Manual of Birth Control* (New York: Buchholz Publishing Co), p. 147.
133. Bergeret, *The Preventive*, p. xvii.
134. Bergeret, *The Preventive*, p. xv.
135. Stopes, *Contraception*, p. 48.
136. Kardamates, *Peri Aunanismou*, pp. 4–5.
137. Sygkelakes, *E Apokryfe*, p. 53.
138. Gr. Stefanou (1927) *O Eros. Fysiologikos kai para Fysin* (Athens: Georgiou Vasileiou), p. 352.
139. Stefanou, *O Eros*, p. 354.
140. Moyseides, *Malthousianismos*, p. 47. The same author, in his treatise on masturbation, remarked that mutual masturbation was much more destructive than self-masturbation partly because of the 'moral corruption'

and partly because of the need it creates for 'artificially repeated sexual needs' (Moyseides, *Aunanismos*, p. 8).

141. Kardamates, *Peri Aunanismou*, pp. 6, 10. This is a side effect also mentioned by Bergeret, *The Preventive*.
142. Anonymous, *Egkyklopaideia tes Ellenidos*, p. 306.
143. M. Yioel (1938) *Steirosis e Egkymosyne kata Voulesi*, 2nd edn, 1st edn 1936 (Athens: Vasileiou), pp. 20–1, citing French and British medical authors, referred to the 'syndrome des frauduleuses'. The symptoms mentioned here were also listed by Bergeret in *The Preventive*.
144. N.N. Drakoulides (1936) *E Sexoualike Leitourgia* (Athens: n.p.), p. 11; Georgios Zouraris (1957) *Sexoualike Orme*, 3rd edn, first edn 1950 (Athens: Melissa), pp. 53–60.
145. Moyseides, *Malthousianismos*, p. 47.
146. Paulides mentioned that semen was useful for the woman's body, while douching 'deprived' the woman of 'a tonic' (Paulides, *Teknopoiese*, p. 29); Anonymous (7 February 1951) 'O Gynaikologos Apanta: Reply to Mia Dystehismenen Syzygo pm', *E Gynaika*, 2(27), p. 49; Anonymous (21 March 1951) 'O Gynaikologos Apanta: Reply to Neopantremene V. Mika', *E Gynaika*, 2(30), p. 49. Interestingly, in his reply the gynaecologist refrains from explicitly naming coitus interruptus, unlike all other methods.
147. Anonymous (21 March 1951) 'O Gynaikologos Apanta: Reply to Agnoia', *E Gynaika*, 2(30), p. 49.
148. Gyras, *Prin*. Similar claims were made in 1980 associating the lack of 'resorption of seminal content during sexual act' with an increased frequency of breast cancer (Arne N. Gjorgov (1980) *Barrier Contraception and Breast Cancer* (Munich: S. Karger), p. viii).
149. Anonymous, 'Dia ten Praxin', 188; Zouraris, *Sexoualike Orme*, pp. 53–60; Moyseides, *Malthousianismos*, pp. 46–9. Evaggelos An. Averof (1939) *Symvole eis ten Ereunan tou Plythesmiakou Provlematos tes Ellados* (Athens: n.p.), p. 72, citing a number of foreign and Greek authors.
150. Kardamates, *Peri Aunanismou*, p. 9; Moyseides, *Malthousianismos*, p. 45; Zouraris, *Sexoualike Orme*, p. 64, emphasis in the original; Yioel, *Steirosis*, p. 13. According to Averof coitus interruptus was the most commonly used method in the late 1930s (Averof, *Symvole*, p. 72). For post-World War II Greece, similarly, the elderly obstetrician interviewed by Arnold in the early 1980s indicated that withdrawal was one of the three most widely used methods, adding that this was detrimental to the woman's health, causing her to become 'hysterical and nervous' (Arnold, 'Childbirth', pp. 171–2).
151. Yioel, *Steirosis*, pp. 13, 19–20.

152. Vasilios Valaoras, A. Polychronopoulou, D. Trichopoulos (1965) 'Control of Family Size in Greece (The Results of a Field Survey)', *Population Studies,* 18(3), 271.
153. Valaoras et al., 'Control', 277.
154. No. 16 Mykonos.
155. No. 20 Mykonos, female, married in 1927, born in rural area of Mykonos, lived while married in the town of Mykonos, worked as a servant in Athens throughout her teenage years.
156. No. 4 Mykonos.
157. Hionidou, 'The Adoption', 67–83.
158. No. 1 Mykonos.
159. No. 10 Hios, married in 1921; the extended family resided in a Hios village and the informant worked as a servant in Hios town between 1915 and 1921.
160. Jane C. Schneider and Peter Schneider (1996) *Festival of the Poor: Fertility Decline and the Ideology of Class in Sicily, 1860–1980* (Tuscon: The University of Arizona Press), pp. 261, 246.
161. No. 12 Mykonos made a similar comment.
162. No. 3 Mykonos.
163. No. 3 Mykonos.
164. Angin and Shorter, 'Negotiating reproduction'.
165. Himes, *Medical History*, p. 94, citing *Aëtios, Des Affections de la Matrice, ou Discours seizième*, edition Skevos Zervos (Leibzig 1901). Interestingly, it was Moyseides who provided Himes with the text.
166. Similar ideas are expressed in books published at the time: see, for example, Zouraris, *Sexoualike Orme*, pp. 65–6.
167. Anonymous (29 November 1950) 'O Gynaikologos Apanta: Reply to SAPFO', *E Gynaika*, 1(22), p. 61.
168. Anonymous (20 June 1951) 'O Gynaikologos Apanta: Reply to Mia Poly Eroteumene', *E Gynaika*, 2(37), p. 49.
169. Zouraris, *Sexoualike Orme*, p. 64, emphasis in the original. Zouraris argued against the use of coitus interruptus due to its health implications.
170. Valaoras et al., 'Control', 270.
171. Valaoras et al., 'Control', 271.
172. Abortion was incorrectly classified as one of the contraceptive methods in the presentation of the results (Valaoras et al., 'Control', 275).
173. This appears to have been written sometime in the 1950s. The translated version I consulted does not indicate the precise date of its publication (Elisabet Sjövall (1964) 'Coitus Interruptus', translated by Christopher Tietze, in Calderone, *Manual of Contraceptive Practice*, p. 202).
174. Sjövall, 'Coitus Interruptus', p. 202.
175. Sjövall, 'Coitus Interruptus', pp. 204–5.

176. Elphis Christopher (1980) *Sexuality and Birth Control in Social and Community Work* (London: Temple Smith), p. 148.
177. Rogow and Horowitz, 'Withdrawal', 150.
178. World Health Organization (2000) *Improving access to quality care in family planning: Medical eligibility criteria for contraceptive use* (Geneva: WHO), 'Coitus Interruptus', p. 1; 'Overview', p. 2.
179. Kate Fisher and Simon Szreter (2003) '"They Prefer Withdrawal"': The Choice of Birth Control in Britain, 1918–1950', *The Journal of Interdisciplinary History*, 34(2), 280.
180. Valaoras et al., 'Control', 277.
181. Fisher and Szreter, '"They Prefer Withdrawal"', 271.
182. See for example Yioel, *Steirosis*, p. 24; Gyras, *Prin*; Paulides, *Teknopoiese*, pp. 19–31; Georgios K. Zouraris (1947) *E Steirosis eis tous andras kai tas gynaikes kai to thauma tes syllepseos*, 2nd edn (Athens: n.p.), pp. 19–29; Tsakires, *Megale Sexologia*, p. 537; Anonymous (21 March 1951) 'O Gynaikologos Apanta: Reply to Agnoia', *E Gynaika*, 2(30), p. 49; Anonymous (27 February 1952) 'O Gynaikologos Apanta: Reply to Mikre Afrikana', *E Gynaika*, 3(55), p. 60.
183. Anonymous (27 February 1952) 'O Gynaikologos Apanta: Reply to Mikre Afrikana', *E Gynaika*, 3(55), p. 60.
184. Zouraris, *E Steirosis*, pp. 19–29; Anonymous (16 February 2001) "'Efuge' o Zouraris", *Rizospastes*, 11(7901), p. 8.
185. Serafeim Papakostas (1947) *To Zetema tes Teknogonias (To Demografiko Provlema apo Hristianikes Apopseos)* 2nd edn (Athens: Adelfotes theologon 'E Zoe'), pp. 122–3.

CHAPTER 9

Contraception and Its Methods, II: Appliances and the Pill

Earlier discussions of birth control methods for England referred to the 'effective appliance methods' and the 'less effective non-appliance methods', though acknowledging that the use of appliance methods by the working class prior to 1910 was only 'slight'.[1] Emphasis was also put on the financial inaccessibility of such methods for the working-class couples.[2] By the early 1990s Woods was arguing that coitus interruptus was, 'most likely', the 'popular' birth control method among the British working class, though Seccombe assumed that the use of appliance methods had been instrumental among the working-class couples.[3] By 2003 Fisher and Szreter in turn showed that their informants—contraceptive users in the post-WW I Britain—did not trust the 'modem' appliance methods of birth control and preferred withdrawal.[4] While this view is in line with Peel, who was writing in the 1960s, Peel also discussed the significant retail presence of many appliance contraceptives in the first half of the twentieth-century England.[5] Such a mixed view on the possible role of appliance contraceptives re-enforces the need for an assessment of the use of such methods in Greece.

V. Hionidou, *Abortion and Contraception in Modern Greece, 1830–1967*, Medicine and Biomedical Sciences in Modern History,
https://doi.org/10.1007/978-3-030-41490-0_9

Using Contraception: The Users' View

Douche

In the early nineteenth-century USA and in late nineteenth-century England, Charles Knowlton's recommended method was 'syringing' of the vagina. This involved purchasing a female syringe, which Knowlton informed his readers could be found in an apothecary's shop for 'a shilling or less'.[6] Knowlton also suggested the use of some kind of solution, rather than just water, in order to act as a spermicide. He saw many advantages in douching (though that term was not yet in use): cheap contraceptive protection; simplicity of use; cleanliness, which protected against disease; and a remedy for specific conditions, such as uterine prolapse, for which syringing was prescribed as a treatment. Uterine prolapse was a rather common condition, as might be expected given the repeated childbearing of women at the time, and is frequently mentioned in midwifery manuals. In 1894 the *Wife's Handbook* similarly suggested syringing morning and night for the same condition.[7] However, douching had also been recommended as a treatment for a wide range of ailments in Greece and elsewhere in both the nineteenth and the twentieth centuries. So, in his 1840 *Medical Handbook*, the Greek physician, priest and author Pyrros Dionysios o Thettalos attributed women's sterility to a good number of conditions, including the suspension of menstruation, leucorrhoea, cachexia, fatness, syphilis, the size of the clitoris, 'great weakness' and the blocking of the fallopian tubes, and douching was one of his recommended treatments for all these conditions and ultimately for sterility.[8]

In the same decade Nikolaos Kostes, the eminent German-educated royal obstetrician, wrote in his *Obstetrics Manual* about how he used douching when performing an abortion in order to save the mother's life.[9] At specific points during the procedure he recommended the use of vaginal 'injections' (eneseis) with various solutions, one of which was infusion of Peruvian bark.[10] A. Vitsares, too, in his 1874 publication on women's diseases repeatedly refers to douching (diaklysmoi) as a therapy or part of a therapy,[11] and Kindynes also referred to douching as part of the therapy for many illnesses, including gonorrhoea and vaginitis. However, the focus of his book was sterility, and he stressed that, as douching killed sperm, a patient who wanted to get pregnant would need to discontinue this practice.[12] M. Venizelos, like Nikolaos Kostes, referred to douching in relation to facilitating natural abortion, where 'warm injections' assisted the removal of the embryo.[13] For gonorrhoea he recommended injections with astringent solutions.[14] Frederick Hollick, writing at the same time as Vitsares, argued for the use of douching or vaginal washings (kolpikes plyseis) or injections (ekhyseis), as the translator M. Meliareses calls them, for contraceptive purposes.[15] Like Knowlton, Hollick declared douching the best contraceptive method, although he pointed out that some of the substances added to the douching water were poor spermicides or were harmful to the woman.

The word Meliareses used for douching was the colloquial word used at the time for enema (klysma).[16] Enemas were widely employed in the nineteenth and the first half of the twentieth century by physicians, but also as a home remedy,[17] and employing the same term for both procedures made douching readily understandable to whoever happened to come across it. Similarly, in the 1840s Pyrros had used the same word for both enemas and douches (klysterio), although occasionally he distinguished douches by using the term 'frontal'.[18] In 1881 Venizelos was referring to 'injections of the vagina' that were to be performed with the 'usual enema-pump (klysterio)'.[19] Across the Atlantic in the same year, Ezra Heywood defended himself in court when accused of advertising a douching syringe as a contraceptive method, arguing that it had a multitude of purposes aside from the contraceptive one.[20]

In the first half of the twentieth century douches were commonly recommended both for specific illnesses and conditions and for reasons of cleanliness:[21] some authors suggested that after *every* coital act the woman should have an antiseptic douche, and that she should also have two such douches every day, irrespective of whether she had coitus or not.[22] Even single women, Drakoulides suggested, should have one such douche daily in order to protect themselves from various afflictions.[23] Again, a good number of authors stressed that antiseptic douches should not be performed when a woman wanted to become pregnant, clearly indicating the contraceptive effect of douches.[24] Recommendations to the readers of the magazine *E Gynaika* to use douches for a range of gynaecological reasons also abound in the mid-twentieth century, suggesting the continued use of douches in medicine.[25] But it was not only physicians employing and recommending douches: midwives did too, as Nikolaos Gyras suggested rather disparagingly, referring to childless patients who were treated by midwives with douches.[26] Similarly, in the late 1940s A. Raymond Mills mentioned that the empirical midwife who was assisting mothers birthing in Rhodes would perform a vaginal douche post-partum, signalling that sexual intercourse was permitted thereafter.[27]

Over and above such numerous references, equally common were the references to douching as a contraceptive, either on its own or in combination with another method.[28] In all the references spanning the period 1920–1960 it was indicated that some kind of spermicidal was needed, though some physician–authors indicated that using a vinegar solution would be sufficiently effective. A good number of authors recommend douching as the best possible contraceptive method, while others indicated the spermicidal properties of antiseptic douching.[29] M. Yioel, for example, recommended douching with antiseptics as the 'most practical and harmless' method, rejecting all other methods as 'useless and dangerous', with the exception of the 'safe period' one.[30] However, many authors, if not a majority, considered douches unsafe and ineffective as a contraceptive method, while a number of health concerns were raised for men, women and potential children too.[31] Stopes vehemently objected to the use of douching as a contraceptive, both for physiological reasons and for emotional ones, as she found the necessity for the woman to get up straight away against her ideals of marital sex.[32] The post-World War II western literature on contraception is devoid of references to douching.[33]

But was this method actually used by women? It was hardly mentioned in Valaoras' 1962 survey, while Moyseides, writing in 1925, suggested that the lower classes, who 'suffered from hydrophobia', did not use it, whereas the rest of the female population—presumably the middle and upper classes—were 'suffering from excessive use' of it.[34] Although his comment should perhaps be taken with a pinch of salt, it could be concluded that this was not a working-class method, certainly not in the late 1920s. However, in later decades this was not necessarily true. Richard and Eva Blum observed in their anthropological research in late 1950s mainland Greece that the only 'modern' female contraceptive used in the villages they studied was 'lemon juice and quinine douches', while the rest of the responsibility for contraception lay with men.[35] Among my informants, two women referred to employing douches after coitus: one lived near the town of Mykonos in a farming family; the other lived in town and ran a coffee shop. While these women's families were not among the poorest on the island, they could not be considered middle class either. Considering the serious doubts expressed by academics about the ability of working-class women to use douches, because of the lack of privacy and running water, these two cases are particularly interesting:[36]

Q. Why did you have only four children and not twelve like [your parents]?
A. Ohhh Christ and Virgin Mary! … Every five years I had one [laughs].
…
Q. And you were careful not to have too many children?
A. I don't know about that. He was a steady man and I myself was careful … many children are a torture for the mother. They suffer and the mother suffers. As I told you, we had wealth/property but we worked. Work is work!
….
Q. How did you manage to have them five years apart, one from the other?
A. ….The man was not demanding. You would say no to him, no. A reasonable person (synennoemenos) …
Q. Where did you find out from? Who talked to you about being careful? You mentioned you were careful.
A. Douches. You get up, have a douche with the syringe (klysma). You cleanse. But it needs to be done immediately. If you leave it, pff [miming a swollen tummy].
Q. Who told you that? Where did you find out from? Your sister?
A. Once I got married, one hears this and that. When you are single, there is none of that [discussion]. Anyway, let's say [female] friends, a midwife, whatever. Because we were many children, I did not want to have many children. But as many as God wants to send, I don't know …
…
Q. Did the other women do the same? Or did they do something different?
A. What else? Except for the condom. But he was not using them. Only I was getting up and getting cleansed, and it is the best too. He is not a man, let's [do it] every night, like other men. Let me tell you, apologies for saying this, once a week and *if* it happened. They work, they get tired those people. It depends on the person too, I see others, God save me, can you bear a man like that? I am not, I did not like it [sex] so much. But since I am his wife I cannot deny it to him, not completely.[37]

The husband of this informant—for whatever reason—did not appear to have taken the initiative or shouldered the responsibility for contraception. The couple seems to have had a knowledge of condoms, but he did not use them. The informant stated this matter-of-factly and without any grievance. For much of this interview the husband was in fact present, although, unlike in interview situations with other couples, he never volunteered answers himself. When I started asking questions about contraception the informant became guarded and her husband, appearing somewhat irritated, left the room. As soon as he was out of the room his wife, in a lowered voice, proceeded to discuss sexuality and contraception. This was a pattern repeated at least once, suggesting—along with the concrete information offered by the wife—that there were issues with the sexuality of the couple.

The second case, the coffee-shop manager, was somewhat different, in that both husband and wife wanted only a few children—she had three—and both employed a contraceptive method—respectively, condom and douche. While this worked very well in the 1930s, in 1939/1940 she became pregnant again because 'she was not careful'.

Q. May I ask how come you had nine years between the second and third [birth]? How come you did not have the third sooner?
A. It was me who did not take precautions.
Q. You did not take precautions? So, did the third one arrive accidentally?
A. Yes.
Q. Was it you who did not take precautions or was it your husband who did not?
A. Eh, one out of the two.
Q. How was the woman taking precautions?
A. All that is secret [laughter].
Q. For us young to learn too.
A. Now it is fashion to have as many children as they want.
Q. That is why I ask. Because you too had as many as you liked, more or less. And I would like to know how. Today we have many and varied [methods]. What methods did exist then for women to have as many [children] as they wanted?
A. There were methods. There were prophylactic [contraceptive] methods.
Q. Like what? What we call today condoms for men?
A. Yes.
Q. And did they sell them here on Mykonos?

A. They would bring them here.
Q. So whoever man wanted, he could find them?
A. Yes.
Q. And did the husband use them?
A. [nodded yes].
Q. Anything else?
A. No.
Q. Have you not heard anything else [other methods]? How did the woman take precautions? Let's say the man did not want to put it on [the condom]. What could the woman do?
A. She did her own things.
Q. Such as?
A. To pull out, to do something.
Q. The woman?
A. Yes.
Q. To stop [him]? Not let the husband to approach her? These kinds of things?
A. Yes.
Q. Was that happening too? Did you do that?
A. No.
Q. But the woman would pull out? Would the woman pull out or the man would pull out?
A. And the woman after the [coital] act will get up and wash herself.
Q. Is that what you did?
A. Yes.
Q. Was it not that he took precautions, but it was that you did that [the reason for the few children]?
A. He did not want children either.
Q. So he was careful too?
A. He was lazy, he did not want children.
Q. Was he careful?
A. Yes.
Q. And you were careful too with that method? Is that how you managed not to have [children] after the second but the third came accidentally?
A. Yes.[38]

While the informant assumed full responsibility for her pregnancy here, it is almost certain that there were no condoms available from 1939 onwards, when World War II started, since condoms were imported. Thus the absence of condoms and a lapse on the informant's part led to a pregnancy. It should be added here that the informant's mother was a midwife, and might have been a further source of information for the informant, although she rejected that suggestion, saying that her mother was extremely 'secretive'.

Both informants were particularly keen to avoid accidental pregnancies and used a combination of methods to achieve their aims. Neither raised any issues relating to their living conditions in relation to employing douches. Until the 1950s all the inhabitants of Mykonos—rural and urban, rich and poor—obtained water from artesian wells that were scattered throughout the town or on neighbouring farms.[39] While some upper-class housing had had separate bathrooms from the start of the twentieth century, middle- and working-class dwellings acquired a separate bathroom only from the 1950s onwards.[40] Nevertheless, what most urban houses did offer was a degree of privacy to the couple, as they usually had a separate bedroom, in which any infant would also sleep.[41] Older children would sleep in the adjacent room, which also was the main living space for the family. Thus, privacy was available but other facilities were not, something that did not deter those women who were determined not to have too many children. Clearly, these Mykonos women did not follow the instructions set out by Moyseides in either his 1925 or his 1932 publications, where he recommended the use of the douche can and copious amounts of water.[42] But, it seems, the informants' more simple and easy approach was good enough to provide contraceptive results. The informant used the work *klysma*, the same one, as noted above, used by Meliareses in 1875 and meaning enema in vernacular Greek.[43] Performing enemas was common and women would have been familiar with the technique and the appliance employed, whether they used it for their children or close relatives.[44]

The frequent references made by the various authors to douching, most of them discussing cleanliness primarily, suggest that it was certainly used for such reasons by upper-class women and would have also been used for contraceptive reasons, usually along with another method. In the late 1940s rather explicit advertisements appeared in women's magazines showing the actual douching devise explicitly named 'kolpó' (a word that closely resembles the Greek word for vagina—kolpos) (Plate 9.1). The text explained that this was 'for every woman' and it was lifesaving, effective and preventive. This is the most explicit advertisement of a female

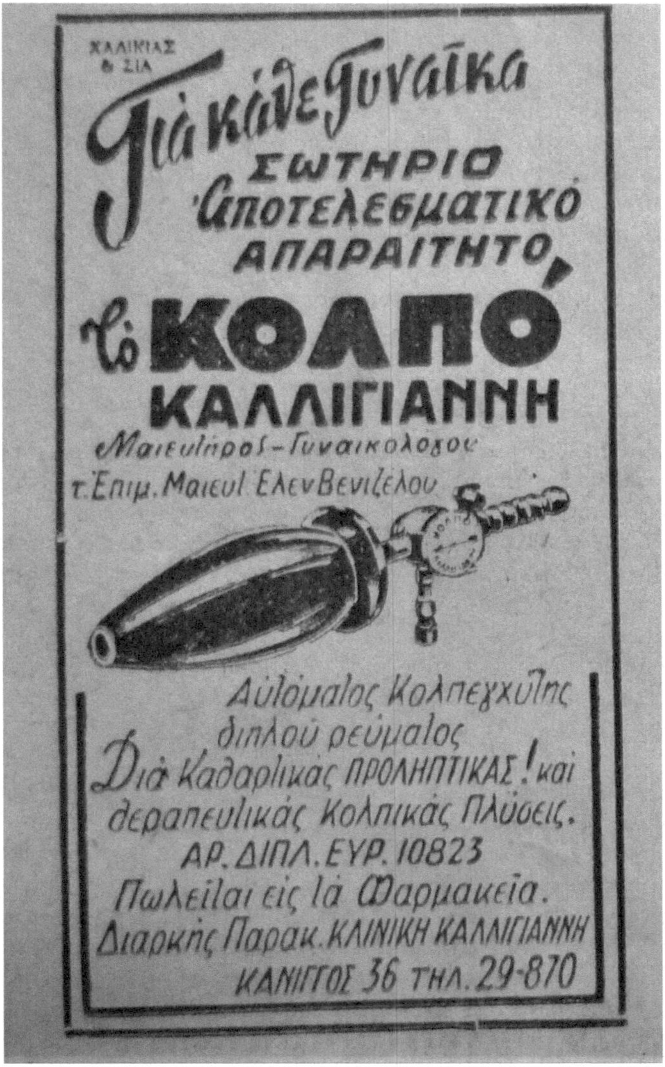

Plate 9.1 Advertisement of a Douche: 'For every woman: LIFESAVING, effective, NECESSARY KOLPO KALLIGIANNE, by the Obstetrician/Gynaecologist, formerly employed in the Maternity Hospital Elen [sic] Venizelou. Automatic douche of double current. For cleansing PREVENTIVE! and therapeutic vaginal douches. LICENSE NUMBER 10823. Sold in pharmacies. Permanent sale KALLIGIANNE CLINIC 36 KANIGGOS STREET TEL 29-870'. (Source: Anonymous (13 October 1946) 'Kolpo Kalligianne', *Thesauros*, 9(411), p. 50)

contraceptive in the post-World War II Greece. Frequent references by physicians to douching, as a contraceptive method now, continued in the 1950s in books and magazines.[45] Marlene Arnold's retired obstetrician informant in Crete commented that douching was one (out of three) of the most commonly used contraceptive methods in the past, although his view was that it was both unreliable and inconvenient. Interestingly, Arnold reported that the method, using water with lemon juice, was still widely used for contraceptive purposes among 'village women' as late as the early 1980s.[46]

The Sponge and Other Plugs/Pessaries

Early twentieth-century contraception pioneers, and historians too, were keen to ignore the sponge as simply another 'unscientific', old-fashioned method. However, this was not the case with those writing about contraception in the nineteenth century. Francis Place, the first person to publicly—although anonymously—write on contraception, discussed and gave clear instruction on the use of the sponge.[47] Shortly afterwards Richard Carlisle went so far as to put his name to his recommendation of the sponge as the best contraceptive method, articulating in detail what was to be reproduced, almost word for word, many times in the century to follow.[48] However, only two years later Robert Dale Owen's 1830 publication rejected the sponge as a method of 'doubtful efficiency' and 'physically disagreeable', banishing it to a footnote.[49] Knowlton discussed the sponge too, along with coitus interruptus, the condom and his recommended method of douching. It was, he said, a method that had been recommended by some 'with considerable confidence', and involved inserting a 'very delicate piece of sponge' into the vagina prior to coitus and removing it immediately afterwards. He advised that, rather than moistening the sponge with plain water, as it was usual, a chemical solution that would destroy the semen should be used.[50] This would increase its effectiveness, although he believed this method to fall short of douching. An anonymous author who published a pamphlet in 1860 entitled *Poverty: Its cause and cure* suggested as a solution to poverty the use of 'preventives', several of which had already been adopted in England, and yet more on the continent.[51] The first contraceptive the author recommended was the sponge, 'being perfectly harmless, easy of adoption, and at the same time not in the least diminishing the enjoyment of the act of coition'. The sponge itself was to be soaked in water and inserted into the vagina so that it would act as a barrier to the sperm. The author indicated that it should be of 'sufficient size, in such a way as to guard the womb', essentially acting as a barrier or capping method.[52] In 1866 the sponge was again mentioned, this time by an American physician, Dr Trall, in his publication *Sexual Physiology*, where, following his discussion of the sponge as a 'mechanical obstruction', he stressed that he approved only of abstinence as a method of preventing pregnancy.[53] In 1885 H.A. Allbutt's *The Wife's Handbook* dedicated a paragraph to the sponge, explaining how it should be used and what its size should be, and noted that it could be highly effective, especially when the sponge was soaked in quinine solution or 'lathered with Quinine Soap (Allbutt's)'.[54] Allbutt's support for the sponge was strong, though the promotion of his own product might be a contributing factor in this; however, this was not the only contraceptive method that he had financial interests in.

Among nineteenth-century Greek writers, only Meliareses discussed the use of the sponge, but he did not recommend its use as it prevented the sperm from reaching the womb and offering its beneficial properties.[55] However, both the sponge and the plug (made from cotton wool or lint) were ever present in most obstetric manuals and habitually employed by obstetricians. Nikolaos Kostes, for example, refers to the use of the 'expansive' sponge or a sponge impregnated with vinegar, alcohol, an astringent or quinine solution in order to stop the bleeding of varicose veins around the vulva, while on other occasions he advocates its use to externally cleanse the vulva of the labouring woman.[56] When the vagina was obstructed, he recommended the 'expandable' sponge, which would have been used internally.[57] Kostes also employed 'capping' (pomasma) for bleeding pregnant women in the hope of saving them from miscarrying, or after they had miscarried in order to stop the haemorrhage.[58] The 'cap' would be made of cotton wool or lint. Vitsares and later Venizelos also recommended capping for a wider range of therapies, suggesting the use of either impregnated sponge or lint-pad.[59] Alavanos also described the method in detail, instructing the use of cotton balls with a string attached, impregnated in potassium permanganate and mercury dust.[60]

Sanger, outlining what she considered to be all the worthwhile methods in the 1914 edition of her volume *Family Limitation*, did mention the sponge, which—she informed her readers—could be found at pharmacies. This she described as having a tape (Knowlton and Allbutt referred to a string) attached to facilitate its removal. Unlike some of the earliest commentators, but like Allbutt, she recommended the use of antiseptic solutions, such as carbolic or boric acid, prior to their use. Sanger argued that this was a widely used method in France and among the middle and upper classes in America, while some 'of the peasants in Europe use the cotton plug soaked in vinegar for the same purpose'. Some physicians in fact recommended the use of cotton plug instead of a sponge.[61] Sanger concluded her short discussion of the sponge (and the plug) by recommending them as 'perfectly safe, if followed by an antiseptic douche before the removal of the plug or sponge'.[62] Interestingly, tampons made of 'lint, fine wool, cotton, flax, or what may be at hand' were also mentioned in Place's manuscript handbill; however, they were omitted from the published version.[63]

By 1918, in her *Wise Parenthood*, Stopes had recommended the use of sponges and pads of cotton wool, soaked in quinine or soap and vaseline, respectively. However, these were not recommended as stand-alone methods but rather as ones providing 'further insurance'.[64] Her own recommendation was the rubber pessary along with quinine pessaries[65]—the latter to be replaced by the sponges or pad only if the user was not keen to employ quinine pessaries or if she felt they did not dissolve. As far as Stopes was concerned, these old methods had validity only insofar as they might enhance the effectiveness of her preferred method.

By 1922, while the sponge continues to be mentioned in the relevant manuals, it seems that it had become a back-up method to the 'modern' rubber pessary, as Stopes had already advised. However, Ettie A. Rout, whose brief biography indicates that she had travelled extensively, advises her reader that if she had 'mislaid the rubber pessary, a small sponge, a piece of clean cotton-wool, or even a piece of soft tissue paper can be used'. Thus, these items that could be easily found in someone's home could be used in cases of emergency. She added that when a sponge or cotton wool was used they should be saturated in 'contraceptive lotion or smeared with contraceptive ointment' before insertion.[66] Though Rout concludes with an emphasis on the superiority of the rubber pessary, the fact that she acknowledges the potential usefulness of the older methods, with which many of her readers would presumably have been familiar, is an important point. Such methods, utilising materials that were easily accessible in a home setting and simple to use, could not be easily rejected when the recommended method was similar to these old ones. Interestingly, Rout also added that 'Native women in different countries use seaweed, moss, sponge, etc., and Japanese women use rice-paper', suggesting the use of a wide range of natural materials in different settings.[67] Similarly,

Norman Himes refers to the use of 'linen rags' or 'cloth' inserted into the vagina as preventives measures by diverse populations such as that in the Styrian Oberland, Slovak women and the inhabitants of Kasai Basin in central Africa.[68]

Returning to this subject in the early 1920s, Stopes discussed the sponge with or without spermicides, as well as plugs and tampons, in her manual for physicians *Contraception (Birth Control): Its Theory, History and Practice*.[69] Her introductory sentence indicated its accessibility and the extent of its use: 'Specially prepared sponges in great variety are now on sale and in use …', and she added later on that some practitioners 'still consider it the very best method for general use'.[70] Unusually for Stopes, who generally vehemently attacked all methods except her preferred one, she went on to offer a catalogue of the sponge's advantages: it was 'cheap, generally safe, very easy to manipulate, easily understood even by a stupid woman'. This last attribute was extremely important for Stopes, since she considered that it was these women who were in most need of contraceptives. She elaborated on the fact that the sponge needed no 'accurate adjustments', in contrast to her favourite method, the cap—adjustments that would have involved the woman in visits to clinics or physicians.[71] Like others, she recommended that the sponge on its own was not sufficient, and that immersing it in a spermicidal substance would significantly improve its efficiency. She discussed in detail the various possible spermicides (alum, quinine powder, soap powder and 'some other of the many possible spermicides', as well as a vinegar and water solution).

Stopes also devotes a significant amount of attention to plugs, usually made with cotton wool or lint and impregnated or not with a spermicidal. She explains that the plug is used in a similar way to the sponge, with the added advantage that it is thrown away after one use and therefore does not require storage or disinfection.[72] Stopes also discusses in some detail the *Specially modified tampons*, which were 'widely used for other purposes'. Her suggestion was to actually modify ordinary tampons offered in the market so that they would be suitable for contraceptive use by shortening them and using ichthyol ointment to prepare them. Her view was that many doctors would recommend this to their patients, presumably because they were already recommending modified tampons for 'definite ailments'. However, she also realised that these would have been expensive for the majority of women.[73]

That the use of a sponge or a cotton plug seemed 'natural' is seen not just in Stopes' writings but also in Antoinette F. Konikow's 1923 pamphlet *Voluntary Motherhood*: 'The very first thing that would come to one's mind is a piece of cotton or a sponge placed into vagina in front of the cervix.'[74] Despite this, though, she notes that '[v]ery few use this method since it gives very poor results'.[75] The same author, addressing physicians in 1931, shuns the method completely, finding it 'entirely unsatisfactory', as a small sponge would be dislodged and therefore lead to pregnancy, while a large one would interfere with coitus.[76] Indeed, the bulk of Konikow's book *Physician's Manual of Contraception* was dedicated, rather, to the rubber pessary and various intrauterine devices (IUDs).

The sponge and other non-rubber pessaries and tampons were, as noted above, largely ignored in the writings of recent historians and demographers,[77] and as much of the recent focus has been on the twentieth-century literature and collected oral histories, the probable earlier use of these methods has been somewhat neglected. Moreover, the female pioneers of contraception, and especially the physicians, focused on the modern version of this method, namely the rubber pessary. Sanger's *Family Limitation* and Stopes' *Contraception* are probably the last writings by such women to present the method in neutral terms.[78] The focus of writers in the first half of the twentieth century on the rubber pessary and the arguably better protection it afforded ignored the extreme simplicity of the earlier pessaries and their wide availability in the private sphere as objects with a number of purposes in the household aside from any association with sex and contraception, as well as their easy maintenance and unobtrusive presence in the house. In their simplest use they—especially the sponge—required nothing more than a bit of water or, as some Greek informants indicated, some lemon juice.

Among Greek publications there are numerous twentieth-century references to sponges. Jean Marestan discussed the use of the sponge as a protection against both venereal diseases and pregnancy, emphasising that its use—just as that of the occlusive (pessaries)—did not require the husband's co-operation.[79] Using the sponge as a contraceptive method was also mentioned by Moyseides, who referred to it as 'a very old' method and not one he would recommend for regular use, owing to its high failure rate and many side effects.[80] Brief mentions, too, come from A. Sygkelakes, who mentioned in addition the cotton plug; the medical journal *Klinike*, which referred to the rubber pessary as well and declared both to be problematic; Yioel, who warned about the side effects and low efficiency of the impregnated sponge; Gyras, who referred to the sponge as impregnated with 'lemon or acids that sting'; and Metropoulos, who mentioned that the sponge and the cotton plug should be followed by a douche.[81] Despite such repeated rejections of the method, in the 1950s the use of pessaries—sponge, cotton and rubber—was listed in the *Encyclopaedia of the Greek Woman*,[82] although the author pointed out that the rubber pessary was difficult to use and expensive, and hardly ever employed in Greece, echoing earlier concerns and observations made by Moyseides.[83]

Among my Greek informants, only one indicated any knowledge of the sponge as a contraceptive method, adding that they were available to purchase from the local pharmacy but that she had never used this method:

Q. Before [you met] your husband, did you know anything [about contraception]?
A. No. I used to hear … I heard that, that woman … there are some kind of sponges in the pharmacy, with a thread and they get it moist with lemon and they insert it inside them and that would destroy the sperm.
Q. When did you hear that?
A. Many years, in my youth. When I was married. I gave birth to my first child in 1920, 1925, 1922 [she was unable to remember the exact year].
Q. Did you discuss such things with your female friends?
A. She told me that she [a third person] did this deed.[84]

The informant confirmed later that she heard about the use of the sponge prior to World War II. Heather Paxson also noted the pre-war use of a sponge with a string and lemon juice, reported to her by her informant Eleni, who had overheard a conversation between her mother-in-law and her own daughters: 'She explained how you take a small piece of sponge—natural, of course—douse it in lemon juice, tie it to a string, and insert it into the vagina. It was effective, as effective as today's sponge.'[85] Eleni's mother-in-law was a midwife who had received a midwifery diploma in 1904 and her own mother was a midwife too, though in all probability an untrained one. A British physician working in Rhodes immediately after World War II also noted a similar use of the sponge by the local women: 'A small piece of sponge soaked in olive oil is used by the woman as a tampon.'[86] Arnold's informants mentioned that a local physician was recommending this contraceptive method to them until the mid-1960s and women were using it.[87] Exactly the same method was in use among the women of Constantinople in the mid-nineteenth century[88] and, considering the presence of Greeks in Constantinople up to the 1950s and the strong links sustained between the people of Greece and those of Constantinople, such information would have been easily circulated.[89]

Sponges were a part of everyday life for islanders, as for some of the Dodecanese islands sponge fishing was the predominant occupation of men from the mid-nineteenth century onwards. They had a number of uses in the household and would have been a familiar household object, as would have been cotton fabrics. The fluids used, such as lemon juice or oil, were equally familiar and widely available items in any Greek household, rural or urban, rich or poor. The use of sponges, cotton plugs or a piece of cloth would have been one of the easiest, most accessible methods of contraception that Greek women could have employed at this early stage in fertility control.[90]

It is worth noting that even in the 1960s, international contraceptive advice included the sponge, which by that time was impregnated with a spermicidal powder or liquid that would foam before its insertion in the vagina. The guidelines were now more specific about the size of the sponge (it should be a circle with a diameter of slightly more than two inches) and the timing of its removal.[91] Edward Tyler emphasised the issue of personal preference in choosing a specific method and mentioned the unusual popularity of this particular method among the clients of the Los Angeles Planned Parenthood Center.[92] In the early 1960s the method was seen as providing a 'reasonably high degree of protection', although not as high as the diaphragm and jelly.[93] The author emphasised its 'simplicity and cheapness', which made it a perfect method for mass distribution.[94] Clarence Gable, writing in the same *Manual of Contraceptive Practice* as Tyler, discussed the impregnation of the sponge with 'household spermicides' such as vinegar and lemon, as well as tampons composed of 'a pad of wool or cotton, with or without a thread tied to it for subsequent removal, a piece of soft cotton cloth folded several times or a number of pieces of cloth … stitched together in the middle'.[95]

Still, the question is how would women make the necessary conceptual leap to consider using a cotton plug or a sponge as pessary? The answer is that both had been in use by physicians and midwives—trained and untrained—throughout the nineteenth century and possibly earlier. So, when in the late 1930s Yioel discusses the use of the sponge and the rubber pessary he refers to the 'capping of the womb', an expression that was rarely used at the time by his fellow physicians but was in wide use in the obstetric manuals throughout the nineteenth century. His use of such an 'old-fashioned' medical expression was perhaps the result of his lack of a Greek medical education. This same expression is widespread in most, if not all, nineteenth-century Greek obstetric and midwifery textbooks in referring to a variety of surgical operations and surgeries, as already discussed.[96] On some occasions 'capping' was used to stop bleeding following, for example, a miscarriage or a curettage.[97] In others, 'gradually thicker' sponge pessaries were inserted into the vagina in order to cure vaginal stenosis.[98]

Employing pessaries and ointment inserted into the vagina for therapeutic reasons was common throughout nineteenth-century Greece, both among traditional healers and physicians. Pyrros, for example, in discussing metritis and the obstruction of the womb, cited as possible causes for these two afflictions the use of pessaries and vaginal ointments by midwives.[99] Pessaries were also extensively recommended and used to treat uterine prolapse.[100] Significantly, pessaries were described in many of the popular medical books, signifying their employment by lay practitioners and unqualified midwives too.[101]

The sponge and cotton plugs were widely employed and recommended for therapeutic, as opposed to contraceptive, reasons by obstetricians outside Greece too. The 1929 description by the physician William J. Robinson of how to treat leucorrhoea locally is revealing: he suggests that '[t]he insertion of a suppository or douching can be easily done by the patient herself'.[102] He goes on to describe in detail how to make such a tampon, how to treat it and how to employ it, all tasks to be performed by the patient herself. Stopes, in her discussion of tampons, alluded to their widespread use for therapeutic, non-contraceptive use.[103] That the availability and use of pessaries was not something new in the nineteenth or twentieth centuries is underlined by Smellie's discussion of them in 1752 in which he refers to pessaries used for uterus prolapse and lint or wool pessaries immersed in powders, wax and oil or in astringent compounds to be used as suppositories, indicating that the latter were recommended by Hippocrates.[104]

The Condom

Withdrawal was one important contraceptive method available to men; another was the condom. Condoms are among the oldest contraceptives, although their earlier use was associated with prostitution and protection from venereal diseases.[105] This historic association, according to Christopher Tietze, meant that there was a reluctance to accept their use within marriage. For that reason, but also because the expectation of the early contraception advocates was that women were those most interested in practising contraception, condoms were rarely recommended in contraception clinics, whether in Britain or the USA.[106] Such an outlook, along with the admission by Tietze and the authors of the *Manual of Contraceptive Practice* in the early 1960s that condoms were one of the most widely available contraceptives and the most used in the USA, raises significant questions about the misunderstandings between contraception providers and users in pre-Pill western societies.[107]

The history of the condom is an interesting one.[108] The earliest condoms were produced from the caeca of various animals.[109] From the late nineteenth century, and with the vulcanisation of rubber, rubber condoms were introduced to the market. By the 1960s these were in use almost exclusively. Production processes also changed. From the early 1930s the latex process permitted the quick, automated production of condoms, presumably reducing their price. Other improvements in technology meant that, by the 1960s, the quality of condoms had significantly improved compared with those of the early twentieth century.

Virtually all writers who discussed contraception mentioned condoms, although not always in a positive light. Knowlton refers to them as the 'baudruche', and dismisses them as not meant for general use but rather for protection from syphilis.[110] Allbutt refers to them as the 'Letter' and explains in detail how they should be used 'by the husband', emphasising their use within marriage.[111] He warned his readers that 'the least hole' in the 'Letter' would enable the semen to escape, resulting in pregnancy. However, beyond that, Allbutt appears to have taken a neutral stance on the method, neither presenting any negative aspects nor advocating its use. In a similar light, Sanger in her *Family Limitation* advised where condoms could be purchased and how much they cost ('two dollars a dozen for the skin gut tissues to one fifty a dozen for the rubber tissue').[112] She warned about the fear of breakage and how the user should take measures to avoid that. In contrast, Stopes did not recommend the condom for 'normal healthy people'.[113] Her main objection to the method, and one that she was at pains to articulate in detail, was that the woman's vagina and womb would be devoid of the semen that was necessary for their health.[114] She also argued that it was detrimental to men's physiological ability to have sex, while 'sensitive women' found the smell of the 'rubber condom disgusting'.[115] She forcefully argued her point of view, though recognising that the recommendation of the condom by 'the medical profession has been weighty' and virtually universal.[116]

Beale, in her 1922 *Wise Wedlock*, was a supporter of the condom who managed an objective presentation of its qualities. She admitted that its drawback was the prevention of 'the perfect closeness of contact', but argued that it was 'better to content oneself with something a shade less than the ideal' in exchange for security against pregnancy. She recommended the use of the better-quality ones, which would 'make themselves little, if at all, felt by the wearer'.[117] The use of a good-quality sheath would also protect its users from the much-feared breakages, Beale suggested.[118]

Writing in the same year, Ettie Rout commented that sheaths were 'apt to break' and 'destroy contact' between husband and wife, and that some users would become 'nervous wrecks'. Rather than blaming condoms for that directly, she added that the users would recover when they stopped using condoms.[119] Rout listed the condom in her appendix under 'Other methods of contraception', separately from the recommended method of the rubber cap and soluble suppositories.[120] Antoinette Konikow, just a year later, echoed Rout's views on their unreliability: 'Condoms tear, leak and slip off.'[121] She did 'not recommend them', as she found them 'neither safe, nor normal'. For those who insisted on using them, however, she suggested the parallel use of chemical methods in order to increase their effectiveness. Writing almost a decade later, she continued to find condoms 'highly disagreeable', 'neither reliable nor normal'.[122] However, in contrast to others, she did not refer to the 'effects' of the condom on the nerves of the users.

While these earlier authors emphasised the unreliability of condoms to the degree that a supplementary method or, as some couples did, the use of two condoms at once was recommended, Tietze, in his 1960 appraisal of the condom, emphasised their reliability. In the USA at the time the proportion of defective condoms was placed at 0.29%—evidently a result of the Food and Drug Administration's quality controls imposed on condoms produced in the USA from 1938 onwards,[123] after an early 1930s study in the USA had shown only 42% of condoms in perfect condition, which led physicians to class them as unsafe. By 1960 Tietze argued that even if semen went through small holes it would not be sufficient to impregnate the woman; there was no reason for consumers to test the condoms before using them; and that they could be reused, if the necessary steps were taken.[124] The overall assessment of the condom was that it was a highly effective method, lagging behind only oral contraceptives.[125]

In comparison to many of their counterparts, especially the British and American specialists of the 1920s and 1930s, Greek writers (and physicians) were much less negative towards the condom. While some authors raised concerns about some negative aspects of the condoms in relation to women, overall, and especially for men, the use of condoms was seen in a positive light.[126] Physicians and authors strongly recommended their use to young men when engaging in sex prior to marriage. Though some authors recommended complete abstinence prior to marriage for men, most authors conceded that this would not be possible, and as single women were expected never to engage in pre-marital sex, the implicit—and often explicit—understanding was that single men would experience pre-marital sex with prostitutes only. Such societal conventions and the fear of venereal diseases in the first half of the twentieth century meant that advice on the issue of protection for young men was imperative and explicit, and invariably included the recommendation to use a condom.[127] Thus, as early as 1901 Filaretopoulos was strongly recommending the condom, along with other potential protective practices.[128] However, it was the 1921 publication by Foteinos, sponsored by the directorate of public health of the Ministry of the Interior Affairs, that brought the issue squarely into the public sphere. In a clear message articulated in simple language (demotike), the author, with a large number of photographs, illustrated the dangers of venereal disease and put forward the condom as the main solution in preventing infection.[129] The government's campaign against venereal disease continued in the 1930s, with further explicit publications in which prophylaxis, including the condom, was mentioned.[130]

The numerous advertisements for specialists in venereal diseases in the daily press were a stark reminder of the presence of such diseases in Greek society.[131] Greece's continuous engagement in conflict from 1912 to 1922 and the apparent increase of prostitution in the 1920s and during the years of the 1941–1944 occupation meant a wider anxiety about venereal diseases, the partial answer to which was the condom.[132] A positive image was promoted by physicians—'We, the physicians, say that [the condom] is spider's web against pleasure and fortress against danger'[133]—and some eagerly refuted what others had presented as possible side effects: 'It is said that condoms weaken man's strength over time. I do not believe that.'[134] While some simply found their use 'ugly', such assessment probably did not put off many from using them, as none of the other methods could be or were classed as pretty.[135] In 1932 Moyseides summed up the overall stance of experts towards the condom: 'if it is a good quality one, [it] is the simplest, the safest, the most perfect, the ideal contraceptive.'[136] He also offered advice, in case the reader was in need, as to which condom was the best and how the user could identify these. Those made from intestines were the best, as they were the finest, but he also acknowledged that in recent years the quality of the rubber ones had improved. Before using the condom, the author urged, the condom should be tested by filling it with water: 'because safety depends on the results of the test'.[137] Not only must the test be carried out before the use of the condom, but the storage of the condom was significant: 'the habit many have to keep the condoms in their pocket contributes to their rapid brittleness and permeability.' After use, we are told, the condom needs to be washed with soap and water or a chemical solution, dried and sprinkled with talcum powder.[138]

That most urban single men in the 1920s and 1930s were familiar with, if not well versed in, the use of condoms is clear. For example, Sygkelakes remarked that recently married men, when advised to use a condom within marriage, 'will laugh—we used to use it when single, will we [have to] use it when married too?'[139] Advertisements in the press presented a young, modern and well-dressed man purchasing his holiday tickets to the countryside and urged him to take a few 'boxes of Mpempeka' (the specific brand of condoms) because he might not find these at his holiday destination. He might find other brands there, the advert advised, but these would be of inferior quality.[140] In places such as Mykonos town pharmacies were selling condoms in the 1930s, although smaller, more remote places did not enjoy such access.[141] The societal expectation in 1930s Greece was that urbanite single men would experience sex with prostitutes, while rural young men would remain chaste because of the difficulties in accessing prostitutes.[142] While this was almost certainly true while they were in the countryside, it ignores the fact that many of them, and virtually all in the post-World War II years, went to work in Athens/Piraeus or in other urban centres and, prior to the mid-1920s, also travelled to the USA and other destinations overseas. Even if their urban stay was a short one, it is likely that for most of them it included a visit to a prostitute.

Q. How did you take precautions? Did you say you used the condom?
W. Didn't I tell you? [I used] condom.
Q. From the beginning [of the marriage]?

W. From the beginning.
Q. Who told you about condoms?
W. My husband. They, men cannot not to go with a woman [cannot abstain]. And he was scared of the diseases. That's why [he knew about condoms]. Because there always were diseases.[143]

The belief that men could not abstain and therefore had to visit prostitutes continued to be part of the 'initiation' experience for young men in the 1960s and beyond. Such young men were equipped with the knowledge and understanding of the usefulness of condoms, which if they had rural roots, they could take back to their place of origin after their city sojourn. Equally knowledgeable were those who spent time as sailors.[144] Male working groups, whether young or old, were ideal venues for individuals to display such sexual knowledge and thus assert their own masculinity while, inadvertently, informing those who were not yet knowledgeable:

Q. You must have been doing something since you did not have an abortion and you did not have nine children [as her mother did].
W. We must have been doing something. Those condoms that were always [available], that's what we did.
Q. Where did you find out about those things?
W. How do I know where my husband found out!
Q. [Addressing the husband] Did you find out? Where from? From friends?
W. He used to go to Chora [the Mykonos town], he had acquaintances.
Q. Did you talk to your friends [about those things]?
W. He does not have many [friends].
H. I had no idea about friends. The others [co-workers] would be chatting, I would …
W. Maybe from my sisters, may be from my sisters-in-law. Maybe, I don't know.
Q. Did you talk to relatives [about these things]?
H. I would listen to the workers, when working for others [as a paid day-labourer]. One would say one thing, the other …, the other another, the other another …
W. He worked for others [not in a family farm], [spending] all the time with men. Each of them would be saying something …
Q. Did you then hear about it before you got married?

H. Of course.
Q. [Addressing the wife] When you got married, had you heard about it? Did you hear that ... ?
W. Did I know [anything]? Leave me now. Did I know? [I did not know anything].[145]

The name of the condom brand 'Mpempeka', mentioned above, expresses a further change in Greek society: it refers to a young, single and liberal—in sexual terms—woman who would enter into sexual relationships. Such relationships did exist among upper-class liberal men and women; however, the condoms plainly had a much wider use.[146] Another brand that was on sale before World War II, and possibly the first to be sold in Greece, was advertised in the 1920s in a book offering infant-caring guidance to mothers.[147] The three-word advert reads 'Antigon προφυλακτικά preservatifs (Antigone prophylactics condoms)'—only the second word was in Greek, while the other two were in French. The name of the condom, through its association with the protagonist of Sophocles' ancient tragedy, expressed ideas of raising children that were 'worthy' of their parents, thus fitting well with the theme of the book in which the advertisement was placed.[148] Another advertisement depicts an elegant box of condoms, clearly imported from Germany, with text explaining that this is the 'condom of the aristocracy of the whole world' and is sold only in 'the aristocratic pharmacies'.[149] All condoms during the examined period appear to have been imported from either the USA or Germany.[150] The main post-World War II brands were 'Assos', 'Kleidi' and 'Stop'.[151]

Greek physicians who dealt with contraception in the first half of the twentieth century presented the condom either in neutral or mostly positive terms, with such statements as 'the most perfect method' or as 'the best method today'.[152] Another suggested that the condom was the best means of contraception, to be combined 'with douche when [the condom] breaks'.[153] Even in the 1950s, gynaecological advice via the columns of women's magazines was promoting the use of condoms as the 'most effective and less harmful' of all methods.[154] It comes as no surprise, therefore, that the condom was found to be the method most often employed among my informants, with nine of them indicating its use (two of whom referred to the 1950s). As an informant from Mykonos remarked, the condoms would be purchased from the two local pharmacies 'sealed, in a box', unlike 'nowadays that the single men have them and they have them openly, as if it is not an issue [having the condoms]'.[155] However, those who travelled regularly to Athens preferred to purchase them from there, thus ensuring more privacy and probably lower prices.

Q. Where did you buy them?
A. From the pharmacy, they used to get them.
Q. Here on Mykonos?
A. They had them here but also [he bought them] from Athens.
Q. When he [her husband] used to come and go [as a private postman between Mykonos and Athens]?
A. Yes.[156]

Condoms seem to have been widely available—at least in Athens—in the 1920s and 1930s and, unlike any other contraceptive, they were advertised in the press, as they served the purpose of protecting men from venereal diseases.[157] Adverts that appeared in the national press were clear and simple, but also effective: 'Mpempeka. Condoms, thin, silky, solid'.[158] Ensuring protection against venereal diseases is how most men learned about condoms and the protection they offered—knowledge that they brought to their marriage when, at a later stage, it was required:

Q. May I ask you where did you find out [about condoms]?
A. Where did I find out? Since I was single … We took prophylactic measures. Even though I was a womaniser, I never caught any disease. Then there were …
Q. Were they expensive? Or could you not find them [when he and his wife had an accidental pregnancy]?
A. It was more due to negligence. Because there was of course, a cost involved in order to get the condom but mostly it was negligence. Mostly I attribute it to negligence.[159]

Condoms began to be in widespread use on Mykonos in the 1930s. Couples who admitted using condoms had not started using them before that date even if they were married before 1930. One reason may have been that imports to the island had not started until then. Beyond that, there was also a cost involved, one that many couples were probably not able to afford, as was the case with the previous informant:

> I did not want to … I had the self-awareness, I did not want to have [many] children because I knew that I can't … I had the feeling [understanding]

> that in order to have them, you must be in the position to feed them, to educate them. But poverty is a reason why people have children. You do not have [cannot afford] the prophylactic measures to take as a male. You do not have the prophylactic measures. There were no appropriate prophylactic measures to take in order not to have many children.[160]

Although this informant seems to be referring to the absence of *any* measures, he meant those male methods that involved an expense, one that the poor could not afford even if they wanted to use them. The importance of such expense is emphasised by the fact that he and his wife avoided it while she was amenorrhoeic during the 1941–1943 famine, thinking that she would not fall pregnant; however, she did.

Furthermore, condoms reduced the pleasure of the act to a varying degree. While for some this was just an inconvenience, for others it was a reason to avoid their use.

Q. Who told you about precautions? When you got married, did you know about precautions?
A. How would we know? He used to go to the [village] square from time to time, my [deceased] husband, and he was finding out [about precautions] from friends I suppose.
Q. And later, years after the wedding, he told you what and how?
A. Half way through the marriage [he told me].
Q. If you had known earlier, would you have started earlier [controlling your childbearing]?
A. How do I know? [laughter] Do you think men liked it [using contraception/condom]?
Q. May I ask what were you using? What kind of precautions you took?
A. Those things that have come out [become available] now, those that men put on.
Q. Was that all?
A. Yes.[161]

Similarly, though much later, another informant attributed their repeated accidents to the husband's distaste for condoms: 'He did not want [to use] condoms. He did not find it pleasurable.' Instead, they used withdrawal throughout their reproductive lives.[162]

While in the 1930s both availability and awareness were relatively high, by the early 1950s condoms were used even in villages.[163]

> I thought I lost the world! Because I was breastfeeding, I did not have my period; then when my period came, I was careful. It was a devil's moment and I was tricked. I remember with [daughter] Elene I was using condom and I was tricked ... I got Elene with a condom! That's why I went to the doctor and I said 'is that possible? How did that happen to me?' He said that if one goes through, it is enough. Sperm. A lot of worries.[164]

This informant was born and raised in the village and got married at the age of 19. Her husband, however, who was also born and raised in the village, spent time in the town of Hermoupolis and in Athens. His knowledge would most certainly have been a result of his urban connections and, although the couple resided and raised their family in the village, they would also have had access to condoms purchased in the pharmacies of Hermoupolis. Here she also raises the issue of unreliability and the 'accidents' that could, and did, occur with condoms. The possibility of such accidents was well known, although clearly not to this informant until she had her first 'accident'. Those who were determined not to have such accidents would adopt a second method in order to maximise the chances of successful contraception.[165]

The work of Valaoras and his colleagues provides us with a picture of the extent of the use of condoms by age but also by place of residence (urban or rural). As the study refers to the methods its subjects had ever used, it informs us not only of the situation in the early 1960s but also in the two or three preceding decades. Significantly, the urban sample did not cover the early contraceptors but rather the second or even later generations of urban contraceptors. The informants were asked whether they had attempted to limit their family size and whether they had used the rhythm method, coitus interruptus, condoms, the diaphragm, douches, suppositories/jellies, abortion or another method. The condom was the second most popular contraception method, varying from 9% to 26% in rural areas depending on the age of the wife, and between 18% and 41% in urban areas.[166] In urban areas, 18% of those wives aged 42 used condoms either as a sole method or in combination with others, while among the younger ones the percentage was 30 or above. Therefore, among the urbanites below age 42, around a third were employing the condom. Condoms were most popular among the youngest wives—that is, those aged 20 or less—with 26% and 40% employing them in rural and urban areas, respectively. The lower percentages among the rural population were attributed by the authors to the cost and/or unavailability of condoms in small villages.[167]

Thus, the role of the condom in facilitating the fertility decline in Greece seems to have been extremely important throughout. To what extent condoms were used certainly depended on the access the population had to them, the availability of a local pharmacy being a minimum requirement. The age of the couple seems also to have been important, at least in the early 1960s; the youngest urbanites relied heavily on condoms (40% as opposed to 43% employing withdrawal among those wives aged 20 or less). Young men presumably found the self-control necessary to effectively practice withdrawal difficult, hence their significant reliance on condoms. The fear of venereal diseases and permission to advertise condoms meant that knowledge of their existence and effectiveness spread quickly. Unlike in the West, and despite single men's use of them with prostitutes, not one informant or writer rejected or negatively commented on the use of condoms within marriage.

The Pill

As it became available in the early 1960s in the USA and in Europe, the Pill was also introduced into the Greek gamut of medicines. From 1963 it was imported and has been on sale in pharmacies without requiring a prescription.[168] In addition, it was prescribed to patients as a therapeutic medicine, specifically for menstrual irregularities, and it was advertised as such.[169] However, although, as with other contraceptives, it was not illegal to advertise the Pill, it was never advertised as a contraceptive or publicly discussed in the press as such, and physicians did not have a thorough knowledge of it. In December 1966, in a round table organised by lecturers of the Athens Medical School, significant new medicines and their side effects were discussed, including the hormonal contraceptive Pill. At the round table it was introduced dispassionately by A. Komnenos, who discussed its various uses, including that of contraceptive, outlining both the positives and its side effects.[170] The round-table discussion was published three months later in a significant medical journal, providing medics with the basic knowledge they may have required.[171] However, it seems that it was very rarely recommended to women as a contraceptive and its uptake was never significant (certainly below 5% of all users, almost certainly below 1% in the 1960s).[172] Both Paxson's and Georges' informants expressed their strong disaffection for the Pill.[173]

Discussion and Conclusions

This extensive discussion of the various contraceptive methods available in nineteenth- and twentieth-century Greece and elsewhere reveals a continuity in the use of methods. All methods had been employed for other purposes before they were used to prevent conception. Some of the materials and techniques—sponge, cotton plugs, douching—had been employed by obstetricians and midwives as part of their everyday practice and prescribed therapies. Women were familiar with them, as such materials and techniques had been used on them or they themselves had used them. Among the pre-existing methods, they seem to have chosen those that were most conspicuous and the materials that were the most accessible, such as sponge in preference to cotton plugs. Condoms had also been available for a while before they were used as contraceptives. Although they were advertised and promoted as offering protection from venereal diseases, their usefulness in preventing conception was evident and thus, when the need arose, they were easily repurposed as such. Withdrawal—or conjugal onanism—was also known, but was considered a perversion rather than a 'normal' sexual activity among married couples. It seems to have taken some time, almost a generation, for its employment as a contraceptive method to become acceptable within marriage, as well as for men to be 'trained' in its use. Within the first cohort of contraceptors among the Mykonos informants, women were practising withdrawal as often as men did, indicating that it may not always have been intuitively clear to men what was needed to be done. Similarly, people were widely aware of the effects of breastfeeding in delaying conception. This ready-made natural method was put into use when women/couples desired to somehow control—albeit to a limited degree—their fertility. Still, not *all* women who knew this made an effort to use it as a contraceptive method.[174]

Thus, contraceptive methods existed, although were not used for this purpose, before the demand to control fertility appeared. These had to be repurposed once the need for contraceptives existed. It also took time for individuals to become familiar with, let alone expert users of, a method. Timing also seems important in terms of when each of the methods was employed. The evidence here suggests that women were most concerned and interested among the earlier contraceptors, using breastfeeding, the sponge and female-controlled withdrawal, as well as encouraging their husbands to use condoms and limiting the days on which coitus took place. It is among the later/second generation of contraceptors, when men became accustomed to withdrawal and accepting of the notion of fewer children, that they took over most of the responsibility for contraception. They did so with passion and pride, trumpeting their ability to 'control' their flow and serve the family aim of a smaller number of children.[175] Fisher and Szreter's findings are not surprising, therefore, as their subjects were part of the later wave of the decline.[176] During the first part of the decline, control was achieved primarily through female methods, as was widely understood at the time. It was that understanding that led the advocates of birth control at the time to focus their attention almost exclusively on female methods and to ignore men as unwilling collaborators in the fertility control project. However, such advocates had failed to detect the change that had occurred among men entering marriage in the 1910s and 1920s in Britain and the USA. Interestingly, in the Greek case there seems no major conflict between the written and oral sources. The evidence from the oral histories covers the period from the mid-1920s to the 1940s, with the data more numerous from the 1930s onwards. There is a very close correspondence between what the informants said they were aware of and used, and the information conveyed in the 1930s literature. For example, the discussions of the rubber cap by Greek authors suggested that this method was virtually never employed in Greece, something that was confirmed by the existing oral evidence as well as Valaoras' study. However, breastfeeding forms an exception to this rule, as only one of the written sources referred to it, while six informants, among them three males, explained that women intentionally used breastfeeding to delay conception. The written sources argue that coitus interruptus was the most popular method in the 1930s, although on Mykonos condoms seem to have been used more widely.

As far as barrier methods are concerned, they were argued by Szreter and Fisher to be 'not self-evident or obviously safe'.[177] Greek women in the 1920s, however, were familiar with some of these, such as pessaries, sponges and (partly because of the popularity of enemas) douches. Because they were familiar with their use, employing them in order to prevent conception *was* self-evident to them. Moreover, women were familiar with handling their own genitalia, a necessity when employing pessaries. Cleanliness and the availability of running water in houses—as articulated by historians but also by Stopes—were preoccupations of contemporary upper-class birth control advocates as well as those of today. Most women in 1920s Mykonos had to manage a household without a toilet and with very little water, all of which was carried from a well. Just as they were able to bring up children, cook and clean under those conditions, they also managed to perform douches and to use a sponge. While their level of cleanliness would not approximate what is considered acceptable today, for them it was performing the task within the available parameters. Significantly, using a condom or withdrawal in such conditions would not have been any easier or cleaner than using a sponge or douche.

That *all* methods were not foolproof and that pregnancy would eventually result was known to all and regularly repeated in the writings of the physicians, and the expectation of most couples was that 'accidental' pregnancies would occur and a reduced number of children—compared with their parents or siblings—was all they aspired to.[178] Before World War II, couples had no specific number of children in their minds.[179] None of the informants expressed a wish or could even engage in a discussion about how many they actually wanted. It would have been strange indeed if they had done so, as for this generation the unreliability of the available methods and the population's reluctance to employ abortion extensively meant it was not possible to achieve a desired number. The most they could do when assessing their reproductive performance during their old age was to articulate whether they would have wanted more or fewer children, assigning to divine forces the actual outcome. Almost all pre-World War II couples were using one contraceptive method and occasionally none. However, there were also some 'determined' contraceptors who were very rigorous in their use of their chosen method. Some were 'determined' contraceptors for a short period of time, others throughout their reproductive lives.[180] Among those couples, some did consider an abortion when a pregnancy occurred. However, such determined contraceptors were a minority in my oral history sample. The majority accepted that 'accidental' pregnancies were inevitable and the baby or babies were welcomed.[181] The 1950s and 1960s were drastically different, as the wider availability of abortion allowed couples to determine the number and timing of children, although this was not the case for all just yet. Still, abortion, through curettage, facilitated the implementation of the new desire for full control.

Fisher and Szreter, in their discussion of withdrawal, stressed the emphasis placed by contraception campaigners in the first half of the twentieth century on the unreliability of coitus interruptus as a contraceptive method.[182] They rightly argued that coitus interruptus was actually more 'reliable' than it was claimed, but also that the couples who employed the method did not actually expect a foolproof method.[183] In the Greek case, the existing published advice did not emphasise the unreliability of withdrawal more than that of the other existing methods. More significant in the Greek writings on contraception was their emphasis on the considerable side effects, psychological and physiological, of withdrawal. Fisher and Szreter noted, however, that their working-class sample ignored 'the putative psychological effect' mentioned in the guides and embraced the method.[184] The Greek working and middle classes continued to use the method for decades, even when the Pill was available, ignoring the warnings of the physician–authors. However, its use probably increased from the 1930s to the early 1960s, especially in the rural areas.[185] It could be that the use of withdrawal increased over time, as the threat of venereal disease had been virtually removed by the 1960s, while a number of other factors may have encouraged the increase in its use. For example, throughout the 1940s it was impossible to get hold of condoms, thus encouraging the use of alternative methods, the cheapest and most easily available being coitus interruptus. If the 'forced' trial of withdrawal during the 1940s proved to individuals its efficiency and lack of side effects, they may have continued with its use beyond the 1940s.[186] However, by the early 1960s it seems that fewer urbanites than rural couples were using this method, favouring condoms instead—possibly suggesting that the middle classes, concentrated in urban areas, were moving slowly away from coitus interruptus, possibly owing to the significant improvements of the quality of condoms by then.

To address Carlsson's question, raised at the beginning of Chap. 8, contraceptive methods did exist before the secular decline in fertility, although, except for abstinence, most required a period of repurposing and experimentation. This phase lasted for some time—probably up to a generation in the case of Greece—during which the control of fertility would have been neither complete nor free from frequent 'accidents'.

Notes

1. Robert Woods (1987) 'Approaches to the Fertility Transition in Victorian England', *Population Studies*, 41(2), 291, 311.
2. Woods, 'Approaches', 297.
3. Robert Woods (1992) 'Debate: Working-Class Fertility Decline in Britain', *Past & Present*, 134, 203–4; Wally Seccombe (1993) *Weathering the Storm: Working-Class Families from the Industrial Revolution to the Fertility Decline* (New York: Verso), p. 181.

4. Kate Fisher and Simon Szreter (2003) '"They Prefer Withdrawal": The Choice of Birth Control in Britain, 1918–1950', *The Journal of Interdisciplinary History*, 34(2), 271.
5. John Peel (1964) 'Contraception and the Medical Profession', *Population Studies*, 18(2), 115.
6. Charles Knowlton (1877) *Fruits of Philosophy. A Treatise on the Population Question, edited by Charles Bradlaugh and Annie Besant*, 1st edn 1832 (London: Freethought Publishing Co), http://www.gutenberg.org/files/38185/38185-h/38185-h.htm#link2H_APPE (accessed 7 July 2019), Chap. 3.
7. H. Arthur Allbutt (1894) *The Wife's Handbook. How a woman should order herself during pregnancy, in the Lying-in Room, and after Delivery with hints on Management of the baby and on other matters of importancy, necessary to be known by married women*, 1st edn 1886[?] (London: R. Forder), p. 44.
8. Pyrros Dionysios o Thettalos (1840) *Egkolpion ton Iatron. Etoi Praktike Iatrike, Periehousa ten Ylen tes Iatrikes, ten Farmakopoiian, ten Ygieinen*, vol. 1 (Athens: Aggelou Aggelidou), pp. 191–3.
9. Nikolaos Kostes (1849) *Egxeiridion Maieutikes* (Athens: S.K. Vlastos), pp. 265–7, 289–90, 310, 331, 334, 382, 395.
10. Kostes, *Egxeiridion*, p. 333.
11. A. Vitsares (1874) *Nosoi ton Gynaikon*, vol. 1 (Athens: Ermou), pp. 51–2, 54, 59–60.
12. Antonios I. Kindynes (1889) *E Steirosis para te Gynaiki kai Therapeia Autes* (Athens: Vlastos Varvaregos), p. 181; M. Moyseides (1925) *E Gyne: Ygieine tou Gamou kai tes Eggamou Gynaikos* (Alexandria: A. Kasigone), p. 72.
13. M. Venizelos (1881) *Maieutike* (Athens: n.p.), p. 301. For a similar use see also K.N. Alavanos (1900) *Odegos pros Exetasin Egkyou Gynaikos* (Syros: P. Printezes), p. 96.
14. Venizelos, *Maieutike*, pp. 267, 301, 303, 557–8.
15. M. Meliareses (1875) *O Odegos ton Eggamon.* By Frederick Hollick M.D. part b, translated by M. Meliareses (Vraila: M. Pestemaltziogou), p. 95.
16. Meliareses, *O Odegos*, p. 96.
17. See Kostes, *Egxeiridion*, pp. 327, 331, 382, for example.
18. Pyrros, *Egkolpion ton Iatron*, p. 192.
19. Venizelos, *Maieutike*, p. 558.
20. Andrea Tone (2001) *Devices & Desires. A History of Contraceptives in America* (New York: Hill and Wang), pp. 37–8.
21. Elias I. Oikonomopoulos (1902) *O Gamos* (Athens: O Kadmos), p. 68; Moyseides, *E Gyne*, pp. 52, 57–9, 74–80. Outside Greece, see William

J. Robinson (1929) *Woman: Her Sex and Love Life*, 21st edn (New York: Eugenics publishing company), https://archive.org/details/womanher-sexlovel00robiuoft/page/1, Chap. 8; Ettie A. Rout (1922) *Safe Marriage: A Return to Sanity* (London: William Heinemann (Medical Books) Ltd.), http://www.gutenberg.org/files/16135/16135-h/16135-h.htm, Chap. II. However, see Stopes' strong rejection of the argument for douching for cleanliness (Marie Stopes (1923) *Contraception (Birth Control): Its Theory, History and Practice* (London: John Bale), p. 117).

22. N.N. Drakoulides (1956) 'Ygieine Genetesiou Omilias', in Paulos Drandakes (ed.) *Megale Ellenike Egkyklopaideia*, vol. 8, 2nd edn (Athens: Phoenix), p. 187. Similar recommendations were made by the physician Sygkelakes (A. Sygkelakes (1927) *E Apokryfe Ygieine tes Gynaikas* (Alexandria: Grammata), p. 46). Sygkelakes rejected the use of antiseptics as injurious to the woman.
23. Drakoulides, 'Ygieine Genetesiou Omilias', p. 187.
24. Drakoulides, 'Ygieine Genetesiou Omilias', p. 187; Moyseides, *E Gyne*, pp. 58, 72; Dem. Antonopoulos (1926) *E Steirosis para te Gynaiki* (Athens: Koronaiou, Denaxa and Co).
25. Anonymous (15 November 1950) 'O Gynaikologos Apanta: Reply to *Anypomone P. Korinthon*', *E Gynaika*, 1(21), p. 25; Anonymous (20 November 1950) 'O Gynaikologos Apanta: Reply to Anesyhe Nea', *E Gynaika*, 1(20), p. 31.
26. Nikolaos Gyras (1939) *Prin kai Meta ton Gamo*, 4th edn (Athena: G. Vallianatou); there were further editions of this work in 1944 and 1956 and eight editions by 1956 (p. 106).
27. A. Raymond Mills (1948) 'Peasant Remedies from the Greek Islands', *Bulletin of the History of Medicine*, 22, p. 443.
28. Jean Marestan (1920) *To Vivlio tes Agapes. E Ygieine tou Gamou*, translated by P. Paulides from the 110th edn, 1st edn 1910 (Thessalonike: P. Paulides), pp. 76, 139, 145, 148–50; Anonymous (1925) 'Dia ten Praxin=Katheg. A. Forel Mesa di on Kanonizetai e Parakolyetai h Syllepsis', *Klinike*, 1(6), 187–9; Antonopoulos, *E Steirosis*, p. 15; N.N. Drakoulides (1933) *E Vlennoroia ston Andra kai ste Gynaika. Synepeies-Profylaxis-Therapeia* (Athens: K. Papadogiannes), p. 38; Mihael Nik. Kaires (1939), *Akindynos Erotas. E Ygieine ton Neon Syzygon kai e Ygieine Profylaxis ton Neon* (Athens: Anatole), pp. 44, 64; M. Yioel (1938) *Steirosis e Egkymosyne kata Voulesi*, 2nd edn, 1st edn 1936 (Athens: Vasileiou), p. 24. For his fascinating life see Rena Molho (ed.), *Oi Anamneseis tou Giatrou M. Yioel*, 2nd edn (Athens: Patakis, 2010); Gyras, *Prin*, p. 106; Anonymous (1954) *Egkyklopaideia tes Ellenidos. Iatrike ton Oikogeneion, Diaitetike, Gynaikeia Provlemata, Kallone, Symperifora* (Athens: Papademetriou), p. 307. See also Margaret Sanger

(1915) *Family Limitation* (New York: n.p.), who in her early editions of this work recommended douching as a contraceptive, as long as antiseptics were used. However, by the time of the 18th edition, in 1922, she believed that douching was good only for cleansing purposes (pp. 8–10), https://archive.org/details/39002086349256.med.yale.edu (accessed 25 April 2019).

29. Marestan, *To Vivlio*, p. 145; Anonymous, *Egkyklopaideia tes Ellenidos*, p. 307; Gyras, *Prin*, p. 91; Anonymous (27 December 1950) 'O Gynaikologos Apanta: Reply to Mellousa Kyria', *E Gynaika*, 1(24), p. 41, where the gynecologist's recommendation to the reader was that douching with an acidic solution was a good means of preventing conception but that it 'needs to take place immediately and not hours or even days after'.
30. Yioel, *Steirosis*, p. 24. This is the Ogino-Knaus method.
31. M. Moyseides (1932) *Malthousianismos Allote kai Nyn. Eleghos Genneseon kai Aposteirosis* (Athens: Gerardon Bros), pp. 62–4; Antonopoulos, *E Steirosis*, p. 32; Yioel, *Steirosis*, p. 24; Alexandros Tsakires (1954) *Megale Sexologia. Anikanotes, Steirosis kai e Syghrone Therapeia ton*, 3rd edn, 1st edn 1947 (Athens: n.p.), p. 582; Sygkelakes, *E Apokryfe*, p. 46.
32. Marie Stopes (1918) *Wise Parenthood. A Sequel to 'Married Love'* (London: n.p.), pp. 26–30. A similar position was taken by Courtenay Beale (1922) *Wise Wedlock. The Complete Treatise on Birth Control & Marriage* (London: Health Promotion), pp. 130–1, who rejected its efficiency as a contraceptive method and also regarded it as a romance killer.
33. See, for example, Mary S. Calderone (ed.), *Manual of Contraceptive Practice* (Baltimore, MD: The Williams & Wilkins Company).
34. Vasilios Valaoras, A. Polychronopoulou, D. Trichopoulos (1965) 'Control of Family Size in Greece (The Results of a Field Survey)', *Population Studies*, 18(3), 265–78; Moyseides, *E Gyne*, p. 57.
35. Richard Blum and Eva Blum (1965) *Health and Healing in Rural Greece* (Stanford, CA: Stanford University Press), p. 76. It is a pity that the authors did not consider it interesting to explore what methods men were using. Quinine was a very commonly recommended addition to the douching solution (see, for example, Allbutt, *The Wife's Handbook*, p. 49).
36. Szreter, for example, refers to the 'expense and impracticality' of female appliance methods in the 'crowded, unplumbed working class houses typical before the later inter-war years', referring to douches, pessaries, caps and diaphragms (Simon Szreter (1996) *Fertility, Class and Gender in Britain, 1860–1940* (Cambridge: Cambridge University Press), p. 427). Seccombe, discussing the apparent increase in the use of female appliance methods in the 1920s, refers exclusively to caps and diaphragms, emphasising the major difficulties in using them in the absence of indoor plumbing but also the 'aversion of touching their own genitals' (Wally

Seccombe (1990) 'Starting to Stop: Working-Class Fertility Decline in Britain', *Past & Present*, 126(1), 169).

37. No. 19 Mykonos, born in 1915, from a farming family.
38. No. 22 Mykonos, female, married 1930, gave birth in 1930, 1931 and 1940.
39. There was a consensus on the part of all informants on this: see, for example, Nos 1, 2, 3, 5, 7, 8, 9, 11 and so on.
40. No. 5 referred to always having a WC on the balcony (elite); No. 3 had had one since the mid-1930s because it was a 'very good house'; No. 17 had had a WC even when they were children (upper class). Most rural residents did not have a designated WC space until the 1950s and beyond (No. 11, No. 12, No. 16, No. 21, No. 26); some urban inhabitants acquired a separate space from the late 1920s, but these did not have running water (No. 7, No. 9, and so on). Urban inhabitants without a WC in their house would use a pot that they would empty into designated holes in the street or in nearby empty spaces (No. 23, referring to her grandmother; No. 18, referring to others).
41. See, for example, No. 4, No. 12, No. 13, No. 14. In rural areas at times there would be only one main living area, with the younger children sleeping in the wooden loft of that room and the older ones, from around the age of 15, sleeping in the barn (see, for example, No. 7, No. 11). These were what some authors referred to as 'monospita', described by Aris Konstantinides, *Mykonos*, cited in Panagiotes Kousathanas (2018) *Paramileta Δ* (Athens: Indiktos), p. 837.
42. M. Moyseides, *E Gyne*, pp. 74–80. Similarly complex and elaborate guidelines were offered by Allbutt, *The Wife's Handbook*, pp. 48–9. Rout made the point that the use of the 'Douche Can' was better than syringing but also acknowledged that its use in most houses would be 'inconvenient' (Rout, *Safe Marriage*, Appendix I). Sanger suggested that 'Every woman should possess a good two quart rubber douche bag called fountain syringe' (Sanger, *Family Limitation*, http://www.gutenberg.org/files/31790/31790-h/31790-h.htm, accessed 7 July 2019).
43. No. 19 Mykonos; Meliareses, *O Odegos*.
44. See, for example, Giannes, who was 14 years old when his mother had to perform twenty-five enemas on him during the famine because of the low quality food they had to consume (No. 9 Hios, male, born approx. 1928).
45. Anonymous (21 March 1951) 'O Gynaikologos Apanta: Reply to Agnoia', *E Gynaika*, 2(30), p. 49. Anonymous (13 December 1950) 'O Gynaikologos Apanta: Reply to D.I.M.O.', *E Gynaika*, 1(23), p. 19.
46. Marlene Sue Arnold (1985) 'Childbirth among Rural Greek Women in Crete: Use of Popular, Folk and Cosmopolitan Medical Systems' (unpublished PhD thesis: University of Pennsylvania), pp. 171–2.

47. Francis Place (1823) *Contraceptive Handbill: To the Married of both Sexes*, Form A and Form B, cited in Norman Edwin Himes (1936) *Medical History of Contraception* (London: G. Allen & Unwin), pp. 214–5. According to Himes, as early as 1797 Jeremy Bentham had also advocated its use (*Medical History*, p. 211). Himes mentions that the sponge is also mentioned as a contraceptive in the Talmud, dated to the second or third century (Himes, *Medical History*, p. 217). The sponge appeared in all three handbills published by Place (Himes, *Medical History*, pp. 217–8).
48. Robert Carlisle (1828) *Every Woman's Book or What is Love?* (London: R. Carlisle), pp. 38–9, https://digital.library.lse.ac.uk/objects/lse:diz789zox/read/single#page/1/mode/2up, accessed 7 July 2019.
49. Robert Dale Owen (1831) *Moral Physiology*, 2nd edn (New York: Wright & Owen), p. 66.
50. Knowlton, *Fruits of Philosophy*, pp. 33–6.
51. M.G.H. (1860) *Poverty: Its cause and cure. Pointing out a means by which the working classes may raise themselves from their present state of low wages and ceaseless toil to one of comfort, dignity, and independence; and which is capable of entirely removing, in course of time, the other principal social evils* (London: Truelove), p. 12, https://www.jstor.org/stable/60203639, accessed 7 July 2019.
52. M.G.H., *Poverty*, p. 13.
53. Halliday G. Sutherland (1922) *Birth Control. A Statement of Christian Doctrine against the Neo-Malthusians* (London: Harding & More), citing R.T. Trall (1895) *Sexual Physiology and Hygiene* (New York: Fowler & Wells Co).
54. Allbutt, *The Wife's Handbook*, p. 49.
55. Meliareses, *O Odegos*, p. 96.
56. Kostes, *Egxeiridion*, pp. 267, 161, 171, 177, 179, 216–7, 220.
57. Kostes, *Egxeiridion*, p. 267. An identical use of the sponge is also mentioned by Venizelos, *Maieutike*, p. 354.
58. Kostes, *Egxeiridion*, pp. 306, 307, 331–3. The term 'pomasma' is used by Yioel in 1938, where he explicitly refers to the use of a sponge or a cap inserted in the vagina (Yioel, *Steirosis*, p. 13).
59. Vitsares, *Nosoi*, pp. 49, 54, 56–8; Venizelos, *Maieutike*, 555; Anna Katsigra (1908) *E Maieutike en te Praksei* (Athens: Auge Athenon), pp. 231–2; Venizelos refers to it as a 'very new method, first applied by Shole in 1842' (*Maieutike*, p. 555). Interestingly, Kostes warned that using 'capping' (pomasma)—i.e., inserting a sizeable piece of sponge, cotton wool or lint high into the vagina—would endanger a pregnancy, if the woman happened to be pregnant (Kostes, *Egxeiridion*, p. 332).
60. Alavanos, *Odegos*, pp. 97–8.

61. Sanger, *Family Limitation*, p. 14.
62. Sanger, *Family Limitation*, p. 14.
63. Place, *Contraceptive Handbill*, cited in Himes, *Medical History*, p. 217.
64. Stopes, *Wise Parenthood*, pp. 16–18.
65. Pessaries are items inserted into the vagina for therapeutic purposes.
66. Rout, *Safe Marriage*.
67. Rout, *Safe Marriage*. Stopes also mentions this (*Contraception*, p. 136).
68. Himes, *Medical History*, p. 182, citing O.V. Hovorka and A. Kronfeld (1908, 1909) *Vergleichende Volksmedizin* (Stuttgard: Strecker & Schröder), vol. 2, p. 523.
69. Stopes, *Contraception*, pp. 51, 132, 135–8.
70. Stopes, *Contraception*, pp. 132–3.
71. Stopes, *Contraception*, p. 133.
72. Stopes, *Contraception*, p. 136.
73. Stopes, *Contraception*, pp. 136–8.
74. Antoinette F. Konikow (1923) *Voluntary Motherhood: A Study of the Physiology and Hygiene of Prevention of Conception* (n.p.), p. 18, https://archive.org/details/23KonikowVoluntarymotherhood/ (accessed 31 March 2019).
75. Konikow, *Voluntary Motherhood*, p. 18.
76. Antoinette F. Konikow (1931) *Physician's Manual of Birth Control* (New York: Buchholz Publishing Co), p. 71.
77. Szreter cites R. Roberts (1971) *The Classic Slum: Salford life in the first quarter of the century* (Manchester: Manchester University Press), where Roberts described the use of home-made sponge plugs in Salford in the first quarter of the twentieth century (Szreter, *Fertility*, p. 439).
78. Szreter mentions that plugs and pessaries were associated with prostitution and therefore their use within marriage was not acceptable (Szreter, *Fertility*, p. 396). However, writings of the early twentieth century do not suggest so, or perhaps at least by the twentieth century this was not the case. The association of such methods with prostitution seem to have originated with Hime (Jane C. Schneider and Peter Schneider (1996) *Festival of the Poor: Fertility Decline and the Ideology of Class in Sicily, 1860–1980* (Tuscon: The University of Arizona Press), p. 144).
79. The occlusive pessary refers to the rubber vaginal pessary (Marestan, *To Vivlio*, pp. 76, 136–7).
80. Moyseides, *Malthousianismos*, pp. 72–4.
81. Sygkelakes, *E Apokryfe*, p. 53; Anonymous (1925) 'Dia ten Praxin', 187–9; Yioel, *Steirosis*, pp. 13, 21; Gyras, *Prin*, p. 91; Konstantinos Metropoulos (1954) *Ygieine tes Egkyou. Enas Polytimos Odegos gia ten Ygieine Diaviose tes Egkyou* (Athens: Papademetriou), p. 146.
82. Anonymous, *Egkyklopaideia tes Ellenidos*, p. 307.

83. Moyseides, *Malthousianismos*, pp. 65–71. Moyseides mentions that the rubber pessary was first used in 1838 for pelvic stenosis. The same pessary was later modified to become the contraceptive Dutch or Mensinga pessary (p. 64). There is a further mention of the rubber pessary in a medical journal, although this is a translated piece from an English article. The effectiveness of the rubber pessary is given as 96 per cent. However, the instructions for its use are very complicated, with many health warnings (Nik. K. Kerameus (1930) 'Bauer. Profylaktika Mesa kata tes Syllepseos', *Ellenike Iatrike*, 4(11), 1226).
84. No. 4 Mykonos. Marestan also mentioned the immersing of the sponge into lemon juice or acidic solutions (Marestan, *To Vivlio tes Agapes*, p. 89).
85. Heather Paxson (2004) *Making Modern Mothers: Ethics and Family Planning in Urban Greece* (Berkeley: University of California Press), p. 45. Paxson interviewed Athenians but this does not necessarily mean that the mother-in-law practised midwifery in Athens. Unfortunately this is not made clear.
86. Mills, 'Peasant remedies', p. 444.
87. Arnold, 'Childbirth', pp. 173, 252. Arnold's fieldwork took place between the late 1970s and the early 1980s (pp. 8–14).
88. Himes, *Medical History*, p. 182–3, citing Lorenz Rigler (1852) *Die Turkei und Deren Bewohner in Ihren Naturhistorischen, Physiologiscen, und Pathologischen Verhältnissen vom Standpunkte Constantinopels* (Wien: C. Gerold).
89. Women from Hios and Tenos were working as servants in Constantinople even in the inter-war years (Violetta Hionidou (2005) 'Female domestic service on three Greek islands in the later 19th and early 20th centuries', *The History of the Family*, 10, 473–89; Violetta Hionidou (in press) 'Yperetries sten Ellada, 19os-20os aionas: Morfes kai sheseis ergasias' in Panagiota Mene, Anna Staurakopoulou, Konstantina Georgiade and Ioulia Pipinia (eds) *Yperetries kai Yperetes: Istorika Ypokeimena kai kallitehnikes anaparastaseis ston ellenofono horo (19os-21os aionas)* (Crete: University Press of Crete); Jill Dubisch (1972) 'The Open Community: Migration from a Greek Island Village' (unpublished PhD thesis: University of Chicago)).
90. Arnold's informants indicated the use of a cloth as a barrier method 'in earlier times', presumably referring to the 1950s and before (Arnold, 'Childbirth', p. 173).
91. Edward T. Tyler (1964) 'Sponge and Foam' in Calderone, *Manual of Contraceptive Practice*, p. 196.
92. Tyler, 'Sponge and Foam', p. 195.
93. Tyler, 'Sponge and Foam', p. 196. The diaphragm here refers to what before the 1940s was called the rubber cap (one of which was the

Messinga) as well as to the coil-spring ones (Robert L. Dickinson (1964) 'The Diaphragm' in Calderone, *Manual of Contraceptive Practice*, p. 165).

94. Tyler, 'Sponge and Foam', p. 196.
95. Clarence J. Gable (1964) 'Sponges and Tampons with Household Spermicides' in Calderone, *Manual of Contraceptive Practice*, pp. 197–8.
96. Kostes, *Egxeiridion*; Venizelos, *Maieutike*; Vitsares, *Nosoi*.
97. Katsigra, *E Maieutike*, pp. 231–2; Kostes, *Egxeiridion*, pp. 306, 307, 331–3.
98. Oikonomopoulos, *O Gamos*, p. 68.
99. Pyrros, *Egkolpion ton Iatron*, §220 Metritis, p. 142, §108, p. 69.
100. Venizelos, *Maieutike*, p. 257; Kostes, *Egxeiridion*, p. 325; Vitsares, *Nosoi*, p. 56.
101. Katsigra, *E Maieutike*, pp. 231–2; Blum and Blum, in *Health and Healing*, p. 76, refer to traditional methods of abortion, including suppositories; see Chap. 4 above; Pyrros attributed the obstruction of the uterus to, among other causes, the insertion of pessaries into the uterus by midwives (*Egkolpion ton Iatron*, p. 69). Inserting leeches into the vagina was also recommended in the nineteenth century by some obstetricians as therapy for some conditions.
102. Robinson, *Woman*, Chap. 20.
103. Stopes, *Contraception*, pp. 136–8.
104. William Smellie (1752) *A Treatise on the Theory and Practice of Midwifery*, 2nd edn (London: D. Wilson and T. Durham), pp. 424, v, vi.
105. See Szreter, for example (*Fertility*, p. 396).
106. Christopher Tietze (1964) 'The Condom' in Calderone, *Manual of Contraceptive Practice*, p. 181. See also Christopher Tietze (1960) *The Condom as a Contraceptive* (New York: National Committee on Maternal Health).
107. Tietze himself admits that the condom was at the time 'the most widely used mechanical contraceptive not only in the United States, but throughout the world' (Tietze, 'The Condom', p. 181). Similarly, Sanger referred to it as 'one of the most commonly known preventatives in the United States' (*Family Limitation*, p. 9).
108. Eric Chevallier (1995) *The Condom: Three thousand years of safer sex* (London: Viking); Aine Collier (2007) *The Humble Little Condom: A History* (Amherst, NY: Prometheus Books); Wolfgang König (2016) *Das Kondom: zur Geschichte der Sexualität vom Kaiserreich bis in die Gegenwart* (Stuttgart: Franz Steiner Verlag); Tietze, *The Condom*.
109. Tietze, 'The Condom', p. 182.
110. Knowlton, *Fruits of Philosophy*, Chap. 3.
111. Allbutt, *The Wife's Handbook*, p. 49.
112. Sanger, *Family Limitation*, pp. 6–9.

113. Stopes, *Wise Parenthood*, p. 24.
114. Stopes, *Contraception*, p. 127.
115. Stopes, *Contraception*, p. 127.
116. Stopes, *Contraception*, pp. 128–31.
117. Beale, *Wise Wedlock*, p. 135.
118. Beale, *Wise Wedlock*, p. 136.
119. Rout, *Safe Marriage*, p. 69.
120. Rout, *Safe Marriage*, pp. 32–50.
121. Konikow, *Voluntary Motherhood*, pp. 11–12.
122. Konikow, *Physician's Manual*, pp. 147, 46.
123. Tietze, 'The Condom', p. 184.
124. Tietze, 'The Condom', pp. 186–7.
125. Mary S. Calderone (1964) 'Theoretical Effectiveness Ratings of Nonsurgical Contraceptive Methods' in Calderone, *Manual of Contraceptive Practice*, p. 232.
126. The *Encyclopaedia of the Greek Woman* focused exclusively on the effects of the use of condoms on the women: vaginal irritation and inflammation, irritation to her nervous system and ultimately frigidity (Anonymous, *Egkyklopaideia tes Ellenidos*, p. 304). Yioel also referred to the ulcers and inflammations of the uterus caused by the use of the condom (Yioel, *Steirosis*, p. 21).
127. I.N. Anninos (1926) *Profylaxis kai Therapeia ton Afrodision Noson* (Athens: Tzakas-Delagrammatikas).
128. G.L. Filaretopoulou (1901) *E Profylaxis ton Afrodision Pathon* (Athens: Anestes Konstantinides), p. 38.
129. Georgios Th. Foteinos (1921) *Sotheitai apo ta Afrodisia Pathe!* (Athens: Ethniko typografeio), p. 57—a publication of the Ministry of the Interior Affairs, Directorate of Public Health, reissued subsequently a number of times, including in 1939.
130. Drakoulides, *E Vlennoroia*, p. 38, published as part of the series Propaganda of Social Hygiene.
131. For example, two advertisements of named Athens-based physicians who cured syphilis and gonorrohoea but also impotence and women's illnesses (Anonymous (1 March 1898) *Skrip*, 3(903), p. 3; Anonymous (1 April 1900) *Skrip*, 5(1658), p. 6); in *Rizospastes*, the newspaper of the Communist party of Greece, there were five advertisements on 30 January 1927 for individual physicians or clinics who offered treatment for venereal diseases (p. 2); Anonymous (27 October 1946) 'Gynaikologika-metadotika-Sexoualika HRHSIS PENIKILLINHS (Gynacological-infectious-sexual USE OF PENICILLIN)', *Thesauros* Θ(413), 60; identical advertisements had appeared in earlier issues of *Thesauros* on 13 October 1946 and 16 August 1946.

132. Euaggelou, *O Kindynos*, pp. 46–52. Antonios Gregoriades (1949) *Afrodisia Nosemata kai Anikanotes. Ygieina Paraggelmata kai Profylaxis ton Neon* (Athens: n.p.), pp. 24–5, recommending the condom for protection against syphilis. Kaires, *Akindynos Erotas*, pp. 68–80.
133. Euaggelou, *O Kindynos*, p. 49.
134. Sygkelakes, *E Apokryfe*, p. 83.
135. Gyras, *Prin*, p. 89.
136. Moyseides, *Malthousianismos*, p. 60.
137. Moyseides, *Malthousianismos*, p. 60.
138. Reusing the condoms was recommended even in the early 1960s (Tietze, 'The Condom', p. 187).
139. Sygkelakes, *E Apokryfe*, p. 83.
140. Thomas Sitaras (2012) *Pothoi kai Pathe sten Palia Athena 1834–1938* (Athens: Okeanida), p. 17, indicating that the advert was published in 1934 but without any further reference to the sources except to say that most were newspapers and magazines.
141. Mykonos in the 1920s and even more so in the 1930s had a stream of summer visitors. Some were visiting the ancient cite of Delos, which had to be accessed via Mykonos. Others were Mykoniates residing in Athens who returned for the summer to visit family and relatives. Others yet were visiting friends who were Mykoniates, enticed by the beauty of the island.
142. Euaggelou, for example, stated that 'continence does not harm the young; look at the young men in villages, nothing happens to them due to continence' (Euaggelou, *O Kindynos*, pp. 46–7).
143. No. 10 Mykonos, year of birth 1916, year of marriage 1936, two children; born in rural Mykonos, lived in Athens after the wedding.
144. No. 14 Hios. However, not all sailors were keen on using birth control (see, for example, No. 5 Hios).
145. No. 21 Mykonos, wife born 1923, husband born 1911, married in 1946, farmers, lived in rural Mykonos all their lives.
146. That this was indeed happening can be seen in the published biographies and diaries of, usually affluent, men. See, for example, Giorgos Theotokas' diary ((2005) *Tetradia Emerologiou 1939–1953*, 4th edn, ed. Demetres Tziovas (Athens: Estia), pp. 348–51, 358, 363, 549, 557–8, 563–4).
147. Anonymous (8 August 2013) 'Apo te Mpempeka sto Life. Ellenika profylaktika. Ena proion me istoria apo to 1950', *iefimerida.gr*, https://www.iefimerida.gr/news/468581/hokingk-zivansi-aritha-franklin-mpoys-milos-forman-ta-megala-antio-toy-2018, accessed 2 January 2019; Apostolos Doxiadis (1926) *Grammata pros Meteras* (Athens: Greka).
148. Doxiadis, *Grammata pros Meteras*, no numbered page.
149. Sitaras, *Pothoi*, p. 195 (no date is given, although it was certainly prior to 1939).

150. Anonymous, 'Apo te Mpempeka'. The article is an interview of Iordanes Kanonides, whose grandfather set up the first post-World War II company producing locally packaged condoms. On the dominance of the USA and Germany in the production of condoms see Tone, *Devices & Desires*, pp. 183–202.
151. Anonymous, 'Apo te Mpempeka'.
152. Sygkelakes, *E Apokryfe*, p. 13.
153. Anonymous, 'Dia ten Praxin', 187–9.
154. Anonymous (13 December 1950) 'O Gynaikologos Apanta: Reply to Mnestera [male]', *E Gynaika*, 1(23), p. 19.
155. No. 2 Mykonos, born 1911, rural resident all her life. Also No. 22 Mykonos, female, born 1905, married approx. 1929. She started using them after the birth of her first child.
156. No. 13 Mykonos, born 1906, married in 1926, lived in rural Mykonos all her life.
157. Books referring to venereal diseases explicitly mentioned the condom as one of the few protective mechanisms against it (Foteinos, *Sotheite apo ta afrodisia pathe*, p. 59; Drakoulides, *E Vlennoroia*, p. 38).
158. *Ethnos*, 2 May 1936, p. 4.
159. No. 14 Hios. The informant is referring to his wife getting pregnant during the famine years. As, owing to the famine, she was amenorhoeic, they believed that they were not in danger of conceiving. Moreover, condoms were scarce during the occupation years, another reason why he did not use one. A similar response was forthcoming from No. 10 Mykonos on venereal diseases.
160. No. 14 Hios, male, born 1914, married in 1938.
161. No. 13 Mykonos, female, born 1906, married in 1926.
162. No. 11 Athens, born in 1938, informant lived most of her life in mainland Greece in one of the Epirus towns, married in 1959. Interviewed in Athens.
163. No. 22 Hios, born 1925, married 1955: she was aware of condoms; No. 22 Mykonos, born 1905, married approx.1929: she was aware that condoms were available on Mykonos; the couple used condoms after their first child was born in 1930 at the husband's suggestion, and she also douched; No. 21 rural Mykonos, born 1923, married 1946: used condoms; No. 22 Syros, born 1927, married 1947, village of Vari: used condoms.
164. No. 22, rural Syros, married 1945, daughter born around 1953.
165. No. 22 Mykonos did exactly that: they combined the use of condoms with douching (No. 22 Mykonos, wife born 1905, husband born approx. 1896, married approx.1929).
166. Valaoras et al., 'Control', 277–8.

167. Valaoras et al., 'Control', 277.
168. George Siampos (1975) 'Law and Fertility in Greece' in Maurice Kirk, Massimo Livi Bacci and Egon Szabady (eds) *Law and fertility in Europe: A study of legislation directly or indirectly affecting fertility in Europe*, vol. 2 (Belgium: Ordina Editions), p. 343.
169. See, for example, Anonymous (1967) 'Dia Olas ta Gynaikas ai opoiai ehoun kathemerina provlemata h Norlestrin didei ten lysin', *Iatrike*, 12(3). The advert recommends the medicine for 'menstrual disorders'. Needless to say, some women were informed and did use them as contraceptives.
170. Anonymous (1967) 'Syghrona Provlemeta ek tes Hreseos ton Farmakon', *Iatrike*, 3(11), 235–7.
171. Anonymous, 'Syghrona Provlemeta', 226–43.
172. N. Louros (1967) 'L' Influence des Avortements sur le Problème Demographique de la Grèce', *Praktika Akademias Athenon*, 42, 402; Eugenia Georges (1996) 'Abortion Policy and Practice in Greece', *Social Science Medicine*, 42(4), 509–19; Paxson, *Making*, pp. 103, 106–7.
173. Georges, 'Abortion Policy'; Paxson, *Making*.
174. See, for example, No. 12 Mykonos.
175. See also Schneider and Schneider, *Festival of the Poor*.
176. Fisher and Szreter interpret the male-centred responses of their sample as a correction to the female-centred bias of earlier studies and of the birth control advocates at the start of the century ('"They Prefer Withdrawal"', 280–1). However, I argue that, rather than correcting an earlier bias, their data reflect that women were in fact earliest in attempting to control their fertility, while men were less interested and less inclined to do so during the earlier part of the decline. Needless to say, many men did take measures in the early part of the decline, as many women also did in the later part of the decline, all depending on couple dynamics and information flows.
177. Fisher and Szreter, '"They Prefer Withdrawal"', 272.
178. No. 1, No. 20, No. 27 Mykonos; No. 2 Hios; No. 22 Syros. Fisher and Szreter, '"They Prefer Withdrawal"', 273, argued that for their British sample such an attitude specifically related to the use of withdrawal, rather than other methods.
179. Violetta Hionidou (1998) 'The Adoption of Fertility Control on Mykonos, 1879–1959: Stopping, Spacing or Both?' *Population Studies*, 52(1), 67–83.
180. Fisher and Szreter argued that historiography has presented a simplified situation in which couples are dealt with as either contraceptors or non-contraceptors, thus ignoring the possibility of couples moving from one group to the other (Fisher and Szreter, '"They Prefer Withdrawal"',

275). However, although many have indeed employed such a dichotomous approach, such an assessment is rather simplistic (see, for example, Hionidou, 'The Adoption', 67–83).

181. See, for example, No. 9 Syros, No. 11 Syros, No. 22 Syros, No. 1 Mykonos, No. 10 Mykonos, No. 27 Mykonos. See also Fisher and Szreter, '"They Prefer Withdrawal"', 274, on their informants being 'accepting of the consequences of failure'.
182. Fisher and Szreter, '"They Prefer Withdrawal"', 270.
183. Fisher and Szreter, '"They Prefer Withdrawal"', 270, 274.
184. Fisher and Szreter, '"They Prefer Withdrawal"', 280.
185. Valaoras et al., 'Control', 271.
186. The use of condoms in the 1930s is mentioned in the diary of a middle-class Athenian, Minos Dounias, who, during the occupation years 1941–44, lamented the unavailability of 'elastics and the related hygiene products' that he was using before the war. In early July 1941 Dounias comments that such items had been 'for quite a while completely vanished' (Ntelopoulos, *'Epeita apo 120 Hronia'*, p. 55, entry of 3 July 1941). All such products were imported and thus had become unavailable either from the time Greece became involved in World War II, in October 1940 or, more probably, from the start of the war the previous year.

CHAPTER 10

Physicians and Their Role: 'Medicine Is a Form of Art'

The role physicians may have played in the decline of fertility has been addressed only incidentally in the international literature. In the case of abortion, physicians and their representing bodies have been squarely in the picture, however, and, at times, have been the exclusive focus of writers. For example, both J. Keown and Barbara Brookes discussed at length the positions and attitudes of British physicians and the British Medical Association, and how these affected the practice of abortion in Britain.[1] James Mohr and Leslie Reagan did the same for the USA and the American Medical Association, while also paying attention to individual physicians and their stance towards abortion.[2] The 'fight' against abortion has been interpreted as part of the 'war' of legitimisation carried out by qualified physicians in establishing their moral authority in society.[3] The actual attitudes and sentiments of individual physicians in their dealings with their own patients have also been addressed to a degree in relation to abortion.[4]

No. 5D. The informant explained that medicine is not only a scientific field but it 'borrows from many other fields too', pointing out that a significant part of medicine is the art of engaging with people, understanding their needs and responding to those.

V. Hionidou, *Abortion and Contraception in Modern Greece, 1830–1967*, Medicine and Biomedical Sciences in Modern History,
https://doi.org/10.1007/978-3-030-41490-0_10

However, assessing the role of physicians in relation to birth control, especially before the Pill, has been carried out rarely, with the exception of John Peel and some recent works outside the West.[5] Peel positioned the timing of physicians' changing attitudes towards contraception in the 1920s, a time when a sizeable majority of the British population had already begun to control their fertility.[6] At around this time, Marie Stopes had repeatedly derided the medical profession for its absence from the birth control movement and for their lack of contraceptive knowledge,[7] while in the USA Margaret Sanger played a role in bringing the provision of birth control to the attention of the medical profession in the interwar period. F.W.A. Van Poppel and Hugo Roling examined the fertility of physicians in the Netherlands, ascertaining its early decline,[8] and argued that, despite implementing some kind of control within their own marriage, the position of physicians within Dutch society led them to publicly condemn birth control for the wider population.[9] British physicians, too, were early birth controllers in their own marriages: in the 1911 census they had the lowest fertility among all occupational groups.[10]

We know very little about the situation in Greece. Therefore, this chapter will outline the position of physicians on issues of abortion and birth control in twentieth-century Greece. Unlike in the USA and Britain, the Athens Medical Association (*Iatrikos Syllogos Athenon*) did not have an official line on these subjects and appears not to have given any guidance to its members on what they should or should not be doing with their patients in relation to birth control. While all physicians had to be members of their local Medical Association, the relationship between the members and the Association could be described as loose or even non-existent.[11] One of my physician-informants called the Athens Medical Association 'ornamental', explaining that its main purpose was to keep an updated register of the physicians eligible to practice.[12] By the start of the twentieth century physicians and their representing body were well established and in no doubt as to the value of their contribution to Greek society. Medicine had established its paramount significance as a pillar of Greek society and as a professional discipline was powerful, influential and widely respected, with many physicians holding political positions in both national and local government. While non-trained practitioners operated in rural areas—where physicians were very thin on the ground—the state considered that physicians were the *only* medical professionals who had the right to practice.[13] Moreover, and unlike in the West, physicians who depended primarily on their private clientele—even when affiliated with hospitals—were allowed to advertise their expertise, credentials and place of practice in the national press. Although much of their clientele was attracted by word of mouth, as is still the case, advertisements were regularly placed in nineteenth- and twentieth-century newspapers, popular health publications aimed at a wider readership and women's magazines.[14] Prominent among advertising physicians were specialists in 'shameful' diseases and ones that were not easily discussed among the populace, such as venereal diseases and women's ailments.[15]

Discussion concerning birth control within the Greek context did not take place publicly until after the collapse of the dictatorship in 1974, except for the explicit, but rare, condemnation of its use mostly by religious figures.[16] However, issues concerning population and its future evolution, and whether or not there was a need to adopt and implement a population policy, were discussed widely in the press in the first half of the 1930s, particularly in 1930–1931.[17] Abortion was also discussed extensively at this juncture, as were the possibility of regulating childbearing—something that was already happening among affluent Athenians, in the USA and in Britain—and the policies implemented by Hitler's and Mussolini's governments on augmenting fertility, which were related to the Greek situation.[18] No details on the methods that may have been used to achieve fertility decline, except for abortion, were ever explicitly articulated in the pre-1940 discussions.[19] The individuals initiating or participating in such public discussions had, almost exclusively, medical backgrounds, even if this was not their principal occupation at the time (such as Apostolos Doxiadis, who in the 1930s was better known as a politician). Individuals without medical training engaged in the debates and discussions were very few indeed and were mostly religious figures.

In assessing the importance of the physicians in relation to the debate on abortion and birth control, it is important to emphasise that every medical professional who published on the subject indicated on the cover of their works and next to their name that they were physicians. In one only case did an author declare his non-medical background and add an apologetic explanation as to why he was writing his book—on the sexual education of young men—when he appeared to be unqualified to do so.[20] Moreover, all authors—with one exception—were men. This probably reflects the virtual absence of women from the profession and also the reluctance of the few female physicians to engage with potentially controversial issues. There was a handful of women physicians, almost exclusively specialising as gynaecologists, either working in private maternity or gynaecological clinics or in their own private practice and catering for those who were reluctant to engage with a male obstetrician,[21] but none of those produced publications on their area of expertise. The one published female physician, and a prolific author, was Anna Katsigra, also the daughter and mother of physicians. However, she represented the (ultra) conservative segment of society, advocating sexual education but rejecting the use of birth control and unquestionably disapproving of abortion; her aim was to build a physiologically and morally strong national population.

As discussed in Chap. 6, the contribution of physicians in discussing, encouraging or even taking forward legislation relating to abortion was of paramount importance during the examined period. The law changes reflect physicians' written arguments, and to a degree the views of the populace, suggesting that it was the physicians, rather than the law setting the parameters in this matter. So, despite abortion remaining illegal in principle, therapeutic abortion was permitted in 1872 in order to save the life of the mother. In the 1890s and 1924, therapeutic abortion was permitted in cases where 'the continuation of the pregnancy put in danger the life or *health* of the mother'.[22] Already in 1881, and in line with US and European physicians, M. Venizelos referred to proptosis and a small pelvis as conditions for which physicians might recommend therapeutic abortion in order to protect the mother's life.[23] Such recommendations became gradually more specific and plentiful, especially in the early twentieth century, when they included various types of tuberculosis, heart and kidney diseases, including chorea, blood disorders such as malignant anaemia, bronchial asthma and psychosis.[24] Abortions induced for health reasons—tuberculosis—were recorded at the Athens Maternity Hospital in the early 1920s.[25] While it was readily accepted by all that induced abortion had to take place in such situations, a parallel movement emerged supporting the introduction of pre-nuptial medical certificates that would have ensured that marriages involving individuals suffering from certain diseases would not take place.[26] So in 1925 M. Moyseides was arguing that anyone suffering from conditions such as syphilis, gonorrhoea, chlorosis, tuberculosis, neurasthenia, epilepsy, mental illness, haemophilia or diabetes should be prevented from getting married and thus procreating.[27] N.N. Drakoulides also expressed similar sentiments, although many others disagreed.[28] During discussions in the late 1930s that led to the revision of the civil code, the committee of lawmakers decided that 'lack of health should not be considered an impediment to marriage'.[29] Drakoulides remarked that the committee did not include a single physician who could have enlightened them. As a consequence of the lawmakers' refusal to prevent the marriage of people who were seen, by some, as unsuitable for procreation, procreation had to be controlled within marriage in such cases. This was exactly the advice that a physician, Haralambos Krithares, who practised in the 1940s on the island of Kythera, offered to the wife of a patient who suffered from syphilis and tuberculosis; advice that she followed.[30] Krithares also had to convince the local priest of the value of his advice, so that eventually both supported the woman in using birth control.

Though it may appear here that the issues of therapeutic abortion due to mother's health, eugenic concerns for the unconceived children of diseased parents, and birth control may be disconnected, they were of major concern and the subjects of extensive discourse in interwar Greece, mostly among physicians.[31] Irrespective of the decisions taken by the state, individual physicians felt responsibility towards their own patients and were guided by the medical discourse and their own scientific understanding of what needed to be done, rather than relying on the guidelines of a medical body, since such guidelines appear not to have existed. Tryfon Andrianakos explicitly makes such connections, recommending that physicians should discuss and encourage the use of contraception for spacing reasons when they thought it was appropriate for them to do so.[32]

The 1924 draft law that permitted therapeutic abortion in order to protect the mother's health was widely discussed in medical journals, with debate especially concerning the medical conditions that the law was potentially referring to.[33] Tuberculosis was prominent among them, but a host of others were also added to the list of 'dangerous' conditions. One such condition, widely repeated, was 'excessive' or 'pernicious' vomiting.[34] Another was a low fever of slightly above 37 degrees centigrade, which was perceived as an indication of possible serious illness.[35] It appears that the decision of whether or not to proceed with an abortion in such cases rested exclusively with the physicians: they were the ones with the knowledge to make the judgement, and that comes across unequivocally in all their writings, whether these were addressing medical students or potential patients.[36] Again, Krithares provides a corroborating example in his diary. In the early 1950s he was approached by a pregnant woman suffering from tuberculosis who had already been 'ordered' by specialists and eminent professors to have an abortion. As the couple desperately wanted a child, they entrusted themselves to Krithares, who argued on their behalf, against the insistent experts, that they should proceed with the pregnancy.[37] Fortunately for all, the outcome was positive. This incident, however, outlines the power of the physicians to impose their opinion, in this case, of the necessity of a therapeutic abortion—against which power the only possible solution for the couple was to search for an alternative medical opinion, one that would enable them to fulfil their dreams.[38] Even pronatalist publications in the 1960s referred to abortion as 'compulsory and permissible only for medical reasons'.[39]

Thus, physicians were making full use of the rights they were given by the law in recommending abortion 'for the 'health of the mother'; and, if anything, some of them seemed to have made a liberal use of the law.[40] In terms of contraception, although the Athens Medical Association had no official policy, individual physicians expressed their medical points of view and knowledge carefully in their writings, divulging extensive and technically (mostly) accurate information on birth control to the public but not taking a positive stance on birth control and very rarely explicitly advocating its use—indeed, often eagerly discouraging their readers from using any method. However, if the individual reader was determined that they should use something, then these authors did tentatively suggest the use of those methods which they were most familiar with professionally: that is, douching—known and used by physicians as part of their practice and advocated to women for cleanliness reasons—and condoms, known and recommended for the prevention of venereal disease. In the early 1950s the column 'The gynaecologist replies' in the women's magazine *E Gynaika* ('The Woman') generally answered women's queries on birth control in a clear and informative manner, but, at times, could be opaque.[41] Those replies that referred to abortion were the least explicit, mostly ending with the advice for the reader to visit a gynaecologist.[42] In the late 1930s and1940s and early 1950s the Ogino-Knaus method was openly recommended because it was felt that it did not contravene religious teachings. Other methods were also mentioned at times. However, most physicians felt they could not be seen to advertise and promote attitudes and practices that went against the ethical and religious stance of the wider society—hence why most authors advocated the use of birth control methods only when it was perceived that there were good reasons for their use, such as eugenic considerations or medical problems.[43] For much of the time examined here, being seen to publicly challenge the ethics of society could have brought an end to a physician's medical career.[44]

Starting in the 1930s, but much more commonly seen from the 1950s onwards, physicians began to suggest that when there were impediments prohibiting a couple from procreation it might be best for them to use contraception rather than abortion.[45] However, those voices were not sufficiently strong to be heard over those concerned with the long-term survival and prosperity of the nation, leading many physicians to act privately and discreetly, addressing the issue with their own patients as and when they believed it was appropriate, as in Krithare's case, mentioned above. The oral evidence suggests that this was happening widely rather than just occasionally:

Q. May I ask you how were you taking care?
A. We can't be talking that!
Q. Was it withdrawal? Sponge?
A. Withdrawal, whatever we could. I did not want any more children. I could not any more. And I had only one kidney.
Q. Did you have an operation?
A. Mm, yes. I had one kidney. And still, I had so many children.
Q. Did the doctor tell you not to have children?
A. Yes, after Yannis I had [1940] ... Four children and [I had them] with one kidney. The other was rotten/decaying, it became a tumour ... Then I had an operation and I had it removed.
Q. Did the doctor say ... ?
A. He told us, yes, to be careful because we did not know if the one kidney would hold on. But it did hold on.
Q. Did he tell you how to be careful?
A. Eh, he could not tell us! But we understood. What can the doctor tell me? The doctor told me 'be careful because we don't know if the kidney will hold on'.[46]

Thus, the physician's advice in this case, given around 1940, was instrumental in alerting the couple to the need to use birth control, while the mere fact of his suggestion conferred automatic approval of its use. While the physician did not necessarily divulge information on how to control fertility, couples did not seem to have had any difficulty in finding methods: condoms and female withdrawal. Other physicians—or possibly the same one—not only advised a temporary halt in one couple's childbearing for a specific period but also recommended condoms to the husband and told him where to find them:

A. Every two years I had one [baby], every two years. As soon as the two years passed, I gave birth [in 1947]. I had the four [children],[47] then I got an umbilical hernia. I would have [liked to have] had two more children. And what did the doctors say? Afterwards, they had me opened [operated] from here to down there, I was in pain .... I had umbilical hernia and I had an operation. And the doctors tell me after six years to have a child [wait for six years before having another child]. And I take precautions for six years. That doctor told him [the husband] how to be careful. Of course, six years, it wasn't [just] a year ... and in six years I had Manolis, my last child I had him after six years. I had the three and then him.

Q. Did the doctor tell you how to take precautions?

A. He [the doctor] told him [the husband] that those things exist ... how do they call them?

Q. Condoms.

A. Condoms ... Did we know anything my dear? Whatever God send us.

Q. So, you didn't know?

A. We did not know anything!

Q. Did you not want?

A. Not [that we] did not want. And [if you wanted] to ask, who could you ask? Since the old women, the village women here [did not know] ... He, since the doctor told him, he [the doctor] had to tell him how to take precautions during the six years. And indeed, the six years passed. Because, they said the tummy will open ..., it was forbidden to have another child then.

Q. And where did he buy the condoms?

A. At the pharmacy.

Q. Did they have them here?

A. Yes, he did not know. The doctor told him that the pharmacies have them.[48]

Physicians, therefore, not only recommended the use of birth control but when they felt it necessary they would divulge all the necessary details to their clients in order to facilitate its implementation. In this case, the informant had expressed her desire to have a couple more children; with her high age at marriage there would probably have been no need for this couple to have used birth control at any point in time under normal circumstances.[49] Nevertheless, and despite their desire for more children, the couple followed the physician's instructions for the good of the wife's health.

In other instances, physicians were eager to put a complete end to childbearing through a hysterectomy. When one informant, at the age of

36, was experiencing heavy bleeding, possibly as a result of an abortion, the physician suggested a hysterectomy: 'I went to the doctor and he tells me "you have that disease [possibly cancer?]. Have an operation to remove it." He says to my husband, "have you got children? Do you want to have [more] children?" He says, "children I have". And I had a general cleansing.'[50] The operation took place in Athens around 1938, while the informant was living there. By the 1950s recommendations to curtail reproduction became more forceful. Some physicians not only advised but also took decisive steps towards curtailing the fertility of individuals without necessarily informing them in detail:

A. We had a doctor here [on Mykonos] ... he gave me some injections [for the wife] ... I bought them in Piraeus and I go to the pharmacy and they say 'Who gave you this paper [prescription]?' I said the doctor. 'Why' I asked [the pharmacist]. He says 'She will become sterile'.
Q. From whatever [medicine] she was taking?
A. Those injections, the medicines she was taking. I find the doctor, well-known doctor, good [i.e., one with a good reputation on the island]. He says, 'the point is that she should not have children ....' But why, doctor? For us to have another child? We had two children [already]. 'It doesn't matter', he says. 'They are good/enough.'
Q. Did he ask your wife? Did your wife know anything [about it]?
A. Not about that.[51]

This was not an isolated incident. Similar injections were employed on other women too, as the midwife who practised concurrently with the physician discussed above also mentioned their use. This was the main contraceptive method this midwife informant was aware of: her reply to my question 'when you became a midwife, did you learn what you could do to avoid having children, if you wanted to?' was 'then [at the time] there were some injections. And we [she and the physician] did these occasionally to women, so that she would not have a child'. The results of such injections were not always successful: 'they worked for some women, they did not for others.'[52] The midwife made it clear that she never recommended such injections herself—it was 'the doctor who knew the prescription'—thus indicating that she was simply aware that this was the physician's established practice. The physician's request that the husband purchase the medicine himself in Athens, rather than ordering it via the local pharmacy, suggests that he wished to ensure a measure of secrecy to protect himself, and removing some of the responsibility from the physician in the case that the law was involved. Such careful planning on the part of the physician demonstrates an actual fear of the law, while at the same time demonstrating his determination to promote fertility regulation even in the absence of an explicit request by the couple.

Mykonos is a small island, and it should not be assumed that such advice was not provided more widely. The approach to fertility regulation among local physicians more generally seems concerted, almost certainly reflecting wider beliefs among physicians in the country at the time. So, an informant from Ano Mera on Mykonos, following two rather difficult deliveries, was 'advised' by a physician not to have another child:

Q. You said that at some point you decided that you did not want to have as many children as your parents had. When did you decide that?
A. The physicians too forbade me to have [more] children.
Q. After the second?
A. After the second they forbade me.
Q. Had you not decided earlier that? Not to have many [children]?
A. But he [the physician] told me … and in four years it happened [to be pregnant], what should I do? To go and get rid of it? And he told me, 'I will oversee your delivery'. But then [during the delivery] the midwife did not want to call the physician and I ended up suffering for two days and nights.
Q. So did you take the decision when after the second they told you that you should not have any more or did you decide earlier?
A. No.
Q. Before then, were you not careful?
A. We were careful but in the early years … in seventeen months I had two children.
Q. And so, when did you take the decision about how many children to have? Did you discuss it when you got married?
A. Listen, we did not discuss it. Since the physician told me after the second one, not to have another, and I have the third with such difficulties, how can I have another one?
Q. Before that [the third], did you not do anything [to prevent another pregnancy]? Whatever came?
A. Er—we did, but we got fooled too.
Q. You got fooled. Which one? In the second or in the third?
A. In the second and in the third![53]

When the informant became pregnant for the third time, she sought help not from the physician who advised her not to have any more children but from the one who was consulted by informant No. 6. This physician promised to help the patient go through the delivery and have her third child safely, as the informant had emphatically said that she did not want an abortion and the physician had not recommended one, despite the perceived threats to the woman's health. The informant stressed that it was the recommendation of the physician following her second pregnancy and her difficult third delivery that led to the couple's decision not to have any more children. Whatever birth control method they employed after the third appears to have been highly effective, unlike their earlier efforts.

Most informants who were advised by physicians not to have further children did follow the advice, despite their evident and usually explicitly expressed desire for more children:

A. My first daughter was born in 1941. My son was born in 1943 and the other [child] in 1947.
Q. And you got married [when]?
A. My wife was of a sickly disposition let's say and I did not have [many] children.
Q. That's why you did not have many children. Did you want many children? Would you have liked more children?
A. The more you have the better it is.[54]

The involvement of a physician is indicated by the informant's use of the term *filasthene* (of a sickly disposition), which is one that would have been used by a physician rather than by a peasant. Moreover, for the first two births physicians were involved and the wife was taken to the local maternity hospital, suggesting that the couple were advised by physicians of the wife's fragile health.

That many of the informants, especially those reproducing in the 1940s and 1950s, would have liked more children than they actually had is revealed in the work of Valaoras and his colleagues, undertaken in 1962–1963.[55] Only urban women aged 39 and over would have liked to have had fewer children than they actually had. In contrast, the rural women interviewed and the urbanites below the age of 39 all wanted more than the live children they had at the time of the survey.[56] This is easily explained for the younger women, who had not, as they saw it, completed their family. It is more difficult to explain for the older rural women.

It could be that physicians 'intervened' in similar ways to those presented above, or that the extensive war, occupation and civil war years had not allowed those women to have as many children as they wanted, signalling that part of the fertility decline was in fact attributable to external factors rather than individuals' conscious efforts.

Midwives and physicians were seen by the Greek public as the most appropriate sources of information and advice on the subject of birth control. These were the experts to whom they would turn for advice if they ever felt overwhelmed by a pregnancy or the prospect of one.[57] And this was widely understood at the time: for example, when a social scientist at the time—and a major politician in later years—decided to examine the question of population control in rural Greece in the second half of the 1930s he turned to the local obstetricians, because 'it is them that people almost always address when they want to curtail their fertility; it is them [obstetricians] who have the most opportunities compared to anyone else to discuss with their compatriots issues concerning the fertility of each one of them,'[58] and as a result they were the most knowledgeable about the actions their clients were taking.[59] Physicians advocated in their writings, if anything, condoms and douches. Thus, much of the population did not in fact need to consult them, as they could 'find' such methods without their help. Ultimately, however, physicians could be approached and questions *could* be asked, though for a fee, and one that not many rural inhabitants could afford.[60] The interactions of informants with physicians and the matter-of-fact provision of necessary information by physicians, seen in the interviews referring to the late 1940s onwards, are indications that physicians were able and willing to provide birth-control information for health reasons, but not for *social* reasons. Nevertheless, after World War II physicians seemed eager to encourage family limitation among their patients, provided that this could be framed around the *medical* needs of the patient, and would respond to specific questions when asked. For example, when one informant heard from a female friend that she was using (emmenagogic) pills to bring on her menses when they were delayed, the informant sought the physician's advice. He explained the treatment to the informant and prescribed some of the pills to her, which she used on a couple of occasions.[61]

That ordinary people were increasingly turning to physicians for advice and guidance could suggest the increasing power and influence of medicine in Greece.[62] However, for Greeks it was not so much the increasing power of medicine that mattered but rather the numbers of physicians and the access that patients had to them. Athens, as the largest city, was amply equipped throughout the twentieth century with physicians who had graduated either from the Athenian university or abroad.[63] Moreover, it acquired a significant number of hospitals in the first half of the twentieth century, making physicians accessible and affordable to the poorer classes of Athens.[64] Those informants from Mykonos who lived in Athens for part of their lives prior to 1940 did use the medical facilities available there despite their low socioeconomic status.[65] For the middle classes, the involvement with the medical profession was much closer and advice and guidance was sought from physicians and followed routinely.[66] For such women pregnancy would be monitored by the physician and advice would be provided and mostly followed by the patient.[67]

The creation in 1942 of Greece's second medical school, in Thessaloniki, augmented significantly the number of qualified physicians from the 1950s onwards, in turn increasing their availability in the provinces and thus to the poorest sections of the population.[68] The most significant change that occurred in the 1950s and 1960s was the increasing numerical presence of gynaecologists, who made up 8% of all physicians in 1962.[69] This was facilitated by both the increased university intake of medical students and the secure income that abortions were known to offer to the medical professional:

Q. Did you know anything about curettage and abortions?
A. Well we knew that there existed always a … gynaecologists earned a lot of money.
Q. Because of that [abortion]?
A. Because of that.[70]

While not all of those who chose gynaecology did so because of the potential earnings from abortion, the overwhelming majority did so.

Q. At university, did you know any fellow students who chose gynaecology [as their specialisation]?
A. Yes of course, many colleagues, many colleagues.
Q. And the reason they chose it, if I may ask?
A. They liked it as a specialty. Just as I liked cardiology, he liked gynaecology. Some did not succumb to that temptation, some did not succumb, that is known. We knew them. They were the ones who did not succumb. 'I cannot do that, religious and moral reasons do not

allow me'. Gynaecologists did it [performing abortions], that is what was said, but not all of them.

Q. What percentage do you think did not do it [performing abortions]?

A. Roughly speaking, I would not say more than 10 per cent [those not performing abortions].[71]

All gynaecologists were trained on how to undertake D&C, as this was one of the main techniques used extensively in their practice:

Q. Where did gynaecologists learn about curettage? Where did they learn the method of curettage?

A. The method of curettage is a therapeutic method. So when a woman is diagnosed with a [specific] problem, she must have curettage in order to undertake an examination of, you know, that material. It is the same method. It is also a therapeutic method. Alas to the gynaecologist who cannot perform a curettage. There are special instruments, special instruments that are specific to this specialty only. It is a method that exists for many reasons. Mostly for diagnostic [reasons] but also when, for example, women had endometriomas or whatever they call them, that caused women to have heavy bleedings, [women] had to have curettage in order for the heavy bleedings to stop.

Q. I see. Which means that they [the physicians] knew the method well.

A. It was … of course they knew it, of course, of course.[72]

However, while gynaecologists were fully trained to undertake curettage, they—and medical students in general—were not taught about contraception while studying at university:

Q. I wanted to ask you about contraception, if you had, were you taught at university anything about contraception?

A. When I was at university, there was no contraception. There were no … those came out around then at the end of 1969, 1970, around then they [became available]. So we were not taught about such things, we did not kn … they did not exist, did not exist [while he was at medical school].

Q. You were taught gynaecology though.

A. Of course, of course.

Q. But contraception, about the Pill you had not …

A. It did not exist, did not exist.
Q. Other methods? Had you not … ?
A. Oh they did not teach us such things. They taught us how to examine the pregnant woman, how we will perform a delivery …. But there wasn't, there was no interest [on teaching contraception], there was no teaching on contraception. That is considered a bit of a taboo, taboo. No one entered there [on that territory], no one entered, it was not taught, it was not written in the gynaecology books, at least the ones I had. It may have been [written] in other [text-books], I don't know. But it was not; it was an area that they did not pick up, they did not touch it.[73]

Many physician-informants, such as the one quoted above, equated contraception essentially with the Pill. They said that when they were in medical school there were *no* contraceptives, and the idea that these appeared later, after their graduation, justified the absence of any teaching on the subject. The Pill was first imported to Greece in 1963 and has been available ever since in pharmacies without prescription; however, it was initially sold as a menstruation regulator and not as a contraceptive.[74] Despite this, it appears that even in the mid-1970s there was still no teaching of modern contraceptives to medical students.[75]

The situation in relation to the provision of birth-control services and information was less straightforward for midwives. In rural Greece untrained midwives were virtually the only ones available until the end of World War II simply because there were not enough trained ones.[76] However, from the nineteenth century, and increasingly in the twentieth century, the desire was expressed by physicians and the authorities to replace those 'uneducated' midwives with trained ones, or physicians.[77] The impossibility of such a task, however, allowed the untrained midwives to continue practising in the rural areas, although some of them seemed to have sought collaboration with the local physician, whom they would consult or send for in the most troublesome deliveries.[78] Midwives in Athens and other cities were regularly accused by physicians of performing abortions, whereas rural midwives, at least in all the material I have consulted, were not.[79] This, almost certainly, is linked to the need for anonymity when performing illegal abortions and the lack of such in rural areas. In such places, where the practice of untrained midwifery was only tolerated, even a rumour would have signalled the end of a midwife's practice. The example of a midwife on one of the islands whose unmarried daughter gave birth to an illegitimate child indicates that the midwife did not perform abortions (or that these were so dangerous that she was not willing to perform it on her daughter). Nevertheless, it was well known among women and midwives that women could travel to Athens or the nearest city to procure abortions from both physicians and midwives,[80] and it is noticeable that on somewhat larger islands with a sizeable town, such as Hermoupolis and Hios Town, midwives did provide such a service.[81] In the immediate post-war period, when transport allowed regular transfer to Athens, rural midwives would have an 'office' in Athens where their rural patients would travel to procure an abortion by their own midwife, protected by the anonymity of the city.[82] Thus, some midwives seem to have been associated with the provision of abortion in urban areas but not with the provision of birth control.[83]

However, by 1969 virtually all abortions were performed by gynaecologists and all were taking place in urban areas.[84] Very rarely general practitioners would have performed abortions, but only in the provinces. By then, it was extremely rare for a midwife to perform an abortion.[85] The method used was invariably curettage. Older rural informants would seek information, advice and moral guidance from 'old ladies' if they felt they needed such advice, but these were replaced by physicians when they became available and/or affordable.

Discussion and Conclusions

Physicians in Greece were instrumental in influencing some people's reproductive histories through their advice to couples not to have more children for health reasons, which would occasionally include guidance on how to avoid pregnancies. Couples invariably followed their advice—although 'accidental' pregnancies might still occur—despite the fact that some of them would have liked more children. This happened to a lesser degree in the 1930s, but much more often from the late 1940s onwards. No such advice came from midwives. It should be reiterated that the evidence presented here comes overwhelmingly from oral interviews of rural residents. In the literature, whether written for physicians or for laypeople—the educated urban population—the focus was on avoiding pregnancy or, if unsuccessful, means of proceeding to abortion in those cases where pregnancy or birth would either endanger the mother's health or result in a dysgenic child. These were acceptable reasons for the medical profession to discuss and recommend both birth control and abortion. If anything, the existence of such cases enabled physicians in discussing birth control and abortion and in educating their readers and clientele on the existing possibilities. Abortions were performed by physicians and some midwives in Athens and other cities in the 1930s, but in the post-World War II years they were increasingly, and by the 1960s exclusively, performed by gynaecologists.[86]

Interestingly, elsewhere in Europe, such as Sweden in the 1930s and Britain in the 1920s and 1930s, 'health issues' surrounding pregnancy became very important in women's and men's arguments as to why they needed to restrict their fertility and/or have abortions.[87] Hera Cook has argued that women reduced the number of children they gave birth to because of the burden of pregnancy,[88] and emphasises the poor health of working-class English mothers in the 1930s, partly as a result of repeated childbearing but also because of their own very low health expectations.[89] Sofia Kling argued that in 1930s Sweden reproductive health was a major factor in the decision-making process of couples in terms of the use of preventive birth control and abortion.[90] What both authors seem to overlook is the fact that fertility decline in both Sweden and England had started in the nineteenth century, long before the 1920s or 1930s. What happened in both countries in those two decades was in fact the extreme control of fertility, pushing it near to or below replacement levels. These decades were the tail-end of fertility decline and those actors who articulated health as an incentive for the use of birth control were not innovators, in terms of either behaviour (fertility control) or methods. They simply articulated what they did—which is what their parents had already done in most cases—in terms of reproductive health.

There is evidence for England that physicians had been influencing their patients' reproductive decisions without necessarily referring to birth control. Evidence presented to the National Birth Rate Commission in 1914 stated that physicians were almost invariably recommending the spacing of pregnancies to their patients, despite the negative stance of the General Medical Council to contraception and abortion.[91] While it appears that they did not reveal to their patients how they could achieve this, they nevertheless steered them in taking action.[92] This was a time when childbirth was becoming increasingly institutionalised, gradually involving physicians whose advice was internalised and mostly followed.[93] In the 1920s and 1930s the letters of mothers and fathers to Marie Stopes seeking help are overwhelmingly constructed around health: the mother's, the child's and sometimes the father's;[94] and the Eugenics Society Medical Committee argued that the health of working-class women who had employed rubber pessaries and suppositories had improved.[95] These factors were not responsible for initiating or sustaining the much earlier fertility declines in Sweden and Britain. Kling suggests that physicians' warnings legitimised and intensified women's fears of childbirth.[96] While this is true, I would argue that for both Britain and Sweden these health-related factors provided women and men with a respectable way of articulating to society at large—in the case of Sweden via the Swedish Association for Sexuality Education—why they should have fewer children. The fact that physicians and their public writings were greatly respected offered those men and women legitimate language to discuss what they were trying to achieve.[97] As Ettie Rout—not a physician herself—stated in 1922, contraceptive information was spread through 'the long and patient efforts of hundreds of doctors, many of them unknown and forgotten'.[98]

For Greece, physicians' help and advice were timely, being given at a period when it could have influenced, and did influence, couples. While their advice was followed, however, the earliest couples 'producing' the decline nevertheless expressed the wish to have had more children. In the post-war era, with more, and more accessible physicians, the arguments of medical professionals that the health of women could be sustained through birth control was a major factor in its uptake. Moreover, their advice left no room for objections to the use of birth control on the part of either the husband or the wife, obliging the couple to unite and shape their birth control plans. In short, medical advice tended to make the receiving couple determined contraceptors, especially after the occasional 'accident'. I can only assume, given the widespread use of abortion at the same time, that women would have been advised to abort on many occasions when their physicians judged that their health was under threat. Health had become an important 'right' in the 1930s for the middle class; after World War II it was becoming so for the working class too.[99] Thus, partly because of the timing of Greece's fertility decline, but also because of physicians' very high status, it appears that they played a significant role in raising awareness of and prescribing the use of birth control, always relating its use to health reasons and thus somewhat accelerating fertility decline, at least for part of the rural population.

The ambivalent stance of physicians in their published material, in which they simply put the essence of their message across (that methods were available, what those methods were, the side effects and their efficiency/inefficiency) while protecting their personal and professional reputation, reflects the varying political and ethical framework of the society in which they were operating. So, for Greece, it is necessary to emphasise not only gender and class relations as important factors in examining the process of fertility change, as Sören Edvinsson and Sofia Kling noted, but also the existing political climate, as it was the case in, for example, 1930s Germany or the USA in relation to abortion.[100] It was the political and social climate that allowed some physicians to discreetly promote contraception at the individual level for 'health' reasons. Equally, it was the political and social climate that provided the appropriate language and reasoning offered for the measures taken by individuals. What individuals say about the measures they take to reduce their fertility at a specific point in time represents how that society 'allows' them to articulate what they are doing.

Notes

1. J. Keown (1988) *Abortion, Doctors, and the Law: Some Aspects of the Legal Regulation of Abortion in England from 1803 to 1982* (Cambridge: Cambridge University Press), p. 166; Barbara Brookes (1988) *Abortion in England, 1900–1967* (London: Routledge). However, Jones focuses on non-physicians (Emma Louise Jones (2007) 'Abortion in England, 1861–1967' (unpublished PhD thesis: Royal Holloway, University of London)).
2. James C. Mohr (1978) *Abortion in America. The Origins and Evolution of National Policy, 1800–1900* (New York: Oxford University Press), pp. 162–70, 238–9. Reagan also outlined how individual physicians reacted—on many occasions—positively to women who sought abortion (Leslie J. Reagan (1997) *When Abortion was a Crime. Women, Medicine and Law in the United States, 1867–1973* (Berkeley: University of California Press), pp. 60–70).
3. Keown, *Abortion*, p. 166; Brookes, *Abortion*.
4. Keown, *Abortion*; Brookes, *Abortion*; Richard Soloway (1982) *Birth Control and the Population Question in England, 1877–1930* (Chapel Hill: The University of North Carolina Press), Chap. 12; Carole Joffe (1991) 'Portraits of Three "Physicians of Conscience": Abortion before Legalization in the United States', *Journal of the History of Sexuality*, 2(1), 46–67.
5. John Peel (1964) 'Contraception and the Medical Profession', *Population Studies*, 18(2), 113–25; Raúl Necochea López (2014) *A History of Family Planning in Twentieth-century Peru* (Chapel Hill: The University of North Carolina Press).

6. Peel, 'Contraception', 137–43.
7. Marie Stopes (1923) *Contraception (Birth Control): Its Theory, History and Practice* (London: John Bale), pp. 6–7.
8. F.W.A. Van Poppel and Hugo Roling (2003) 'Physicians and Fertility Control in the Netherlands', *Journal of Interdisciplinary History*, 34(2), 183–4.
9. Poppel and Roling, 'Physicians', 155–85. A handful of physicians were prepared to offer advice to patients.
10. Peel, 'Contraception', 136.
11. All six physicians who were interviewed by the author attested to that, referring to their post-1950s experience. However, there is no indication that the situation differed in earlier times.
12. No. 6D. The specific informant graduated in 1965.
13. Violetta Hionidou (2016) 'Popular Medicine and Empirics in Greece, 1900–1950: An Oral History Approach', *Medical History*, 60(4), 492–513.
14. *Ygeia* was one such 'fortnightly illustrated magazine', edited by three physicians. The opening page had four advertisements for physicians covering four different specialisations (I. Veglidou, V. Kelemene and M. Moyseides (eds) (1925) *Ygeia. Dekapenthemero Egxromo Periodiko Praktikes Ygieines pros ten Hresin olon ton Koinonikon Taxeon* 2 (Athens: n.p.)). Anonymous (3 November 1946) 'ANTON. A LASKARIS Gynaikologika Metadotika Sexoualika', *Thesauros*, 9(414), 25. In the small set of newspapers available online through the National Library of Greece such advertisements can be found variously from 1898 to the 1960s (http://efimeris.nlg.gr/ns/main.html). See, for example, the advertisement of 30 August 1961 for a female gynaecologist in *Eleutheria*, 17(5196), 5; that for a venearologist of 30 August 1961 in *Eleutheria*, 17(5196), 4; and four separate advertisements for various specialisations of 10 July 1965 in *Makedonia*, 54(17265), 4.
15. Newspapers of all political affiliations are replete with such advertisements. Many have been cited throughout this monograph.
16. One of the earlier public announcements on women's sexuality, unwanted pregnancies and planned motherhood was the 1 May 1976 Proclamation of the Movement for Women's Liberation (*Kinese gia ten Apeleutherose ton Gynaikon*) (Marianna Kondyle and Aggelika Psarra (1986) '1976–1986 EKTROSE. To Hroniko mias Diekdikeses', *Dine*, 1(2), 9–12).
17. See the earlier section on Public Discourse on Population Change.
18. See, for example, Apostolos Doxiadis (11 September 1930) 'Periorismos e diarrythmisis ton genneseon?', *Eleutheron Vema*), and Apostolos Doxiadis (15 March 1931) *Eleutheron Vema*.

19. Post-World War II, articles referring to birth and population control or the Pill were occasionally published in the national press, but these invariably referred to non-Greek populations. See, for example, Robin Smay (12 November 1965) 'O Eleghos ton Genneseon ehei kataste kyrion proeklogikon thema eis Gallian (Birth Control has become the main Election Issue in France)', *Kathemerine*, 47(16325); Anonymous (5 January 1966) 'Tha Epikratese telikos o Eleghos ton Genneseon? (Will the birth control dominate eventually?)', *Kathemerine*, 47(16371); Paul Parizo (26 March 1966) 'Antisylleptika Diskia dia Iatrikous Skopous (Contraceptive Pills for Medical Purposes)', *Kathemerine*, 47(16432). Even those articles were published when the government was liberal.
20. The author instead emphasised his anti-communist credentials. Anastasios V. Antonopoulos (n.d.) *Meta ten Thyellan tou Symmoritismou* (Patras: Synadinou Bros).
21. See, for example, Anonymous (22 June 1901) 'Maieutika kai Gynaikologika Nosemata', *Empros*, 5(1669), 4, referring to 'Doctor Miss Anthe Vasileiadou', who had just returned from Paris; Anonymous (29 September 1930) 'Maieutike Klinike Elenes Stasinopoulou' *Akropolis*, B(600), 6, a much smaller advertisement than those of her male colleagues on the same page; Anonymous (30 November 1961) 'Rousa Plate-Konstantinidou Maieuter-Gynaikologos', *Eleutheria*, 17(5276), 6. In the 1960s *Eleutheria* had advertisements of gynaecologists in almost every issue.
22. V.A. Fotakes (January 1924) 'Ypo poias peristaseis dikaiologetai e iatrike amvlosis', *Iatrike Proodos*, 39(1), 4. My emphasis in the text.
23. M. Venizelos (1881) *Maieutike* (Athens: n.p.), pp. 257–8, 558–9. Similar indications regarding stenosis were given by M. Meliareses (1875) *O Odegos ton Eggamon.* By Frederick Hollick M.D. part b, translated by M. Meliareses (Vraila: M. Pestemaltziogou), pp. 88–90.
24. Fotakes, 'Ypo poias', 3–9. On therapeutic abortion see also Reagan (1997) *When Abortion was a Crime*; and Keown, *Abortion*, pp. 60–6.
25. Tryfon K. Andrianakos (1925) *E Maieytike kai Gynaikologia en Elladi* (Athens: A. Sakellarios), pp. 152–3.
26. See, for example, the relevant discussion in Sevasti Trubeta (2013) *Physical Anthropology, Race and Eugenics in Greece (1880–1970s)* (Leiden: Brill), pp. 233–6.
27. M. Moyseides (1925) *E Gyne. Ygieine tou Gamou kai tes Eggamou Gynaikos* (Alexandreia: A. Kasigone), pp. 12–21, 50–64, 66–80, 83, 86–91. For a thorough discussion of the numerous attempts to introduce legislation on pre-marital health certification and a ban on the marriage of unhealthy individuals see Trubeta, *Physical Anthropology*, pp. 239–46. All such efforts failed during the examined period.

28. N.N. Drakoulides (14–17 February 1932) 'E pro tou Gamou Iatrike Exetasis', *Eleutheros Anthropos*; N.N. Drakoulides (1933) *Ygeia kai Gamos. Me poia mesa prostateuontai. To Progamiaio Pistopoietiko* (Athens: Hronika). There were certainly dissenting voices too (Demosthenes Eleutheriades (1948) *Mathemata Koinonikes Viologias*, vol. 2 (Athens: n.p.), pp. 170–3).
29. Drakoulides, *Ygeia kai Gamos*, p. 20.
30. Haralambos E. Krithares (1996) *Anamneseis enos Giatrou. Apo to Horio, to Nosokomeio, te Zoe* (Athens: Etaireia Kytheraikon Meleton), pp. 148–50. It should be mentioned that neither syphilis nor gonorrhoea were considered to be illnesses necessitating therapeutic abortion (Fotakes, 'Ypo poias', 4) and therefore contraceptives had to be employed in order to avoid childbearing.
31. See, for example, Apostolos Doxiadis (1933) 'Eugonike', *Vibliotheke Koinonikes Ygieines* 2, 47.
32. Tryfon K. Andrianakos (1 May 1930) 'Organosis tes Proleptikes Iatrikes pros Katapolemesin tes Tehnetes Ektroseos kai Prostasian tes Teknogonias kai tes Metrotetos (Anakoinosis en to A Panellenion Synedrion Ygieines)', *Ellenike Iatrike*, 4(10), 1028. In 1954 Metropoulos was advocating that women who were obese and those using cannabis should not have children (Konstantinos Metropoulos (1954) *Ygieine tes Egkyou. Enas Polytimos Odegos gia ten Ygieine Diaviose tes Egkyou* (Athens: Papademetriou), p. 139).
33. Fotakes, 'Ypo poias', 3–9.
34. G.K. Lameras (August 1929) 'Endeixeis diakopes tes kyeseos epi kakoethon emeton', *O Praktikos Iatros* 7(8), 315.
35. Nikolaos Gyras (1939) *Prin kai Meta ton Gamo*, 4th edn (Athena: G. Vallianatou), pp. 122–3. Such induced abortions did take place (Andrianakos, *E Maieytike*, p. 152).
36. Moyseides, *E Gyne*, p. 70.
37. Krithares, *Anamneseis*, pp. 187–8.
38. Similarly, one of Arnold's informants explained how the physician insisted that she should have an abortion because the informant had taken a specific drug during the early stages of pregnancy and while she was unaware of being pregnant. The informant felt she was forced into having an abortion, while the physician informed her that having an abortion under such circumstances was legal as the eugenic clause had been introduced by then (Arnold, *Childbirth*, p. 120).
39. Demetrios Th. Stefanou (1963) *O Plethysmos tes Ges, o Periorismos ton Genneseon kai to Demografikon mas Provlema* (Athens: n.p.), p. 30.
40. One of Arnold's informants mentioned that when she sought an illegal abortion the gynaecologist demanded prior to the operation that she

signed a paper declaring that she was very ill and therefore in need of a therapeutic abortion (Arnold, *Childbirth*, p. 119, referring to the 1960 or 1970s).

41. For example, see Anonymous (27 December 1950) 'O Gynaikologos Apanta: Reply to *Mellousa Kyria*', *E Gynaika*, 1(24), 41; Anonymous (27 February 1952) 'O Gynaikologos Apanta: Reply to Mikre Afrikana', *E Gynaika*, 3(55), 60.
42. The replies of the gynaecologist would frequently suggest that the reader should visit a gynaecologist, encouraging such consultations to take place for a variety of reasons (see, e.g. (29 November 1950) 'O Gynaikologos Apanta', *E Gynaika*, 1(22), 25, where four out of seven replies recommended consulting a gynaecologist).
43. Krithare's disagreement with the local priest, whom he eventually persuaded, is an example in which the physician's concerns about the child that would be conceived by parents in ill-health convinced the priest to accept the use of contraceptives.
44. There are a couple of references to the existence of a law prohibiting the advertising of contraceptive methods (M. Moyseides (1932) *Malthousianismos Allote kai Nyn. Eleghos Genneseon kai Aposteirosis* (Athens: Gerardon Bros), p. 30, referring to Law 18277/2720, 30/3/1928; Heather Paxson (2004) *Making Modern Mothers: Ethics and Family Planning in Urban Greece* (Berkeley: University of California Press), p. 53, indicating that in the 1980s it was 'illegal to advertise contraceptives'). Similar assertions are made by Barmpouti for the 1950s to the 1980s (Alexandra Barmpouti (2019) *Post-War Eugenics, Reproductive choices and Population Policies in Greece, 1950s–1980s* (London: Palgrave Macmillan), pp. 106–7). Neither Paxson nor Barmpouti directly reference such a law. There is no evidence that such a law may have existed. Siampos for example, in his 'Law and Fertility in Greece' overview, does not indicate the existence of such a law. The 1950 Penal Code did indeed prohibit any advertisement of abortion (George Siampos (1975) 'Law and Fertility in Greece' in Maurice Kirk, Massimo Livi Bacci and Egon Szabady (eds) *Law and fertility in Europe: A study of legislation directly or indirectly affecting fertility in Europe*, vol. 2 (Belgium: Ordina Editions), pp. 337–64).
45. Gyras, *Prin kai Meta ton Gamo*, 93; D. Diamantopoulos (1957) *Iatrike Egkyklopaideia tes Gynaikas* (Athens: Gerolympou), p. 134; A. Sygkelakes (1927) *E Apokryfe Ygieine tes Gynaikas* (Alexandria: Grammata), p. 53; Alexandros Tsakires (1954) *Megale Sexologia. Anikanotes, Steirosis kai e Syghrone Therapeia ton*, 3rd edn, 1st edn 1947 (Athens: n.p.), p. 537.
46. No. 1 Mykonos.

47. Later on became clear that the informant had, in total, four children. The third been born in 1947, after which she had health problems, and the last child came six years after the third.
48. No. 2 rural Mykonos.
49. Still, the informant emphasised her lack of knowledge of methods of birth control; if she had known about them, she probably would have be keen to use them for spacing purposes.
50. No. 4 Mykonos. Note that the doctor asked the husband if he wanted any more children. Thus, the recommended operation was, rather, 'optional' and not necessarily imperative for the health of the wife and presumably alternative therapy could be used. That the doctor asked the husband and not the wife indicates the significance and priority of the husband in decision-making, possibly to a degree that had momentous effects on the wife's health.
51. No. 6 Mykonos, referring to the early 1950s.
52. No. 23 Mykonos.
53. No. 21 Mykonos.
54. No. 3 Hios.
55. The study was associated with PIKPA, a national children's health and welfare organisation. Essentially, the sample was drawn from mothers of children who used the PIKPA facilities, meaning that the sample was not representative of the whole female population (Vasilios Valaoras, A. Polychronopoulou and D. Trichopoulos (1965) 'Control of Family Size in Greece (The Results of a Field Survey)', *Population Studies*, 18(3), 270).
56. Valaoras et al., 'Control', Table 9, 274.
57. See, for example, No. 12 Mykonos and No. 22 Syros.
58. Evaggelos Averof (1939) *Symvole eis ten Ereunan tou Plythesmiakou Provlematos tes Ellados* (Athens: n.p.), p. 73.
59. Averof, *Symvole*, p. 72.
60. Violetta Hionidou (2009) '"It Was a Bridge from Life to Death": Hospitals during the Food Crisis, Greece 1941–1944', *Social History of Medicine*, 22(2), 361–85; Violetta Hionidou (2016) 'Popular Medicine and Empirics in Greece, 1900–1950: An Oral History Approach', *Medical History*, 60(4), 492–513; Richard Blum and Eva Blum (1965) *Health and Healing in Rural Greece* (Stanford, CA: Stanford University Press), p. 144.
61. No. 11 Athens, referring to the 1960s in a town in mainland Greece.
62. For Germany and the increasing power of medicine, social hygiene and social medicine see Annette F. Timm, *The politics of fertility in twentieth-century Berlin* (Cambridge: Cambridge University Press, 2010), pp. 7–9.

63. Even at the turn of the twentieth century a visitor referred to the 'hugely overstocked' availability of physicians in the capital city (William Miller (2012) *Greek Life and Country*, 1st edn 1905 (Miami Florida: HardPress), p. 196).
64. Hospitals offered consultations to external poor patients for a nominal fee.
65. No. 4 and No. 24 Mykonos.
66. See, for example, Anonymous (1939) 'O Iatros os Daskalos ton Meteron', *Era, Meniaia Epitheoresis Praktikes Paidokomias, Eugonikes kai Noseleutikes*, 2(2), 26–9.
67. Gyras, *Prin kai Meta ton Gamo*, pp. 122–3.
68. E. Georges (2008) *Bodies of Knowledge: The Medicalisation of Reproduction in Greece* (Nashville, TN: Vanderbuilt University Press), pp. 160–1; Blum and Blum, *Health and Healing*, pp. 140–65. Blum and Blum also emphasised villagers' mistrust of physicians. Similar sentiments of mistrust were expressed by the physician-informants No. 3D, No. 5D and No. 7D, who all practised in rural Greece in the late 1960s.
69. Valaoras et al., 'Control', 278.
70. No. 5D; similar responses from No. 4D and No. 6D.
71. No. 6D, similar comments from No. 5D.
72. No. 6D.
73. No. 6D graduated in 1965; similar comments by No. 5D, who graduated in 1968, No. 3D, who graduated in 1967, and No. 1D, who graduated in 1972.
74. Siampos, 'Law and Fertility in Greece', p. 343.
75. Siampos, 'Law and Fertility in Greece', p. 343.
76. See the section on Law and Abortion earlier in this monograph. Also Metropoulos, *Ygieine*, pp. 138–42; *Nea Mykonos* April 1954; *Nea Mykonos* February 1957; Georges, *Bodies of Knowledge*, pp. 160–4; Blum and Blum, *Health and Healing*, pp. 150–5. However, in the 1950s and 1960s, when a trained state-funded midwife co-existed with an untrained one in many cases the women preferred the latter (Blum and Blum, *Health and Healing*, p. 150). In Rhodes some women preferred the experience of giving birth with the untrained midwife rather than with the physician (Georges, *Bodies of Knowledge*, p. 140).
77. Violetta Hionidou (1993) 'The Demography of a Greek island, Mykonos 1859–1959: A Family Reconstitution Study' (unpublished PhD thesis: University of Liverpool), pp. 28, 37, 38, 160–1; Otto, King of Greece (1836) 'Law on Midwives', *Asklepios*, E, appendix, 84–6; General State Archives of Athens, Mykonos archive, Lyta eggrafa, folder 20, No. 155, 30 December 1834, letter to the municipal authorities of Mykonos.

78. No. 23 Mykonos. Still, informant No. 21 lamented that the midwife did not call the physician despite the fact that her delivery had lasted for two days.
79. The wife of informant No. 7D indicated that abortions were performed by midwives on Hios; No. 24 had an abortion with a midwife in Athens in 1938–39; Blum and Blum, *Health and Healing*, pp. 150–1; in a mainland provincial town, No. 12 Athens had two abortions with two separate gynaecologists in the 1960s.
80. No. 23 Mykonos, explaining that those who could afford the journey had them; the poor did not (referring to the 1930s onwards). No. 20 travelled to Athens in the 1930s to have an abortion.
81. No. 7D, referring to Hios in the late 1950s and early 1960s; No. 5 Syros, referring to early-1940s Hermoupolis.
82. Blum and Blum, *Health and Healing*, pp. 150–1, 154–5. Interestingly, both the trained and untrained midwives saw patients in Athens. The former would secretly see 'troubled unmarried girls in Athens to give them advice', whereas the latter declared that she would provide abortions in Athens.
83. Blum and Blum, *Health and Healing*, pp. 74–7.
84. Ioannes M. Danezes (1969) 'E Tehnete Ektrosis os Diethnes kai Ellenikon Provlema', *Iatrike*, 15(3), 200; Vasilios Valaoras, A. Polychronopoulou and D. Trichopoulos (1969) 'Greece: Postwar Abortion Experience', *Studies in Family Planning*, 1(46), 14.
85. Danezes, 'E Tehnete', 200.
86. In the 1930s abortion was available in Athens and in towns: No. 23 Mykonos became aware that abortions were taking place in the Athens hospital where she was trained as a midwife in the late 1930s; a similar point was made by No. 20 Mykonos; No. 24 Mykonos had abortions with two different physicians in Athens after 1945; No. 10 Hios referred to the physician from the nearby town of Volissos, where abortions could be done; Arnold, *Childbirth*, pp. 117–9, referred to 1960s rural Crete, from where women in need would travel to towns or Athens to have an abortion with a physician; Danezes, 'E Tehnete', 200.
87. Sofia Kling (2010) 'Reproductive health, birth control, and fertility change in Sweden, circa 1900–1940', *The History of the Family*, 15(2), 161–73.
88. Hera Cook (2005) *The Long Sexual Revolution: English Women, Sex, and Contraception, 1800–1975* (Oxford: Oxford University Press), pp. 11–12, 29.
89. Cook, *The Long Sexual Revolution*, pp. 37, 134–5.
90. Kling, 'Reproductive health', 161.
91. Peel, 'Contraception', 136.

92. Peel, 'Contraception', 136.
93. The increasing use of physicians during pregnancy and delivery in the 1910s is shown in the letters from working women collected by the Women's Co-operative Guild (Margaret Llewelyn Davies (ed.) (1978) *Maternity. Letters from Working Women collected by the Women's Co-operative Guild* (New York: W.W. Norton)). Physicians were strongly arguing for the necessity of pre-natal care for all, a novel idea at the time (Diana Palmer (1986) 'Women, Health and Politics, 1919–1939: Professional and lay involvement in the women's health campaign' (unpublished PhD thesis: University of Warwick), p. 100).
94. Marie C. Stopes (ed.) (1929) *Mother England. A contemporary History Self Written by Those who had no Historians* (London: John Bales & Sons). In the index section of the book there are three pages under the heading 'Doctor advised ...'. In most cases these are letters written to Stopes by individuals advised by their physician to avoid another pregnancy for health reasons (pp. 195–7).
95. Soloway, *Birth Control*, p. 275.
96. Kling, 'Reproductive health', 165.
97. Writings concerned with infant mortality, the heath of the nation and maternal mortality are only some of the few that would have certainly come to the attention of some of the readers.
98. Ettie A. Rout (1922) *Safe Marriage: A Return to Sanity* (London: William Heinemann (Medical Books) Ltd).
99. An article in a popular women's magazine opens with the declaration that 'The young woman, in order to be a perfect hostess, needs to be in full health and to know how to sustain her health' (Emma Drake (21 September 1950) 'Ti prepei na xerei e nea Gynaika', *Gynaika*, 1(17), 12–14).
100. Sören Edvinsson and Sofia Kling (2010) 'The practice of birth control and historical fertility change: Introduction', *The History of the Family*, 15(2), 118.

CHAPTER 11

Conclusions

The population of Greece started from a position of demographic devastation in the 1830s after the Greek Revolution, the civil war that ensued and the departure of the Muslim population from what became the Greek state. The Greek state, therefore, always showed a keen interest in increasing the size of the population. But the people of Greece, too, were keen to have sufficiently large numbers of surviving children in order to have working hands—either to work on the family's land or to earn cash wherever they migrated to—and heirs who would inherit the family's land, continue the 'name' of the family and support their elderly into their old age. Sterility and childlessness were abhorrent, representing one of the largest 'disasters' that could befall a family. Childlessness, for both man and woman, was a failure to achieve their purpose in life. Such representations of sterility did not cease within the timeframe of this study.

Women and their advisors had an array of methods and materials that would help them to keep their menstruation—considered to be a sign of reproductive health—in order. These emmenagogues ensured and protected women's fertility, which was what was desired. Traditional emmenagogues—herbals or pessaries—were part of popular culture and were accessible through empirical midwives, empirical female 'doctors' or other knowledgeable women. In the early twentieth century printed sources also provided knowledge of herbal emmenagogues. Over time, physicians provided 'modern' emmenagogues for exactly the same reasons, the Pill being the latest one. John Riddle, when discussing the use of emmenagogues

V. Hionidou, *Abortion and Contraception in Modern Greece, 1830–1967*, Medicine and Biomedical Sciences in Modern History,
https://doi.org/10.1007/978-3-030-41490-0_11

from ancient times to modern, referred to a 'broken chain of knowledge' in the West, the break having happened by the early modern period, after which their use was virtually nonexistent.[1] In Greece the chain of knowledge was unbroken—or, at the very least, it was clearly present in the nineteenth and twentieth centuries and some evidence for earlier times suggests that the link may have been maintained then as well. More research would be necessary to establish that. In the nineteenth and twentieth centuries the population—or individuals within it—had an excellent knowledge not only of emmenagogues but also of ecbolics/expellants, utilised when it was necessary to expel a dead foetus. These would be used as abortifacients when needed. However, at times some emmenagogues were also used as abortifacients, although in many cases they were not effective.

Improvements in childhood mortality towards the end of the nineteenth century—which was quite high in relation to infant mortality—would have visibly increased the number of surviving children.[2] The main demographic release valve, when one was needed, was out-migration—often temporary to begin with, but which became permanent for many.[3] The significant out-migration wave in the decades around 1900 was attributable partly to the economic crisis that affected the country at the time but also, I would argue, to the improving demographic balance of the country. This migratory reaction was sufficient to maintain the fertility status quo; however, the demographic squeeze was becoming visible. The well-known effects of breastfeeding were employed by some in the early decades of the twentieth century in order to delay the arrival of the next child, thus practising deliberate spacing before the onset of the fertility decline.[4] The long-distance migration of some family heads and their infrequent visits home—sometimes a handful over their married life—also curtailed fertility significantly for such families. The concurrent increasing affluence of such visibly small families must have been glaringly clear for all to see in their local communities.

With a government that—most of the time—encouraged procreation, there were no clear avenues leading to fertility change. However, the issues were becoming increasingly visible to individuals and the burden was heaviest on women, who would bear the children, bring them up and have much of the responsibility for getting them—at least their daughters—married too. The decade 1912–1922 was one of war and devastation that was followed by almost a decade of major economic crises. We have no clear understanding of what happened demographically in the

1910s and much of the 1920s, except that this was a period of public health disasters linked to the wars, the incorporation of new areas into the Greek state and the arrival of more than a million destitute refugees. As in all periods of crisis—wars, famines, economic devastation—the population 'reacted' with reduced nuptiality, partly because of the absence and deaths of many young men, but also with reduced coital frequency. One would expect these crises to have resulted in reduced fertility that would have been visible to the population. The economic and food crises of the post-1922 peaceful years further delayed recovery to normality, which was reached only at the end of the decade. Impotence and temporary sterility would have resulted from both psychological trauma and low food intake, at least in parts of the country.[5]

Recent literature has explored fertility during crises in pre-fertility decline settings,[6] revealing that fertility was controlled during such periods despite the background demographic setting. The population groups most severely affected by the economic shock or crisis were the ones whose fertility was most affected. The question, then, is whether this temporary fertility decline reflected a considered desire for control on the part of those affected by the crisis, or whether, rather, it was a reflex, almost involuntary reaction. In the former case, it would be necessary for the population to have had a clear set of birth-control methods that its members could adopt very quickly, such as abstinence, coitus interruptus or abortion—and these could also be abandoned equally quickly, presenting a sharp change in fertility closely responding to the timing of the crisis.[7] In the latter case, psychological and physiological reasons could explain the changes. For example, if sections of the population experienced reduced access to food, physiological changes would include impotence and amenorrhoea, although these would take some time to manifest themselves. Psychological effects, for example, might involve, among other things, loss of libido, reduced coital frequency or even temporary abstinence, which would also be reflected in the fertility rates. This is the most probable explanation for the early fertility decline in South East Asian historical famines, where the decline in conceptions started as soon as the monsoon failed and before hunger was visible.[8] The population was so well versed in the effects of the failed monsoon that fear determined its rapid reproductive responses. Thus, while abstinence may have been the method that created fertility decline in the pre-decline era as a response to crises, we need to be able to identify intention before we can claim that such occasions represent a deliberate control of fertility.

In the Greek case, it seems that for much of the population the reaction was of the latter type in the 1910s and 1920s. The repeated major crises of those years affected the population psychologically and physiologically. However, the upper and some of the middle classes were aware of birth-control methods and, we are repeatedly told by authors, did use them in the 1920s. Curettage, which had been widely used to combat sterility until 1950, was also quickly repurposed to provide abortions for members of the middle classes who required them in the 1920s. During those years, beyond the political and military crises, the economic crisis and high inflation led to the wiping out of all bank savings, something that hit harder those who had such savings—that is, the upper and middle classes and to a degree urban workers. For the poorer classes, the loss of men to the warfront up to 1922, the effects of malnutrition on the desire and the ability to perform sex and, most importantly, the fear for the present and future would have deterred the population from sex and procreation. The 1920s appear to have been for Greece a 'buffer zone' between non-controlled and controlled fertility, a time when birth-control methods were used by some when in crisis but not otherwise.

The demographic squeeze at the turn of the twentieth century and the fertility decline observed by commentators in the 1920s did not necessitate further action by the population in demographic terms. However, as the political and financial situation became stable for a short while in the early 1930s, fertility returned to 'normal'—that is, a 'natural'-looking fertility curve, distinctly high in comparison with contemporaneous European populations and distinctly lower than in earlier years in Greece; emigration came to a halt for external reasons for the foreseeable future; and childhood mortality had experienced significant declines in the preceding decades: all factors leading to a pressing demographic imbalance. This was discussed in the press, commented upon by social observers, leading the working class and the rural population to initiate control of their fertility.

The timing of the secular decline for Greece has been thus resituated by this study: I have argued that it started in the mid-1920s for the urban upper and middle classes and in the early 1930s for the rest. This is a significant realignment from the findings of the Princeton European Fertility Project, which have already been questioned by Brown and Guinnane and Amialchuk and Dimitrova.[9] Moreover, the emerging understanding of the important contribution of spacing in 'natural' fertility situations but also in the reduction of fertility during crises requires a serious re-evaluation of what should be taken as the threshold for the decline.[10] The control of fertility through spacing prior to the secular decline has been demonstrated for Mykonos and elsewhere.[11] A new threshold for the secular decline of fertility will change our understanding of when the declines occurred for various populations: if we cannot be sure of when this occurred it is difficult to meaningfully discuss the how and why, let alone compare populations. Employing the results of the Princeton European Fertility Project as a guide is not sufficient anymore, considering our changing understanding of what uncontrolled fertility was. However, is it meaningful to refer at all to a threshold for the start of fertility decline? A threshold implicates a radical break with the past and the separation of the before and after conditions. I would strongly argue that what research in recent decades demonstrates is that fertility decline was a process of change and adaptation over a considerable period of time, with a buffer zone potentially of a decade or more between the before and the after. During these buffer years, spacing was introduced, emmenagogues started to be treated as abortifacients and populations reacted to crises by controlling their fertility. Exploring what was happening during this buffer period, rather a regimented focus on a date, may lead to a greater understanding of the processes of change.

The means and materials used in controlling fertility among the Greek population were those with which women and men were familiar. These had to be repurposed and adapted to serve this new need to somewhat reduce their fertility. As the methods were imperfect and the users experimenting novices, many 'accidents' occurred. Before World War II only few were unwilling to accommodate accidental pregnancies and so they employed abortifacients or/and curettage. From the 1950s onwards many more were willing to use curettage in order to closely regulate their fertility, especially as urban centres and urban-based gynaecologists became more accessible.

In most cases, the decision to employ contraception was a joint decision made by the couple but initiated in many instances by the woman, or so it appears, as the majority of my informants and those writing to women's magazines were women. In some cases, however, it was a unilateral decision, sometimes made by the man, sometimes the woman. Following another disastrous decade in the 1940s—with war, occupation, famine, economic collapse, hyperinflation and civil war—the population controlled its fertility 'too' stringently, leading to final family sizes below what couples would have liked, as they articulated in the early 1960s. Greece, unlike the West, did not experience the post-World War II euphoria that led to a baby boom.

But how did couples take action and what kind of birth control did they use? Abortion was the simplest, most intuitive solution to the problem of excess fertility. Desperate single pregnant women had always used it, and while it was feared for its possible health consequences and its ethical implications, determined birth controllers in the 1920s and later did use it. Others were aware of its existence but were reticent in employing it, whether it involved abortifacient preparations or other means. Significantly, abortion was often achieved by the consumption of drinks and substances bought from the pharmacist or self-prepared—methods that had been available throughout the nineteenth century and before, and were known to midwives, empirics and married women. Such methods existed primarily in order to treat women's ailments, to bring on menstruation when it stopped and 'put themselves right'—acts aimed at securing their health and ensuring their potential fertility in the face of the ever-present fear of sterility. Thus, emmenagogues had always been readily available, and it was merely a matter of changing attitudes that led women to employ such methods when they did not want to be pregnant. From the 1920s onwards, alongside the 'traditional' emmenagogues medical preparations became available and were prescribed by physicians for the exact same purposes: to bring on menstruation and cure sterility or enhance fertility in the early twentieth century, or to 'cleanse' a woman at the very early stages of a potential pregnancy from the 1920s onwards. However, from the 1960s onwards abortion gradually became synonymous with D&C and was performed in those decades almost exclusively by physicians.

The long-term use and existence of emmenagogues and women's familiarity with them thus made them eminently suitable as means for curtailing fertility when—some—women decided to take this course. As some of them could act as abortifacients, too, using them would also actually have results in some cases. The most determined women could also employ the traditionally available ecbolics/expellants, that is, effective but dangerous abortifacients.

Similarly, condoms were available more widely from 1900, though more so from the 1920s onwards, and were promoted by physicians and the state as a prophylactic against venereal diseases. In the 1930s men, single and married, were knowledgeable about their existence and usefulness, learning about them during conversations in male-only environments such as workplaces, the military and coffee shops, with knowledgeable individuals eager to share their prowess. Condoms were advertised in the press and were readily accessible in pharmacies, so the only obstacle in using them was the absence of the desire to control fertility or personal preference. The first was taken care of by desperate wives who wished to have a different life from that of their mother, or physicians who recommended contraception to protect the health of the mother. Those men who did not like using condoms employed coitus interruptus. However, most men employed coitus interruptus anyway, even if at times they used condoms too, as this was the cheapest and least complicated method from the male perspective. Coitus interruptus continued to be the most widely used method among the Greek population well into the 1980s. Any 'accidental' pregnancies were dealt with by abortion when the couple—or just one of them—was determined not to have more children; otherwise the child was welcomed to the family, as in most cases accidental pregnancies were the expected outcome of imperfect methods. A good number of couples had *only* accidental pregnancies. This was never frowned upon in Greek society; even today, the expectation of such pregnancies is depicted in television family shows. The strict, long-term planning of such issues is still difficult to comprehend in Greek society.

A significant finding of this study was that, unlike today's understanding of coitus interruptus as being a male method, informants implied that it could be female-controlled too, especially in the early stages of fertility control. Similar evidence from Sicily, as revealed by Jane Schneider and Peter Schneider's informants, suggests that this was known more widely.[12] Such a revelation strongly questions our own understanding and perceptions of what are male or female methods of birth control. Similarly, our understanding of abortion as an exclusively female method is challenged by the strong input of husbands in the decision-making process and—at times—the imposition of their decision that an abortion must take place. Negotiations on birth control between husband and wife were—in most cases—explicit rather than tacit, reflecting the real importance of this aspect of their lives. At times, women would take action on their own behalf, especially if there was or was expected to be disagreement from the husband. Or, in situations where the husband was unable to employ coitus interruptus effectively and was unwilling to employ condoms, the woman would take on the responsibility of using a female method such as douching, sponges or vaginal plugs. As childrearing was exclusively a woman's responsibility, and this was the acknowledged female domain, in most cases her views carried more weight. However, this may be a reflection of the fact that the majority of my informants were women. Nevertheless, if the informants presented themselves as being central and instrumental in the decision-making process, this is significant in itself, as it suggests that this is how they perceived their role in family and society. Arnold, too, stressed that among her older informants—referring to the 1940s and earlier—women were taking unilateral decisions as to whether or not they would have an abortion.[13] Other methods were also used to achieve the control of fertility: breastfeeding, douching, sponges, vaginal plugs and menstrual regulation. All these were either methods that were recommended by physicians or involved appliances that were employed by them, in both cases for reasons other than birth control. As physicians and the populace regularly employed the various appliances, so their repurposing was neither revolutionary nor attention-provoking. Similarly, breastfeeding was perceived as a good practice for the health of the baby by both physicians and the population, and so its lengthy employment was not frowned upon.

Greek physicians also adapted to the needs of women when they sought a 'scientific' way to overcome old problems such as menstrual regulation: to achieve this they offered them emmenagogic pills in the late 1940s and 1950s; the contraceptive pill in the 1960s; and D&C as well. D&C became a widespread practice after World War II for a number of reasons: it was practised by physicians and mostly—later exclusively—by gynaecologists, and was therefore perceived as safe; it guaranteed the end of the pregnancy, a success rate that *none* of the other methods could ever match; and it was, as a one-off procedure, much more discreet and convenient compared, for example, with the contraceptive Pill. Physicians, just as they had done with emmenagogues, reacted to what women sought by making D&C widely available in the 1960s in most urban centres, especially in Athens. By then Athens was easy to access whenever a rural resident required such an operation. Just like other birth-control methods, D&C was employed in the early decades of the twentieth century as a therapeutic method for female ailments and was repurposed when abortion was required.

Thus, all birth-control methods, whether contraceptives or abortions, had existed for some time and were already used for other purposes before they were adopted to reduce fertility. Thus, methods did not need to be invented, but they had to be repurposed.[14] The availability of methods may have been less of an issue than the advocates of the innovation hypothesis to fertility decline thought, as Carlsson suggested many years ago.[15]

However, as the methods were not generally publicised, and certainly not in Greece—except for condoms—finding out about them was not immediately possible for all. Neither were negotiations between husband and wife always smooth. This meant that what some couples achieved in the 1930s, others came to do in the 1940s or even in the 1950s. It also meant that at times decisions were taken unilaterally, either by a husband who practised withdrawal and chose to have an 'accident' when he thought it was a good time to have another child, or by a wife when she decided to have an abortion without discussing it with her husband. Unlike ideas that freely circulated in the public arena, were discussed extensively in the press and, as a consequence, were also discussed in groups and privately, fertility and birth control were private matters and people were left to a large degree to their own devices in both exploring the idea of controlling their own fertility and finding a method suitable to them. The political stance of the Greek state towards population—always a pronatalist one although to varying degrees, depending on who governed—did not facilitate the spread of such ideas and practices. In contrast, physicians—especially after World War II—were in the majority pro-control and offered medical advice that did facilitate the spread of knowledge of birth-control methods. Even in earlier times, physicians' practices and views were overwhelmingly encouraging of population control, in many cases indirectly rather than directly. For example, many physicians were prescribing induced abortion to their patients for health reasons in the late 1920s, while some were prescribing birth control for eugenic and health reasons. Considering the high esteem in which their occupation was generally held, such advice was taken in and acted upon. Such advice empowered women further and ensured that the husband would not challenge whatever decisions they made following such advice. The role of physicians in encouraging birth control, mostly for reasons associated with the woman's health, was of fundamental importance to the speed of the fertility decline. Moreover, physicians gave their patients both a 'legitimate' reason to control their fertility and the language to articulate why they were doing so. The legitimacy offered by the physicians to the cause of birth control was enormous. In the case of Greece, the support was only occasionally explicit and public; nevertheless, because of the extremely important position they held in society, even tacit support was significant. In a state where a law which was never observed had forbidden abortion since the early days of the state, but where contraceptives were never publicly discussed and virtually never advertised, despite the fact that no law forbade that, it was left to the respected and powerful profession of physicians to facilitate the transition. To what degree this may have been the case elsewhere remains to be seen.

The control of fertility appears to be an ideational change that occurs when people perceive 'excessive' procreation as undesirable and population levels as no longer controllable by previously employed methods such as migration. It appears that this change—in a good number of cases—happened immediately after periods of national 'crisis': the French Revolution in France, the Civil War in the USA, the war and crisis that affected Greece in the 1910s and 1920s. Whether people who had been through such major social upheavals were more prone to receive and adopt new ideas, whether men's sexual abilities were affected psychologically and possibly physiologically, or whether simply the long-term effects of such disasters encouraged people to continue with practices adopted—voluntarily or involuntarily—during the disasters are questions to be explored in the future.

Notes

1. John Riddle (1998) *Eve's Herbs: A History of Contraception and Abortion in the West* (London; Cambridge, MA: Harvard University Press), pp. 179–80.
2. Violetta Hionidou (1993) 'The Demography of a Greek island, Mykonos 1859–1959: A Family Reconstitution Study' (unpublished PhD thesis: University of Liverpool); Michalis Raftakis (2019) 'Mortality Change in Hermoupolis, Greece (1859–1940)' (unpublished PhD thesis: Newcastle University).
3. See, for example, Violetta Hionidou (2002) '"They used to go and come". A century of circular migration from a Greek island, Mykonos 1850 to 1950', *Annales de Demographie Historique*, 51–77. Migration destinations during the end decades of the nineteenth century and the early twentieth century were the USA, the Danube area, Russia, the Ottoman Empire, Egypt, Africa, South America and even Australia. When such destinations became inaccessible in the 1920s the migration waves turned towards Athens, with similar patterns of single and married men migrating and the family, in many cases, remaining in their place of origin. On the significant effect migration can have on fertility, even when just seasonal, see, for example, Luciana Quaranta (2011) 'Agency of Change: Fertility and Seasonal Migration in a Nineteenth Century Alpine Community', *European Journal of Population*, 27(4), 457–85.

4. Violetta Hionidou (1998) 'The adoption of fertility control on Mykonos 1879–1959: Stopping, spacing or both?' *Population Studies*, 52, 67–83.
5. See Violetta Hionidou (2002) '"Send us either food or coffins": The 1941–43 famine on the Aegean island of Syros' in T. Dyson and C. Ó Gráda (eds) *Famine Demography. Perspectives from the Past and Present* (Oxford: Oxford University Press), pp. 181–203, where both the physiological and the psychological effects of the multiple crises on the fertility of the population are traced.
6. Tommy Bengtsson and M. Dribe (2006) 'Deliberate control in a natural fertility population: Southern Sweden, 1766–1864', *Demography*, 43(4), 727–46; A. Amialchuk and E. Dimitrova (2012) 'Detecting the evolution of deliberate fertility control before the demographic transition in Germany', *Demographic Research*, 27(article 19), 507–42; and Shamma Adeeb Alam and Claus C. Pörtner (2018) 'Income shocks, contraceptive use, and timing of fertility', *Journal of Development Economics*, 131, 96–103.
7. See Alam and Pörtner, 'Income shocks', who argue that the Tanzanian population of the early 1990s adopted 'traditional' methods of contraception to deal with the economic shock. They identify abstinence and the rhythm method as the methods employed.
8. See Hionidou, 'Send us either food or coffins'; Violetta Hionidou (2006) *Famine and Death in Occupied Greece, 1941–1944*, Cambridge Studies in Population, Economy and Society in Past Times Series (Cambridge: Cambridge University Press), pp. 178–86. Also see John C. Caldwell, P.H. Reddy, Pat Caldwell, Indra Gajanayake, Gaminiratne Wijesekere, Indrani Pieris and Bruce Caldwell (1992) 'A note on "conscious planning"', *Health Transition Review*, 2, 105–6.
9. John C. Brown and Timothy W. Guinnane (2007) 'Regions and Time in the European Fertility Transition: Problems in the Princeton Project's Statistical Methodology', *The Economic History Review*, 60(3), 574–95; Amialchuk and Dimitrova, 'Detecting'.
10. D.L. Anderton and L.L. Bean (1985) 'Birth spacing and fertility limitation: A behavioral analysis of a nineteenth-century frontier population', *Demography*, 22, 169–83; Paul A. David and Warren C. Sanderson (1986) 'Rudimentary contraceptive methods and the American transition to marital fertility control, 1855–1915' in Stanley L. Engerman and Robert E. Gallman (eds) *Long-term Factors in American Economic Growth: Studies in Income and Wealth* (Chicago: University of Chicago Press), pp. 307–90; Alfred Perrenoud (1988) 'Espacement et arret dans le controle des naissances', *Annales de Demographie Historique*, 59–78; Simon Szreter (1996) *Fertility, Class and Gender in Britain, 1860–1940* (Cambridge: Cambridge University Press); Jan Van Bavel (2004) 'Deliberate birth spacing before the fertility transition in Europe: Evidence from nineteenth-century

Belgium', *Population Studies*, 58(1), 95–107; Bengtsson and Dribe, 'Deliberate control'.
11. Hionidou, 'The adoption', 73–5.
12. Jane C. Schneider and Peter Schneider (1996) *Festival of the Poor: Fertility Decline and the Ideology of Class in Sicily, 1860–1980* (Tuscon: The University of Arizona Press).
13. Marlene Sue Arnold (1985) 'Childbirth among Rural Greek Women in Crete: Use of Popular, Folk and Cosmopolitan Medical Systems' (unpublished PhD thesis: University of Pennsylvania), p. 118.
14. Similarly, among the Tanzanian population investigated by Alam and Pörtner in the early 1990s, the 'traditional' methods of contraception they chose to use, abstinence and rhythm, were methods that the same population had employed in the past, although for a different purpose: namely, culturally prescribed abstinence during breastfeeding ('Income shocks').
15. Gösta Carlsson (1966) 'The Decline of Fertility: Innovation or Adjustment Process', *Population Studies*, 20(2), 150; Gigi Santow (1995) 'Coitus Interruptus and the Control of Natural Fertility', *Population Studies*, 49(1), 19–43.

Appendix: Background Information of Informants

All interviews were conducted by the author. Only those cited in the book are listed here.

Mykonos, Interviews Took Place in March/April 1994

No 1 Mykonos

Female
Age: 80
Marital status at the time of the interview: Married
Age at marriage: 18
Main occupation: None. Husband was a fisherman/working class
Parents' place of residence: Chora
Informant's place of residence as adult: Chora
Informant's place of residence at interview: Chora
Number of own children: 7
Number of mother's children: 1 (adopted)

V. Hionidou, *Abortion and Contraception in Modern Greece, 1830–1967*, Medicine and Biomedical Sciences in Modern History,
https://doi.org/10.1007/978-3-030-41490-0

No 2 Mykonos

Female
Age: 77
Marital status at the time of the interview: Widow
Age at marriage: 24
Main occupation: Working in own family's agricultural jobs
Parents' place of residence: Dheles/Rural Mykonos
Informant's place of residence as adult: Rural Mykonos
Informant's place of residence at interview: Rural Mykonos
Number of own children: 4
Number of mother's children: 9

No 3 Mykonos

Female
Year of birth: 1908
Marital status at the time of the interview: Widow twice
Year of marriage: 1929
Main occupation: Running a coffee shop with husband and as a widow
Parents' place of residence: Rural Mykonos
Informant's place of residence as adult: Athens/Chora
Informant's place of residence at interview: Chora
Number of own children (two marriages): 2+0
Number of mother's children: 7

No 4 Mykonos

Female
Age: 91
Marital status at the time of the interview: Widow
Age at marriage: 16
Main occupation: Working in own family's agricultural jobs while single, bringing milk to town and selling it. Working on the loom and selling her creations while married. Husband: sailor/Working class
Parents' place of residence: Chora
Informant's place of residence as adult: Chora/Athens
Informant's place of residence at interview: Chora
Number of own children: 5
Number of mother's children: 3?

No 5 Mykonos

Female
Age: 83
Marital status at the time of the interview: Widow
Year of marriage: 1934
Main occupation: None. Husband: Shop owner/upper class
Parents' place of residence: Chora
Informant's place of residence as adult: Chora
Informant's place of residence at interview: Chora
Number of own children: 1 (adopted)
Number of mother's children: 5

No 6 Mykonos

Male
Year of birth: 1909
Marital status at the time of the interview: Widower
Year of marriage: 1945
Main occupation: Butcher-shop owner/middle class
Parents' place of residence: Dheles/Chora
Informant's place of residence as adult: Chora
Informant's place of residence at interview: Chora
Number of own children: 2
Number of mother's children: 10

No 7 Mykonos

Male
Age: 89
Marital status at the time of the interview: Married, earlier Widower
Age at marriage: 24
Main occupation: Farmer
Parents' place of residence: Rural Mykonos
Informant's place of residence as adult: Rural Mykonos
Informant's place of residence at interview: Rural Mykonos
Number of own children: 4+0
Number of mother's children: 10

No 8 Mykonos

Female
Age: 70
Marital status at the time of the interview: Married
Year of marriage: 1943
Main occupation: Working in own family's agricultural jobs while single. Working on the loom and selling her creations while married.
Parents' place of residence: Dheles/Chora
Informant's place of residence as adult: Rural Mykonos/Athens
Informant's place of residence at interview: Rural Mykonos
Number of own children: 1 (adopted)
Number of mother's children: 9

No 9 Mykonos

Female
Year of birth: 1893
Marital status at the time of the interview: Widow
Age at marriage: 23
Main occupation: Domestic servant in Athens while single. Husband was a miller/middle class.
Parents' place of residence: Rural Mykonos
Informant's place of residence as adult: Athens/Chora
Informant's place of residence at interview: Chora
Number of own children: 6
Number of mother's children: 10

No 10 Mykonos

Female
Year of birth: 1916
Marital status at the time of the interview: Married
Age at marriage: 20
Main occupation: None. Husband builder/working class
Parents' place of residence: Ano Mera
Informant's place of residence as adult: Athens
Informant's place of residence at interview: Ano Mera
Number of own children: 2
Number of mother's children: 10

No 11 Mykonos

Male
Year of birth: 1916
Marital status at the time of the interview: Widower
Age at marriage: 30
Main occupation: Farmer
Parents' place of residence: Rural Mykonos/Dheles
Informant's place of residence as adult: Rural Mykonos/Dheles
Informant's place of residence at interview: Rural Mykonos
Number of own children: 1 (adopted)
Number of mother's children: 7

No 12 Mykonos

Female
Age: 1913
Marital status at the time of the interview: Widow
Age of marriage: 17
Main occupation: Working in own family's agricultural jobs, bringing and selling eggs and butter to town to specific customers. Creating thread and selling it to specific customers. All while she was married.
Parents' place of residence: Rural Mykonos
Informant's place of residence as adult: Rural Mykonos
Informant's place of residence at interview: Rural Mykonos
Number of own children: 10
Number of mother's children: 6

No 13 Mykonos

Female
Age: 1906
Marital status at the time of the interview: Widow
Year of marriage: 1926
Main occupation: Seamstress, assisting with own family's agricultural jobs.
Parents' place of residence: Ano Mera
Informant's place of residence as adult: Ano Mera
Informant's place of residence at interview: Ano Mera
Number of own children: 8
Number of mother's children: 2+8

No 14 Mykonos

Female. Husband present throughout the interview. Contributed extensively.
Age: 1916
Marital status at the time of the interview: Married
Year of marriage: 1938
Main occupation: None. Husband farmer.
Parents' place of residence: Ano Mera
Informant's place of residence as adult: Ano Mera
Informant's place of residence at interview: Ano Mera
Number of own children: 6
Number of mother's children: 12

No 15 Mykonos

Female
Age: 90
Marital status at the time of the interview: Widow
Age at marriage: 24
Main occupation: Creating thread, distaff, embroidery and assisting her husband during harvest
Parents' place of residence: Rural Mykonos
Informant's place of residence as adult: Rural Mykonos
Informant's place of residence at interview: Chora
Number of own children: 4
Number of mother's children: 8

No 16 Mykonos

Female
Age: 84
Marital status at the time of the interview: Widow
Year of marriage: 1936
Main occupation: Working in own family's agricultural jobs.
Parents' place of residence: Ano Mera
Informant's place of residence as adult: Ano Mera
Informant's place of residence at interview: Ano Mera
Number of own children: 2
Number of mother's children: 3+6

No 17 Mykonos

Female sisters
Age: 90
Marital status at the time of the interview: Both single
Year of marriage: n.a.
Main occupation: One was seamstress, the other was embroiderer
Parents' place of residence: Chora
Informant's place of residence as adult: Athens/Chora
Informant's place of residence at interview: Chora
Number of own children: 0
Number of mother's children: 7

No 18 Mykonos

Female
Age: 85
Marital status at the time of the interview: Widow
Year of marriage: 1949
Main occupation: Embroidering, carpet-making, assisting family in the family-owned bakery and grocery while single
Parents' place of residence: Chora
Informant's place of residence as adult: Chora
Informant's place of residence at interview: Chora
Number of own children: 0
Number of mother's children: 6

No 19 Mykonos

Female
Age: 1915
Marital status at the time of the interview: Married
Year of marriage: 1939
Main occupation: Working in own family's agricultural jobs.
Parents' place of residence: Rural Mykonos
Informant's place of residence as adult: Chora/Rural Mykonos
Informant's place of residence at interview: Rural Mykonos
Number of own children: 4
Number of mother's children: 13

No 20 Mykonos

Female
Age: 1905
Marital status at the time of the interview: Widow
Year of marriage: 1926
Main occupation: Domestic servant on Mykonos, Syros, Athens while single; Helping run the family coffee shop.
Parents' place of residence: Rural Mykonos
Informant's place of residence as adult: Chora
Informant's place of residence at interview: Chora
Number of own children: 3
Number of mother's children: 10

No 21 Mykonos

Female. Husband was present throughout the interview and at some points contributed.
Year of birth: 1923
Marital status at the time of the interview: Married
Year of marriage: 1946
Main occupation: Working in own family's agricultural jobs.
Parents' place of residence: Ano Mera
Informant's place of residence as adult: Ano Mera
Informant's place of residence at interview: Ano Mera
Number of own children: 3
Number of mother's children: 3+5

No 22 Mykonos

Female
Age: 89
Marital status at the time of the interview: Widow
Year of marriage: Around 1929
Main occupation: Helping run the family coffee shop.
Parents' place of residence: Chora
Informant's place of residence as adult: Chora
Informant's place of residence at interview: Chora
Number of own children: 3
Number of mother's children: 4

No 23 Mykonos

Female
Year of birth: 1907
Marital status at the time of the interview: Widow
Age at marriage: 16
Main occupation: Wet-nurse in Alexandria, Egypt; midwife on Mykonos
Parents' place of residence: Chora
Informant's place of residence as adult: Athens/Chora
Informant's place of residence at interview: Chora
Number of own children: 5
Number of mother's children: 6

No 24 Mykonos

Female
Age: 79
Marital status at the time of the interview: Widow
Year of marriage: 1938
Main occupation: None. Husband's occupation sailor; Father's occupation carpenter
Parents' place of residence: Chora
Informant's place of residence as adult: Athens/Chora
Informant's place of residence at interview: Chora
Number of own children: 3
Number of mother's children: 15

No 25 Mykonos

Male. Wife was present throughout the interview, listened and participated extensively.
Year of birth: 1905
Marital status at the time of the interview: Married
Year of marriage: 1939
Main occupation: Sea captain/upper class
Parents' place of residence: Chora
Informant's place of residence as adult: Chora
Informant's place of residence at interview: Chora
Number of own children: 3
Number of mother's children: 5

No 26 Mykonos

Female
Age: 72
Marital status at the time of the interview: Widow
Year of marriage: Around 1942
Main occupation: Working in own family's agricultural jobs
Parents' place of residence: Rural Mykonos
Informant's place of residence as adult: Rural Mykonos
Informant's place of residence at interview: Rural Mykonos
Number of own children: 1 (adopted)
Number of mother's children: 5

No 27 Mykonos

Female
Year of birth: 1909
Marital status at the time of the interview: Married
Year of marriage: 1933
Main occupation: Domestic servant in Athens while single, husband was a farmer
Parents' place of residence: Rural Mykonos/Dheles
Informant's place of residence as adult: Rural Mykonos
Informant's place of residence at interview: Chora
Number of own children: 7
Number of mother's children: 13

No 28 Mykonos

Male. The informant's wife was present for parts of the interview but did not participate.
Age: 77
Marital status at the time of the interview: Married
Year of marriage: 1960
Main occupation: Seafarer/owner of a caique
Parents' place of residence: Dheles/Chora
Informant's place of residence as adult: Chora
Informant's place of residence at interview: Chora
Number of own children: 2
Number of mother's children: 10

Hios, Interviews Took Place in Winter 1999

No 1 Hios

Female. Husband was present throughout the interview and contributed to it.
Year of birth: 1912 and 1909
Marital status at the time of the interview: Married
Year of marriage: 1939
Main occupation/social class: None. Teacher/middle class.
Parents' place of residence: Thymiana Hios
Informant's place of residence as adult: Thymiana Hios
Informant's place of residence at interview: Thymiana Hios
Number of own children: 3
Number of mother's children: 5

No 2 Hios

Female
Year of birth: 1915
Marital status at the time of the interview: Widow
Year of marriage: Middle of 1930s
Main occupation/social class: None. Husband was a sailor/working class.
Parents' place of residence: Vrontado Hios
Informant's place of residence as adult: Vrontado Hios
Informant's place of residence at interview: Vrontado Hios
Number of own children: 5
Number of mother's children: 6

No 3 Hios

Man
Year of birth: 1909
Marital status at the time of the interview: Widower
Year of marriage: 1939
Main occupation/social class: Farmer-builder.
Parents' place of residence: Ai Georgis Sikousis Hios
Informant's place of residence as adult: Ai Georgis Sikousis Hios
Informant's place of residence at interview: Ai Georgis Sikousis Hios
Number of own children: 3
Number of mother's children: 5

No 4 Hios

Female
Year of birth: Around 1904
Marital status at the time of the interview: Widow
Year of marriage: 1932
Main occupation/social class: None, the husband was a farmer, was a migrant in the USA before marriage/working class.
Parents' place of residence: Ai Georgis Sikousis Hios
Informant's place of residence as adult: Ai Georgis Sikousis Hios
Informant's place of residence at interview: Ai Georgis Sikousis Hios
Number of own children: 2
Number of mother's children: 3

No 5 Hios

Female
Year of birth: 1918
Marital status at the time of the interview: Widow
Year of marriage: 1938
Main occupation/social class: None working class.
Parents' place of residence: Castle in Hios Town.
Informant's place of residence as adult: Castle in Hios Town.
Informant's place of residence at interview: Castle in Hios Town.
Number of own children: 3
Number of mother's children: 5

No 8 Hios

Male
Year of birth: 1908
Marital status at the time of the interview: Married
Year of marriage: 1937
Main occupation/social class: Municipal employee/middle class.
Parents' place of residence: Hios Town
Informant's place of residence as adult: Hios Town
Informant's place of residence at interview: Hios Town
Number of own children: 4
Number of mother's children: 4

No 9 Hios

Male
Year of birth: Around 1928
Marital status at the time of the interview: Married
Year of marriage: 1982
Main occupation/social class: Taxi driver/working class.
Parents' place of residence: Hios Town, the family moved to their own small farm during the occupation situated just outside the town of Hios.
Informant's place of residence as adult: Hios Town
Informant's place of residence at interview: Hios Town
Number of own children: 0
Number of mother's children: 4

No 10 Hios

Female
Year of birth: Around 1899
Marital status at the time of the interview: Widow
Year of marriage: 1921
Main occupation/social class: Domestic servant before and during marriage-engaged in own family's agricultural jobs/working class.
Parents' place of residence: Siderounta Hios
Informant's place of residence as adult: Siderounta Hios
Informant's place of residence at interview: Hios Town
Number of own children: 6
Number of mother's children: 3?

No 13 Hios

Female
Year of birth: 1920
Marital status at the time of the interview: Widow
Age at marriage: 27
Main occupation/social class: Well-off farmer/middle class.
Parents' place of residence: Campos Hios
Informant's place of residence as adult: Campos Hios
Informant's place of residence at interview: Campos Hios
Number of own children: 3
Number of mother's children: 5

No 14 Hios

Male
Year of birth: 1914
Marital status at the time of the interview: Widower
Year of marriage: 1938
Main occupation/social class: Barber-sailor/working class.
Parents' place of residence: Hios Town
Informant's place of residence as adult: Varvasi Hios
Informant's place of residence at interview: Hios Town
Number of own children: 3
Number of mother's children του: 5

No 15 Hios

Man. Wife was present throughout and contributed substantially.
Age: 77 *ετών*. Wife's year of birth: 1922
Marital status at the time of the interview: Married
Year of marriage: 1946
Main occupation/social class: Private employee/working class.
Parents' place of residence: Vrontado Hios
Informant's place of residence as adult: Vrontado Hios
Informant's place of residence at interview: Vrontado Hios
Number of own children: 1
Number of mother's children: 2

No 22 Hios

Female
Year of birth: 1925
Marital status at the time of the interview: Widow
Year of marriage: 1955
Main occupation/social class: None—husband solicitor/middle class.
Parents' place of residence: Vrontado Hios
Informant's place of residence as adult: Vrontado Hios
Informant's place of residence at interview: Vrontado Hios
Number of own children: 3
Number of mother's children: 4

Syros, Interviews Took Place in Summer 2000

No 1 Syros

Female
Year of birth: 1902
Marital status at the time of the interview: Widow
Year of marriage: 1922
Main occupation/social class: None/upper class—husband owner of a factory.
Parents' place of residence: Hermoupolis
Informant's place of residence as adult: Hermoupolis
Informant's place of residence at interview: Hermoupolis
Number of own children: 3
Number of mother's children: At least four

No 5 Syros

Male
Year of birth: 1924
Marital status at the time of the interview: Married
Year of marriage: 1942
Main occupation/social class: Civil servant/middle class
Parents' place of residence: Hermoupolis
Informant's place of residence as adult: Hermoupolis
Informant's place of residence at interview: Hermoupolis
Number of own children: 2
Number of mother's children: 4

No 9 Syros

Male. Wife was present throughout and contributed substantially
Year of birth: 1914
Marital status at the time of the interview: Married
Year of marriage: 1943
Main occupation/social class: Shop servant, factory worker/working class
Parents' place of residence: Ano Syros
Informant's place of residence as adult: Ano Syros
Informant's place of residence at interview: Ano Syros
Number of own children: 5
Number of mother's children: 6

No 10 Syros

Male
Year of birth: 1912
Marital status at the time of the interview: Married
Year of marriage: 1940
Main occupation/social class: White-collar employee/middle-upper class
Parents' place of residence: Hermoupolis
Informant's place of residence as adult: Hermoupolis
Informant's place of residence at interview: Hermoupolis
Number of own children: 2
Number of mother's children: 2

No 11 Syros

Male
Year of birth: Around 1920
Marital status at the time of the interview: Married
Age at marriage: 1943
Main occupation/social class: Carpenter
Parents' place of residence: Hermoupolis
Informant's place of residence as adult: Hermoupolis
Informant's place of residence at interview: Hermoupolis
Number of own children: 3
Number of mother's children: 16

No 22 Syros

Male. Wife was present throughout the interview adding and commenting on what was said; she took over for the questions on fertility and childbearing
Year of birth: 1918 and 1927
Marital status at the time of the interview: Married
Year of marriage: 1945
Main occupation/social class: Farmer
Parents' place of residence: Rural Syros
Informant's place of residence as adult: Rural Syros
Informant's place of residence at interview: Rural Syros
Number of own children: 4
Number of mother's children: 5–4

No 11 Athens, 2011

Female
Year of birth: 1938
Marital status at the time of the interview: Widow
Age at marriage: 21
Main occupation: Working on the loom while single and selling what created, seamstress. None as married. Husband house painter/working class.
Parents' place of residence: Town in Epirus
Informant's place of residence as adult: Town in Epirus
Informant's place of residence at interview: Athens
Number of own children: 4
Number of mother's children: 7

No 12 Athens, 2011

Female
Year of birth: 1933
Marital status at the time of the interview: Widow
Age at marriage: 23
Main occupation: Office work while single, domestic cleaner in Athens while married/working class.
Parents' place of residence: Soviet Union
Informant's place of residence as adult: Soviet Union/Athens
Informant's place of residence at interview: Athens
Number of own children: 3
Number of mother's children: 3

Interviews with Physicians, Interviews Took Place in 2011

No 1D

Male
Year of birth: 1946
Marital status at the time of the interview: Married
Occupation specialisation: Cardiologist
Parents' place of residence: Athens

Informant's place of practice: Athens
Residence at the time of interview: Athens
Year of graduation 1972
University attended: Athens
Place of first rural practice: Samos Hospital

No 3D

Female
Year of birth: 1940
Marital status at the time of the interview: Widow
Occupation specialisation: Paediatrician
Parents' place of residence: Athens
Informant's place of practice: Greater Athens
Residence at the time of interview: Greater Athens
Year of graduation 1967
University attended: Germany/Athens
Place of first rural practice: Aigio Hospital, Peloponnese

No 4D

Female
Year of birth: 1950
Marital status at the time of the interview: Married
Occupation specialisation: Radiologist
Parents' place of residence: Greater Athens
Informant's place of practice: Greater Athens
Residence at the time of interview: Greater Athens
Year of graduation 1974
University attended: Athens
Place of first rural practice: Hospital Soteria (Hospital specialising on chest illnesses, especially tuberculosis)

No 5D

Male
Year of birth: 1940
Marital status at the time of the interview: Married
Occupation specialisation: General practitioner

Parents' place of residence: Athens
Informant's place of practice: Athens
Residence at the time of interview: Greater Athens
Year of graduation 1968
University attended: Athens
Place of first rural practice: Village of Zaverda (and neighbouring villages), Aitoloakarnania

No 6D

Male
Year of birth: 1941
Marital status at the time of the interview: Married
Occupation specialisation: Cardiologist
Parents' place of residence: Thessalonike, Athens
Informant's place of practice: Athens
Residence at the time of interview: Greater Athens
Year of graduation 1965
University attended: Athens
Place of first rural practice: Hospital of a small town in Peloponnese

No 7D

Male. Wife was present for parts of the interview and participated when she wished.
Age:
Marital status at the time of the interview: Married
Occupation specialisation: General Practitioner
Parents' place of residence: Alexandria, Egypt
Informant's place of residence as adult: Hios
Residence at the time of interview: Hios
Year of graduation 1950
University attended: Athens
Place of first rural practice: Small town on Hios

Index[1]

[1] Note: Page numbers followed by 'n' refer to notes.

V. Hionidou, *Abortion and Contraception in Modern Greece, 1830–1967*, Medicine and Biomedical Sciences in Modern History,
https://doi.org/10.1007/978-3-030-41490-0

The manufacturer's authorised representative in the EU is Springer Nature Customer Service Centre GmbH, Europaplatz 3, 69115 Heidelberg, Germany. If you have any concerns regarding our products, please contact ProductSafety@springernature.com

Printed and bound by CPI Group (UK) Ltd, Croydon, CR0 4YY
25/09/2026
02222886-0001